ANATOMICAL CHART COMPANY

ATLAS of PATHOPHYSIOLOGY

ANATOMICAL CHART COMPANY

ATLAS of PATHOPHYSIOLOGY

SPRINGHOUSE

Springhouse, Pennsylvania

Staff

Senior Publisher
Donna O. Carpenter

Clinical Director
Marguerite Ambrose, RN, MSN, CS

Creative Director
Jake Smith

Executive Editor
H. Nancy Holmes

Clinical Project Manager
Lisa Morris Bonsall, RN, MSN, CRNP

Art Director
Mary Ludwicki (design project manager)

Editors
Jennifer P. Kowalak (senior associate editor),
Audrey Selena Hughes

Copy Editors
Catherine B. Cramer, Barbara F. Ritter

Clinical Editors
Shari A. Regina Cammon, MSN, RN, CCRN;
Carol Ann Knauff, MSN, RN, CCRN;
Elizabeth D. McNeeley, BSN, RN;
Lori Musolf Neri, RN, MSN, CCRN, CPNP

Designers
Arlene Putterman (associate design director),
Joseph John Clark, Patsy Cook Graber,
Donna S. Morris

Illustrators
Anatomical Chart Company: Dawn Gorski,
Marguerite Aitken, Diane Abeloff, Liana Bauman,
Ernie Beck, Michael Carroll, Carl Clingman,
Birck Cox, Ruth Daly, Leonard Dank, Brian Evans,
Robert Fletcher, Claudia Grosz, Fred Harwin,
Tonya Hines, William Jacobson, Keith Kasnot,
Jeanne Koelling, Lik Kwong, Mark Lefkowitz,
Noah Lowenthal, Lena Lyons, Kimberly Martins,
Marcelo Oliver, David Rini, Linda Warren,
William Westwood, Christine Young; Bot Roda

Electronic Production Services
Diane Paluba (manager), Joyce Rossi Biletz

Manufacturing
Patricia K. Dorshaw (manager), Otto Mezei (book
production manager)

Editorial Assistants
Carol Caputo, Arlene Claffee, Beth Janae Orr

Indexer
Barbara E. Hodgson

Printed in the United States of America.
AP-D N O S A J J M
05 04 03   10 9 8 7 6 5 4

Library of Congress Cataloging-in-Publication Data

Atlas of pathophysiology.
    p. ; cm.
At head of title: Anatomical Chart Co.
Includes bibliographical references and index.
    ISBN 1-58255-109-X (alk. paper)
    1. Physiology, Pathological—Atlases.
    [DNLM: 1. Pathology—Atlases. 2. Physiology—Atlases. QZ 17
A880398 2001] I. Springhouse Corporation. II. Anatomical
Chart Co.
    RB113 .A87 2001
    616.07'022'2—dc21
                                                        2001031149

Contents

Consultants

Anita M. Bargardi, RN, MA, ACNP, CCRN, CS
Clinical Director, Advanced Practice
  Nursing, Cardiology
Veterans Administration Ann Arbor
  (Mich.) Healthcare System

John M. Bertoni, MD, PhD
Professor and Chair
Department of Neurology
Creighton University
Omaha

Nancy P. Blumenthal, MSN, CRNP, CS
Senior Nurse Practitioner, Lung
  Transplant Program
University of Pennsylvania Medical
  Center
Philadelphia

Cheryl L. Brady, RN, MSN
Adjunct Faculty
Kent State University
East Liverpool, Ohio

Jo Forsythe Dole, RN, PhD
Adjunct Assistant Professor
University of Pennsylvania School of
  Nursing
Philadelphia

DuWayne C. Englert, PhD
Professor Emeritus of Zoology
Southern Illinois University
Carbondale

Lisa K. Hansen, RN, MS, AOCN
Clinical Program Specialist
Autologous Blood and Marrow
  Transplantation
Legacy Good Samaritan Hospital
Portland, Ore.

Nancy H. Haynes, RN, MN, CCRN
Assistant Professor, Nursing
St. Luke's College
Kansas City, Mo.

Marcia J. Hill, RN, MSN
Associate Manager, Professional
  Education
Bertek Pharmaceuticals, Inc.
Morgantown, W.Va.

Shelley Yerger Huffstutler, RN, DSN, CFNP
Director, Primary Care Nurse
  Practitioner Program
Assistant Professor
University of Virginia School of Nursing
Charlottesville

John H. Lohnes, PA-C, MHS
Physician Assistant
University of North Carolina School of
  Medicine
Chapel Hill

Margaret E. Miller, RN, MSN
Clinical Nurse Specialist
Northwestern Medical Faculty
  Foundation
Chicago

Roger M. Morrell, MD, PhD, FACP (P.C.), ABPN
Clinical Neurologist in private practice
Southfield, Mich.

Mary Clare A. Schafer, MS, RN, ONC
Clinical Nurse Specialist, Orthopedics,
  Infection Control Nurse
Graduate Hospital
Philadelphia

Bradley G. Somer, MD
Fellow, Hematology-Oncology
University of Pennsylvania
Philadelphia

David Toub, MD
Medical Director
Newton Interactive
Pennington, N.J.

Catherine Ultrino, RN, MS, OCN
Nurse Manager, Hematology/Oncology
Boston Medical Center

Foreword

As health care professionals, we've all studied anatomy — with lots of pictures to guide us. We've studied physiology and disease, and we carry a raft of facts in our heads. But facts don't always bring the deep understanding that pictures do. For crucial day-to-day disease management in a busy clinical practice, we need not only the facts, but also pictures of what's going wrong in our patients' bodies. When it comes to *pathophysiology*, the pictures aren't always there — in our minds or in our reference books — when we need them.

How does high plasma glucose affect the diabetic patient's blood vessels and nerves? What process is driving disseminated intravascular coagulation? Why does Cushing's disease have such far-reaching clinical implications? Knowing the answers can speed patient assessment, guide diagnostic testing, and make appropriate treatment apparent.

Atlas of Pathophysiology is a stunningly visual reference that provides the answers to guide your clinical steps. For more than 150 diseases, this outstanding reference provides beautifully detailed illustrations of pathophysiology along with comprehensive explanations and clinical guidance side by side — a uniquely helpful arrangement.

The atlas begins with introductory chapters that discuss cell physiology and injury, homeostasis, and the ways disease disrupts the body's equilibrium. Discussions follow of cancer, infection, immune and genetic disorders, and fluid and electrolyte imbalances. Succeeding chapters cover disorders in every body system, and alphabetical arrangement within each chapter makes finding a specific disease easy. Each discussion begins with a brief overview of the disease followed by a framework that describes pathophysiology and lists causes, signs and symptoms, diagnostic tests, and treatments. Bulleted facts provide quick, concise, up-to-date information under each heading.

It's all there — hypervolemia, cardiac arrhythmias, anemias, Crohn's disease, osteoarthritis, leukemia, pneumonia, renal failure, and more. Whether you wish to quickly review an entire disease or to merely update your understanding of the disease process, the facts and illustrations are there, together, for targeted physical assessment and diagnostic testing, appropriate care, and patient counseling.

The layout of the book is extremely well suited for busy professionals. Each disease explanation features clearly labeled, full-color illustrations from the Anatomical Chart Company that provide excellent visual understanding of the anatomical structures and pathologic processes involved. Throughout the book, color logos call your attention to key information about age-related disease incidence and effects plus helpful tips to use in clinical practice. A glossary of common pathophysiology terms provides further information.

In addition to serving as an excellent student reference, *Atlas of Pathophysiology* can greatly simplify patient counseling, as the full-color illustrations make disease readily understandable. Often patients best understand information that is visually presented. This helps to clarify misunderstanding of the disease process — a common clinical problem. The beautiful color and overall visual attractiveness ensure this atlas's use as the perfect teaching aid — regardless of a patient's native language.

In the classroom, as well as in clinical practice, the need exists for clear illustrations of the disease process to use as teaching and learning tools. Anyone who teaches pathophysiology knows that students want a reference that provides them with a quick, easy-to-understand overview and illustrations that make learning easier. Such a book is difficult, if not impossible, to find. Thus, most students accumulate multiple references to supplement their learning.

A book that meets all needs is a rare find. *Atlas of Pathophysiology* is just such a find. I envision that this reference book will soon be found in professional offices, at nursing stations throughout the hospital, in students' book bags, in instructors' offices, on library shelves, and anywhere else that an excellent pathophysiology resource is needed. *Atlas of Pathophysiology,* with its concise, clear illustrations and functional layout, provides a unique way to give professionals quick access to a wealth of information about disease mechanisms.

Kristine A. Scordo, PhD, RN, CS, ACNP
Director, Acute Care Nurse Practitioner Program
Wright State University
Dayton, Ohio

PART I

CENTRAL CONCEPTS

CELLS, HOMEOSTASIS, AND DISEASE

The cell is the smallest living component of a living organism. Organisms can be made up of a single cell, such as bacteria, or billions of cells, such as human beings. In large organisms, highly specialized cells that perform a common function are organized into tissue. Tissues, in turn, form organs, which are integrated into body systems.

CELL COMPONENTS

Cells are complex organizations of specialized components, each component having its own specific function. The largest components of a normal cell are the cytoplasm, the nucleus, and the cell membrane. (See *Cell components*.)

Cytoplasm

The cytoplasm consists primarily of a fluid in which the tiny structures that perform the necessary functions to maintain the life of the cell are suspended. These tiny structures, called organelles, are the cell's metabolic machinery. Each performs a specific function to maintain the life of the cell. Organelles include:

● *mitochondria* — spherical or rod-shaped structures that produce most of the body's adenosine triphosphate (ATP). ATP contains high-energy phosphate chemical bonds that fuel many cellular activities. Mitochondria are the sites of cellular respiration — the metabolic use of oxygen to produce energy, carbon dioxide, and water.
● *ribosomes* — the sites of protein synthesis
● *endoplasmic reticulum* — an extensive network of two varieties of membrane-enclosed tubules:
– *rough endoplasmic reticulum*, which is covered with ribosomes
– *smooth endoplasmic reticulum*, which contains enzymes that synthesize lipids
● *Golgi apparatus* — synthesizes carbohydrate molecules that combine with protein produced by the rough endoplasmic reticulum and lipids produced by the smooth endoplasmic reticulum to form such products as lipoproteins, glycoproteins, and enzymes
● *lysosomes* — digest nutrients as well as foreign or damaged material in cells. A membrane surrounding each lysosome separates its digestive enzymes from the rest of the cytoplasm. The enzymes digest nutrient matter brought into the cell by means of endocytosis, in which a portion of the cell membrane surrounds and engulfs matter to form a membrane-bound intracellular vesicle. The membrane of the lysosome fuses with the membrane of the vesicle surrounding the endocytosed material. The lysosomal enzymes then digest the engulfed material. Lysosomes digest the foreign matter ingested by white blood cells by a similar process, which is called *phagocytosis*.
● *peroxisomes* — contain oxidases, enzymes that chemically reduce oxygen to hydrogen peroxide and hydrogen peroxide to water
● *cytoskeletal elements* — a network of protein structures that maintain the cell's shape

● *centrosomes* — contain centrioles, short cylinders adjacent to the nucleus that take part in cell division
● *microfilaments* and *microtubules* — enable movement of intracellular vesicles (allowing axons to transport neurotransmitters) and formation of the mitotic spindle, the framework for cell division.

Nucleus

The cell's control center is the nucleus, which plays a role in cell growth, metabolism, and reproduction. Within the nucleus, one or more nucleoli (dark-staining intranuclear structures) synthesize ribonucleic acid (RNA), a complex polynucleotide that controls protein synthesis. The nucleus also stores deoxyribonucleic acid (DNA), the double helix that carries genetic material and is responsible for cellular reproduction or division.

Cell membrane

The semipermeable cell membrane forms the cell's external boundary, separating it from other cells and from the external environment. The cell membrane consists of a double layer of phospholipids with protein molecules embedded in it. These protein molecules act as receptors, ion channels, or carriers for specific substances.

CELL DIVISION

Each cell must replicate itself for life to continue. Cells replicate by division in one of two ways: mitosis (produces two daughter cells with the same DNA and chromosome content as the mother cell) or meiosis (produces four gametocytes, each containing half the number of chromosomes of the original cell). Most cells divide by mitosis; meiosis occurs only in reproductive cells. Some cells, such as nerve and muscle cells, typically lose their ability to reproduce after birth.

CELL FUNCTIONS

In the human body, most cells are specialized to perform one function. Respiration and reproduction occur in all cells. The specialized functions are:
● *movement* — the result of coordinated action of nerve and muscle cells to change the position of a specific body part, contents within an organ, or the entire organism
● *conduction* — the transmission of a stimulus, such as a nerve impulse, heat, or sound wave, from one body part to another
● *absorption* — movement of substances through a cell membrane (For example, nutrients are absorbed and transported ultimately to be used as energy sources or as building blocks to form or repair structural and functional cellular components.)
● *secretion* — release of substances that act in another part of the body
● *excretion* — release of waste products generated by normal metabolic processes.

CELL TYPES

Each of the following four types of tissue consists of several specialized cell types, which perform specific functions.

- *Epithelial cells* line most of the internal and external surfaces of the body. Their functions include support, protection, absorption, excretion, and secretion.
- *Connective tissue cells* are present in skin, bones and joints, artery walls, fascia, and body fat. Their major functions are protection, metabolism, support, temperature maintenance, and elasticity.
- *Nerve cells* comprise the nervous system and are classified as neurons or neuroglial cells. Neurons perform the following functions:
  - generating electrical impulses
  - conducting electrical impulses
  - influencing other neurons, muscle cells, and cells of glands by transmitting impulses.

  Neuroglial cells support, nourish, and protect the neurons. The four types are:
  - *oligodendroglia* — produce myelin within the central nervous system (CNS)
  - *astrocytes* — provide essential nutrients to neurons and assist neurons in maintaining the proper bioelectrical potentials for impulse conduction and synaptic transmission
  - *ependymal cells* — involved in the production of cerebrospinal fluid
  - *microglia* — ingest and digest tissue debris when nervous tissue is damaged.
- *Muscle cells* contract to produce movement or tension.
  - *Skeletal (striated) muscle cells* extend along the entire length of skeletal muscles. These cells cause voluntary movement by contracting or relaxing together in a specific muscle. Contraction shortens the muscle; relaxation permits the muscle to return to its resting length.
  - *Smooth (nonstriated) muscle cells* are present in the walls of hollow internal organs, blood vessels, and bronchioles. By involuntarily contracting and relaxing, these cells change the luminal diameter of the hollow structure and thereby move substances through the organ.
  - *Striated cardiac muscle cells* branch out across the smooth muscle of the chambers of the heart and contract involuntarily. They produce and transmit cardiac action potentials, which cause cardiac muscle cells to contract.

 AGE ALERT
In older adults, skeletal muscle cells become smaller and many are replaced by fibrous connective tissue. The result is loss of muscle strength and mass.

PATHOPHYSIOLOGIC CONCEPTS

The cell faces a number of challenges through its life. Stressors, changes in the body's health, disease, and other extrinsic and intrinsic factors can change the cell's normal functioning.

Adaptation

Cells generally continue functioning despite changing conditions or stressors. However, severe or prolonged stress or changes may injure or destroy cells. When cell integrity is threatened, the cell reacts by drawing on its reserves to keep functioning, by adaptive changes, or by cellular dysfunction. If

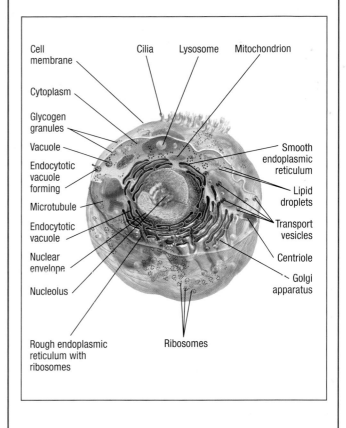

CELL COMPONENTS

cellular reserve is insufficient, the cell dies. If enough cellular reserve is available and the body doesn't detect abnormalities, the cell adapts by atrophy, hypertrophy, hyperplasia, metaplasia, or dysplasia. (See *Adaptive cell changes*, page 4.)

Atrophy

Atrophy is a reduction in the size of a cell or organ due to disuse, insufficient blood flow, malnutrition, or reduced stimulation. An example is loss of muscle mass after prolonged bed rest.

Hypertrophy

Hypertrophy is an increase in the size of a cell or organ due to an increase in workload. There are three types:
- *physiologic hypertrophy* — reflects an increase in workload that is not caused by disease; for example, the increase in muscle size caused by hard physical labor or weight training
- *compensatory hypertrophy* — increase in cell size to take over for nonfunctioning cells; for example, enlargement of one kidney when the other is not functioning or is absent
- *pathologic hypertrophy* — response to disease; for example, thickening of heart muscle as it pumps against increasing resistance in patients with hypertension.

Hyperplasia

Hyperplasia is an increase in the number of cells caused by increased workload, hormonal stimulation, or decreased tissue

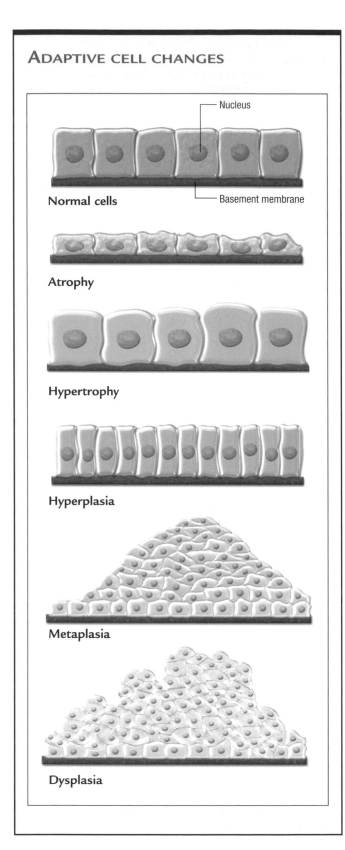

ADAPTIVE CELL CHANGES

Normal cells

Nucleus

Basement membrane

Atrophy

Hypertrophy

Hyperplasia

Metaplasia

Dysplasia

• *Compensatory hyperplasia* occurs in some organs to replace tissue that has been removed or destroyed; for example, regeneration of liver cells when part of the liver is surgically removed.
• *Pathologic hyperplasia* is a response to either excessive hormonal stimulation or abnormal production of hormonal growth factors; for example, acromegaly, in which excessive growth hormone production causes bones to enlarge.

Metaplasia

Metaplasia is the replacement of one cell type with another cell type that can better endure the change or stressor.
• *Physiologic metaplasia* is a normal response to changing conditions and is generally transient. For example, in the body's normal response to inflammation, monocytes migrate to inflamed tissues and transform into macrophages.
• *Pathologic metaplasia* is a response to an extrinsic toxin or stressor and is generally irreversible. For example, after years of exposure to cigarette smoke, stratified squamous epithelial cells replace the normal ciliated columnar epithelial cells of the bronchi. Although the new cells can better withstand smoke, they don't secrete mucus or have cilia to protect the airway. If exposure to cigarette smoke continues, the squamous cells can become cancerous.

Dysplasia

In dysplasia, abnormal differentiation of dividing cells results in abnormal size, shape, or appearance. Although dysplastic cell changes aren't cancerous, they can precede cancerous changes. Common examples include dysplasia of epithelial cells of the cervix or the respiratory tract.

Cell injury

Injury to any cellular component can lead to disease as the cells lose their ability to adapt. Cell injury may result from any of several intrinsic or extrinsic causes:
• *toxins* — may be endogenous or exogenous (Common endogenous toxins include products of genetically determined metabolic errors and hypersensitivity reactions. Exogenous toxins include alcohol, lead, carbon monoxide, and drugs that alter cellular function.)
• *infection* — may be caused by viruses, fungi, protozoa, or bacteria
• *physical injury* — disruption of a cell's structure or the relationships among the organelles. For example, two types of physical injury are thermal and mechanical
• *deficit injury* — loss of normal cellular metabolism caused by inadequate water, oxygen, or nutrients.
     Injury becomes irreversible when the cell membrane or the organelles can no longer function.

Cell degeneration

Degeneration is a type of sublethal cell damage that generally occurs in the cytoplasm and that doesn't affect the nucleus. Degeneration usually affects organs with metabolically active cells, such as the liver, heart, and kidneys. When changes in cells are identified, prompt health care can slow degeneration and prevent cell death. Unfortunately, many cell changes are unidentifiable, even with the use of a microscope, and early detection of disease is then impossible. An example of reversible degenerative change is cervical dysplasia. Examples of irreversible degenerative diseases include Huntington's disease and amyotrophic lateral sclerosis.

density. Like hypertrophy, hyperplasia may be *physiologic*, *compensatory*, or *pathologic*.
• *Physiologic hyperplasia* is an adaptive response to normal changes; for example, monthly increase in the number of uterine cells in response to estrogen stimulation after ovulation.

Cell aging

During the normal process of aging, cells lose both structure and function. Atrophy may reflect loss of cell structure; hypertrophy or hyperplasia; or lost function. Signs of aging occur in all body systems. Aging can proceed at different rates depending on the number and extent of injuries and the amount of wear and tear on the cell.

Cell death

Cell death may be caused by internal (intrinsic) factors that limit the cell's life span or external (extrinsic) factors that contribute to cell damage and aging. When stress is severe or prolonged, the cell can no longer adapt and it dies. Cell death, or necrosis, may manifest in different ways, depending on the tissues or organs involved.

● *Apoptosis* — genetically programmed cell death — accounts for the constant cell turnover in the skin's outer keratin layer and the lens of the eye.

● *Liquefactive necrosis* occurs when a lytic (dissolving) enzyme liquefies necrotic cells. This type of necrosis is common in the brain, which has a rich supply of lytic enzymes.

● *Caseous necrosis* occurs when necrotic cells disintegrate but the cellular pieces remain undigested for months or years. Its name derives from the resulting tissue's crumbly, cheeselike (caseous) appearance. It commonly occurs in pulmonary tuberculosis.

● *Fat necrosis* occurs when lipase enzymes break down intracellular triglycerides into free fatty acids. These free fatty acids combine with sodium, magnesium, or calcium ions to form soaps. The tissue becomes opaque and chalky white.

● *Coagulative necrosis* commonly follows interruption of blood supply to any organ — generally the kidneys, heart, or adrenal glands — except the brain. It inhibits activity of lysosomal lytic enzymes in the cells, so that the necrotic cells maintain their shape, at least temporarily.

● *Gangrenous necrosis*, a form of coagulative necrosis, typically results from a lack of blood flow and is complicated by an overgrowth and invasion of bacteria. It commonly occurs in the lower limbs as a result of arteriosclerosis or in the GI tract. Gangrene can occur in one of three forms:

– *dry gangrene* — occurs when bacterial invasion is minimal. It's marked by dry, wrinkled, dark brown or blackened tissue on an extremity.

– *moist (or wet) gangrene* — is accompanied by liquifactive necrosis — extensive lytic activity from bacteria and white blood cells that produces a liquid center in affected area. It can occur in the internal organs as well as the extremities.

– *gas gangrene* — develops when anaerobic bacteria of the genus *Clostridium* infect tissue. It's more likely to follow severe trauma and may be fatal. The bacteria release toxins that kill nearby cells and the gas gangrene rapidly spreads. Release of gas bubbles from affected muscle cells indicates that gas gangrene is present.

Cell death releases intracellular enzymes, which start to dissolve cellular components, and triggers an acute inflammatory reaction in which white blood cells migrate to the necrotic area and begin to digest the dead cells.

HOMEOSTASIS: MAINTAINING BALANCE

Every cell in the body participates in maintaining a dynamic, steady state of internal balance, called *homeostasis*. Pathophysiology results from changes or disruption in normal cellular function. Three structures in the brain are primarily responsible for maintaining homeostasis of the entire body:

● *medulla oblongata* — the part of the brain stem associated with vital functions such as respiration and circulation

● *pituitary gland* — regulates the function of other glands and, thereby, the body's growth, maturation, and reproduction

● *reticular formation* — a network of nerve cells and fibers in the brain stem and spinal cord that helps control vital reflexes such as cardiovascular function and respiration.

Each structure that maintains homeostasis through self-regulating feedback mechanisms has three components:

● *sensors* — cells that detect disruptions in homeostasis reflected by nerve impulses or changes in hormone levels

● *CNS control center* — receives signals from the sensor and regulates the body's response to those disruptions by initiating the effector mechanism

● *effector* — acts to restore homeostasis.

Feedback mechanisms exist in two varieties:

● *positive* — moves the system away from homeostasis by enhancing a change in the system

● *negative* — works to restore homeostasis by correcting a deficit in the system. Negative feedback mechanisms produce adaptive responses.

DISEASE

Although *disease* and *illness* are often used interchangeably, they aren't synonyms. *Disease* occurs when homeostasis isn't maintained. *Illness* occurs when a person is no longer in a state of perceived "normal" health. A person may have a disease, but not be ill all the time because his body has adapted to the disease.

The cause of disease may be intrinsic or extrinsic. Genetic factors, age, gender, infectious agents, or behaviors (such as inactivity, smoking, or abusing illegal drugs) can all cause disease. Diseases that have no known cause are called *idiopathic*.

The way a disease develops is called its *pathogenesis*. A disease is usually detected when it causes a change in metabolism or cell division that causes signs and symptoms. How the cells respond to disease depends on the causative agent and the affected cells, tissues, and organs. In the absence of intervention, resolution of the disease depends on many factors functioning over a period of time, such as extent of disease and the presence of other diseases. Manifestations of disease may include hypofunction, hyperfunction, or increased mechanical function.

Typically, diseases progress through the following stages:

● *exposure or injury* — target tissue exposed to a causative agent or injury

● *latency or incubation period* — no signs or symptoms are evident

● *prodromal period* — signs and symptoms are generally mild and nonspecific

● *acute phase* — disease reaches its full intensity, possibly with complications; called the *subclinical acute phase* if the patient can still function as though the disease weren't present

● *remission* — a second latency phase that occurs in some diseases and is commonly followed by another acute phase

● *convalescence* — patient progresses toward recovery

● *recovery* — return of health or normal functioning; no signs or symptoms of disease remain.

Cancer

Cancer refers to a group of more than 100 different diseases characterized by DNA damage that causes abnormal cell growth and development. Malignant cells have two defining characteristics: first, they can no longer divide and differentiate normally, and, secondly, they can invade surrounding tissues and travel to distant sites. In the United States, cancer accounts for more than half a million deaths each year, second only to cardiovascular disease.

CAUSES

The healthy body is well equipped to defend itself against cancer. Only when the immune system and other defenses fail does cancer prevail. Current evidence suggests that cancer develops from a complex interaction of exposure to carcinogens and accumulated mutations in several genes. Researchers have identified approximately 100 cancer genes, most of which fall into one of two categories:
- *oncogenes* — activate cell division and influence embryonic development
- *tumor-suppressor genes* — halt cell division.

Most normal human cells contain proto-oncogenes (oncogene precursors) and tumor-suppressor genes, which remain dormant unless they are transformed by genetic or acquired mutation. Common causes of acquired genetic damage are viruses, radiation, environmental and dietary carcinogens, and hormones. Other factors that interact to increase a person's likelihood of developing cancer are age, nutritional status, hormonal balance, and response to stress.

RISK FACTORS

Many cancers are related to specific environmental and lifestyle factors that predispose a person to develop cancer. Accumulating data suggest that some of these risk factors initiate carcinogenesis, others act as promoters, and some both initiate and promote the disease process.

Air pollution

Air pollution has been linked to the development of cancer, particularly lung cancer. Many outdoor air pollutants — such as arsenic, benzene, hydrocarbons, polyvinyl chlorides, and other industrial emissions as well as vehicle exhaust — have been studied for their carcinogenic properties. Indoor air pollution, such as cigarette smoke and radon gas, also poses an increased risk of cancer. In fact, indoor air pollution is considered to be more carcinogenic than outdoor air pollution.

Tobacco and alcohol

A cigarette smoker's risk of lung cancer is more than ten times greater than that of a nonsmoker's by late middle age. Tobacco smoke contains carcinogens that are known to cause mutations. The risk of lung cancer from cigarette smoking correlates directly with the duration of smoking and the number of cigarettes smoked per day. Research also shows that a person who stops smoking decreases his or her risk of lung cancer.

Although the risk associated with pipe and cigar smoking is similar to that of cigarette smoking, some evidence suggests that the effects are less severe. Smoke from cigars and pipes is more alkaline. This alkalinity decreases nicotine absorption in the lungs and also is more irritating to the lungs, so that the smoker doesn't inhale as readily.

Inhalation of "secondhand" smoke, or passive smoking, by nonsmokers also increases the risk of lung and other cancers. Use of smokeless tobacco, in which the oral tissue directly absorbs nicotine and other carcinogens, is linked to an increase in oral cancers that seldom occur in persons who don't use the product.

Alcohol consumption is commonly associated with cirrhosis of the liver, a precursor to hepatocellular cancer. The risk of breast and colorectal cancers also increases with alcohol consumption. Heavy use of alcohol and cigarette smoking synergistically increase the incidence of cancers of the mouth, larynx, pharynx, and esophagus. It's likely that alcohol acts as a solvent for the carcinogenic substances in smoke, thus enhancing their absorption.

Sexual factors

Sexual practices have been linked to specific types of cancer. The age of first sexual intercourse and the number of sexual partners are positively correlated with a woman's risk of cervical cancer. Furthermore, a woman who has had only one sexual partner is at higher risk if that partner has had multiple partners. The suspected underlying mechanism here involves virus transmission, most likely human papilloma virus (HPV).

Hormones — specifically the sex steroid hormones estrogen, progesterone, and testosterone — have been implicated as promoters of breast, endometrial, ovarian, or prostate cancer.

Occupation

Certain occupations, by exposing workers to specific substances, increase the risk of cancer. For example, persons exposed to asbestos are at risk of a specific type of lung cancer, called mesothelioma. Asbestos also may act as a promoter for other carcinogens. Workers involved in the production of dyes, rubber, paint, and beta-naphthylamine are at increased risk of bladder cancer.

Radiation

Exposure to ultraviolet radiation, or sunlight, causes genetic mutation in the P53 control gene. Sunlight also releases tumor necrosis factor alpha in exposed skin, possibly diminishing the immune response. Ultraviolet sunlight is a direct cause of basal and squamous cell cancers of the skin. The amount of exposure to ultraviolet radiation also correlates with the type of cancer that develops. For example, cumulative exposure to ultraviolet sunlight is associated with basal and squamous cell skin cancer, and severe episodes of burning and blistering at a young age are associated with melanoma.

Ionizing radiation (such as X-rays) is associated with acute leukemia, thyroid, breast, lung, stomach, colon, and urinary tract cancers as well as multiple myeloma. Low doses can cause DNA mutations and chromosomal abnormalities, and large doses can inhibit cell division. Ionizing radiation also can enhance the effects of genetic abnormalities. Other compounding variables include the part and percentage of the body exposed, the person's age, hormonal balance, prescribed drugs and preexisting or concurrent conditions.

Diet

Numerous aspects of diet are linked to an increase in cancer, including:
- obesity
- high consumption of dietary fat
- high consumption of smoked foods and salted fish or meats and foods containing nitrites
- naturally occurring carcinogens (such as hydrazines and aflatoxin) in foods
- carcinogens produced by microorganisms stored in foods
- diet low in fiber.

PATHOPHYSIOLOGIC CONCEPTS

The characteristic features of cancer are rapid, uncontrollable proliferation of cells and independent spread from a primary site (site of origin) to other tissues where it establishes secondary foci (metastases). (See *Histologic characteristics of cancer cells.*) This spread occurs through circulation in the blood or lymphatic fluid, by unintentional transplantation from one site to another during surgery, and by local extension. Thus, cancer cells differ from normal cells in terms of cell size, shape, number, differentiation, function, and ability to travel to distant tissues and organ systems.

Cell growth

Typically, each of the billions of cells in the human body has an internal clock that tells the cell when it is time to reproduce. Mitotic reproduction occurs in a sequence called the *cell cycle.* Normal cell division occurs in direct proportion to cells lost, thus providing a mechanism for controlling growth and differentiation. These controls are absent in cancer cells, and cell production exceeds cell loss. The loss of control over normal growth is termed *autonomy.* This independence is further evidenced by the ability of cancer cells to break away and travel to other sites.

Normal cells reproduce at a rate controlled through the activity of specific control or regulator genes. These genes produce proteins that act as "on" and "off" switches. There is no generalized control gene; different cells respond to specific control genes. In cancer cells, the control genes fail to function normally. The actual control may be lost or the gene may become damaged. An imbalance of growth factors may occur, or the cells may fail to respond to the suppressive action of the growth factors. Any of these mechanisms may lead to uncontrolled cellular reproduction.

Hormones, growth factors, and chemicals released by neighboring cells or by immune or inflammatory cells can influence control gene activity. These substances bind to specific receptors on the cell membranes and send out signals causing the control genes to stimulate or suppress cell reproduction.

Substances released by nearby injured or infected cells or by cells of the immune system also affect cellular reproduction. For example, interleukin, released by immune cells, stimulates cell proliferation and differentiation, and interferon, released from virus-infected and immune cells, may affect the cell's rate of reproduction.

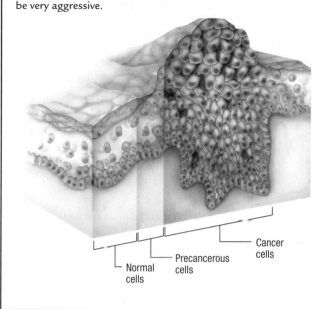

HISTOLOGIC CHARACTERISTICS OF CANCER CELLS

Cancer is a destructive (malignant) growth of cells, which invade nearby tissues and may metastasize to other areas of the body. Dividing rapidly, these cells tend to be very aggressive.

Normal cells

Precancerous cells

Cancer cells

Additionally, cells that are close to one another appear to communicate with each other through gap junctions (channels through which ions and other small molecules pass). This communication provides information to the cell about the neighboring cell types and the amount of space available. The nearby cells send out physical and chemical signals that control the rate of reproduction. Cancer cells fail to recognize the signals about available tissue space. Instead of forming only a single layer, cancer cells continue to accumulate in a disorderly array.

Differentiation

Normally, during development, cells become specialized. That is, they develop highly individualized characteristics that reflect their specific structure and functions. As the cells become more specialized, their reproduction and development slow down. Eventually, highly differentiated cells become unable to reproduce and some, skin cells for example, are programmed to die and be replaced.

Cancer cells lose the ability to differentiate; that is, they enter a state, called *anaplasia,* in which they no longer appear or function like the original cell. Anaplasia occurs in varying degrees. The less the cells resemble the cell of origin, the more anaplastic they are said to be. As the anaplastic cells continue to reproduce, they lose the typical characteristics of the original cell. Some anaplastic cells begin functioning as another type of cell, possibly beginning to produce hormones. Anaplastic cells of the same type in the same site exhibit many different shapes and sizes. Mitosis is abnormal and chromosome defects are common.

Intracellular changes

The abnormal and uncontrolled proliferation of cancer cells is also associated with numerous changes within the cancer cell itself. These changes affect cell components as follows:

● *cell membrane* — affects the organization, structure, adhesion, and migration of the cells. Impaired intercellular communication, enhanced response to growth factors, and diminished recognition of other cells causes uncontrolled growth and greatly increases metabolic demand for nutrients.

● *cytoskeleton* — disrupts protein filament networks, including actin and microtubules. Normally, actin filaments exert a pull on the extracellular organic molecules that bind cells together. Microtubules control cell shape, movement, and division.

● *cytoplasm* — components fewer in number and abnormally shaped. Less cellular work occurs because of a decrease in endoplasmic reticulum and mitochondria.

● *nucleus* — becomes pleomorphic (enlarged and misshapen) and highly pigmented. Nucleoli are larger and more numerous than normal. The nuclear membrane is often irregular and commonly has projections, pouches, or blebs, and fewer pores. Chromatin may clump along the outer areas of the nucleus. Chromosomal breaks, deletions, translocations, and abnormal karyotypes are common and seem to stem from the increased mitotic rate in cancer cells.

Tumor development and growth

Typically, a long time passes between the initiating event and the onset of the disease. During this time, the cancer cells continue to grow, develop, and replicate, each time undergoing successive changes and further mutations.

For a tumor to grow, an initiating event or events must cause a mutation that will transform the normal cell into a cancer cell. After the initial event, the tumor continues to grow only if available nutrients, oxygen, and blood supply are adequate and the immune system fails to recognize or respond to the tumor.

Two important tumor characteristics affecting growth are location of the tumor and available blood supply. The location determines the originating cell type, which in turn determines the cell cycle time. For example, epithelial cells have a shorter cell cycle than connective tissue cells. Thus, tumors of epithelial cells grow more rapidly than do tumors of connective tissue cells.

Tumors need an available blood supply to provide nutrients and oxygen for continued growth, and to remove wastes, but a tumor larger than 1 to 2 mm in size has typically outgrown its available blood supply. Some tumors secrete tumor angiogenesis factors, which stimulate the formation of new blood vessels, to meet the demand.

The degree of anaplasia also affects tumor growth. Remember that the more anaplastic the cells of the tumor, the less differentiated the cells and the more rapidly they divide.

Many cancer cells also produce their own growth factors. Numerous growth factor receptors are present on the cell membranes of rapidly growing cancer cells. This increase in receptors, in conjunction with the changes in the cell membranes, further enhances cancer cell proliferation.

Important characteristics of the host that affect tumor growth include age, sex, overall health status, and immune system function.

Certain cancers are more prevalent in females, others in males. For example, sex hormones influence tumor growth in breast, endometrial, cervical, and prostate cancers. Researchers believe that the hormone sensitizes the cell to the initial precipitating factor, thus promoting carcinogenesis.

Overall health status is also an important characteristic. As tumors obtain nutrients for growth from the host, they can alter normal body processes and cause cachexia. Conversely, if the person is nutritionally depleted, tumor growth may slow. Chronic tissue trauma also has been linked with tumor growth because healing involves increased cell division. And the more rapidly cells divide, the greater the likelihood of mutations.

Spread

Between the initiating event and the emergence of a detectable tumor, some or all of the mutated cells may die. The survivors, if any, reproduce until the tumor reaches a diameter of 1 to 2 mm. New blood vessels form to support continued growth and proliferation. As the cells further mutate and divide more rapidly, they become more undifferentiated, and the number of cancerous cells soon begins to exceed the number of normal cells. Eventually, the tumor mass extends and invades the surrounding tissues. When the local tissue is blood or lymph, the tumor can gain access to the circulation. Once access is gained, tumor cells that detach may travel to distant sites in the body, where they can survive and form a new tumor in the secondary site. This process is called metastasis. (See *How cancer spreads*.)

Dysplasia

Not all cells that proliferate rapidly go on to become cancerous. Throughout a person's life span, various body tissues experience periods of benign rapid growth, such as during wound healing. In some cases, changes in the size, shape, and organization of the cells leads to a condition called dysplasia. Exposure to chemicals, viruses, radiation, or chronic inflammation causes dysplastic changes that may be reversed by removing the initiating stimulus or treating its effects. However, if the stimulus is not removed, precancerous or dysplastic lesions can progress and give rise to cancer.

Localized tumor

Initially, a tumor remains localized. Recall that cancer cells communicate poorly with nearby cells. As a result, the cells continue to grow and enlarge, forming a mass or clumps of cells. The mass exerts pressure on the neighboring cells, blocking their blood supply, and subsequently causing their death.

Invasive tumor

Invasion is growth of the tumor into surrounding tissues. It's actually the first step in metastasis. Five mechanisms are linked to invasion:

● *cellular multiplication* — By their very nature, cancer cells multiply rapidly.

How cancer spreads

Cancer cells may invade nearby tissues or metastasize (spread) to other organs. Cancer cells may move to other tissues by any or all of three routes:

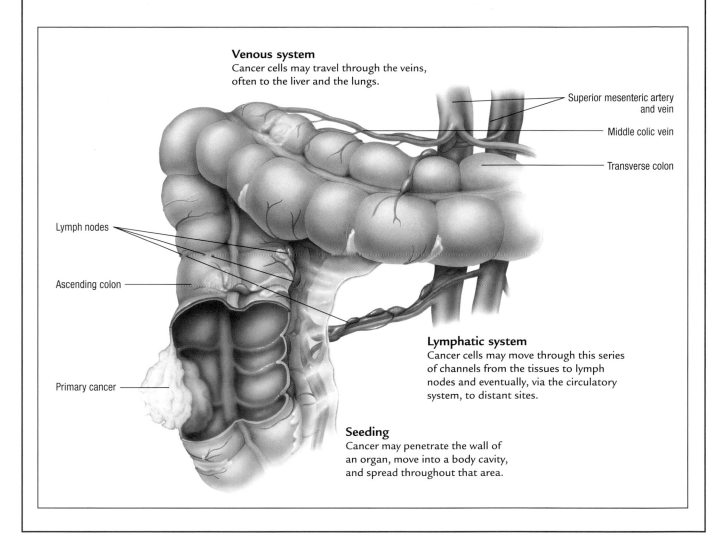

Venous system
Cancer cells may travel through the veins, often to the liver and the lungs.

Superior mesenteric artery and vein

Middle colic vein

Transverse colon

Lymph nodes

Ascending colon

Primary cancer

Lymphatic system
Cancer cells may move through this series of channels from the tissues to lymph nodes and eventually, via the circulatory system, to distant sites.

Seeding
Cancer may penetrate the wall of an organ, move into a body cavity, and spread throughout that area.

● *mechanical pressure* — As they grow, they exert pressure on surrounding cells and tissues, which eventually die because their blood supply has been cut off or blocked. Loss of mechanical resistance opens the way for the cancer cells to spread along the lines of least resistance and occupy the space once filled by the dead cells.

● *lysis of nearby cells* — Vesicles on the cancer cell surface contain a rich supply of receptors for laminin, a complex glycoprotein that is a major component of the basement membrane. These receptors permit the cancer cells to attach to the basement membrane, forming a bridgelike connection. Some cancer cells produce and excrete powerful proteolytic enzymes; other cancer cells induce normal host cells to produce them. These enzymes, such as collagenases and proteases, destroy the normal cells and break through their basement membrane, enabling the cancer cells to enter.

● *reduced cell adhesion* — This is likely the result of damage to the cell membrane.

● *increased motility* — Cancer cells secrete a chemotactic factor that stimulates motility. Thus, they can move independently into adjacent tissues, and into the circulation, and then to a secondary site. Finally, cancer cells develop fingerlike projections called pseudopodia that facilitate cell movement. These projections injure and kill neighboring cells and attach to vessel walls, enabling the cancer cells to enter.

Metastatic tumor

Metastatic tumors are those in which the cancer cells have traveled from the original or primary site to a second or more distant site. Most commonly, metastasis occurs through the blood vessels and lymphatic system. Tumor cells also can be transported from one body location to another by external means, such as surgical instruments or gloves.

Invasive tumor cells break down the basement membrane and walls of blood vessels, and the tumor sheds malignant cells into the circulation. Most of the cells die, but a few escape the host defenses and the turbulent environment of the bloodstream. From here, the surviving tumor mass of cells travels downstream and commonly lodges in the first capillary bed it encounters. Once lodged, the tumor cells develop a protective coat of fibrin, platelets, and clotting factors to evade detection by the immune system. Then they become attached to the epithelium, ultimately invading the vessel wall, interstitium, and the parenchyma of the target organ. To survive, the new tumor develops its own vascular network and, once established, may ultimately spread again.

The lymphatic system is the most common route for distant metastasis. Tumor cells enter the lymphatic vessels through damaged basement membranes and are transported to regional lymph nodes. In this case, the tumor becomes trapped in the first lymph node it encounters. The consequent enlargement, possibly the first evidence of metastasis, may be due to the increased tumor growth within the node or a localized immune reaction to the tumor. The lymph node may filter out or contain some of the tumor cells, limiting their further spread. The cells that escape can enter the blood from the lymphatic circulation through plentiful connections between the venous and lymphatic systems.

Typically, the first capillary bed, whether lymphatic or vascular, encountered by the circulating tumor mass determines the location of the metastasis. For example, because the lungs receive all of the systemic venous return, they are a frequent site for metastasis.

SIGNS AND SYMPTOMS

In most patients, the earlier the cancer is found, the more effective the treatment is likely to be and the better the prognosis. Some cancers may be diagnosed by a routine physical examination, even before the person develops any signs or symptoms. Others may display some early warning signals. (See *Cancer's seven warning signs*.)

Unfortunately, a person may not notice or heed the warning signs. These patients may present with some of the commoner signs and symptoms of advancing disease, such as fatigue, cachexia, pain, anemia, thrombocytopenia and leukopenia, and infection. Unfortunately, these signs and symptoms are nonspecific and can be attributed to many other disorders.

CANCER'S SEVEN WARNING SIGNS

The American Cancer Society has developed an easy way to remember the seven warning signs of cancer. Each letter in the word *CAUTION* represents a possible warning sign that should spur an individual to see a doctor.

C hange in bowel or bladder habits

A sore that doesn't heal

U nusual bleeding or discharge

T hickening or lump in the breast or elsewhere

I ndigestion or difficulty swallowing

O bvious change in a wart or mole

N agging cough or hoarseness

DIAGNOSTIC TESTS

A thorough history and physical examination should precede sophisticated diagnostic tests. The choice of diagnostic tests is determined by the patient's presenting signs and symptoms and the suspected body system involved. Diagnostic tests serve several purposes, including:
- establishing tumor presence and extent of disease
- determining possible sites of metastasis
- evaluating affected and unaffected body systems
- identifying the stage and grade of tumor.

Useful tests for early detection and staging of tumors include screening tests, X-rays, radioactive isotope scanning (nuclear medicine imaging), computed tomography (CT) scanning, endoscopy, ultrasonography, and magnetic resonance imaging (MRI). The single most important diagnostic tool is the biopsy for direct histologic study of the tumor tissue.

- *Screening tests* are perhaps the most important diagnostic tools in the prevention and early detection of cancer. They may provide valuable information about the possibility of cancer even before the patient develops signs and symptoms.
- *X-rays* are most commonly ordered to identify and evaluate changes in tissue densities. The type and location of the X-ray is determined by the patient's signs and symptoms and the suspected location of the tumor or metastases.
- *Radioactive isotope scanning* involves the use of a specialized camera which detects radioactive isotopes that are injected into the blood stream or ingested. The radiologist evaluates their distribution (uptake) throughout tissues, organs, and organ systems. This type of scanning provides a view of organs and regions within an organ that cannot be seen with a simple X-ray.
- *CT scanning* evaluates successive layers of tissue by using narrow beam X-ray to provide a cross-sectional view of the structure. It also can reveal different characteristics of tissues within a solid organ.
- *Endoscopy* provides a direct view of a body cavity or passageway to detect abnormalities. During endoscopy, the physician can excise small tumors, aspirate fluid, or obtain tissue samples for histologic examination.
- *Ultrasonography* uses high-frequency sound waves to detect changes in the density of tissues that are difficult or impossible to observe by radiology or endoscopy. Ultrasound helps to differentiate cysts from solid tumors.
- *MRI* uses magnetic fields and radio frequencies to show a cross-sectional view of the body organs and structures.
- *Biopsy*, removing a portion of suspicious tissue, is the only definitive method to diagnose cancer. Biopsy tissue samples can be taken by curettage, fluid aspiration, fine-needle aspiration, dermal punch, endoscopy, and surgical excision. The specimen then undergoes laboratory analysis for cell type and characteristics to provide information about the grade and stage of the cancer.

Some cancer cells release substances that normally aren't present in the body or are present only in small quantities. These substances, called tumor markers or biologic markers, are produced either by the cancer cell's genetic material during growth and development or by other cells in response to the presence of cancer. Markers may be found on the cell membrane of the tumor or in the blood, cerebrospinal fluid, or urine. Tumor cell markers include hormones, enzymes, genes, antigens, and antibodies.

Unfortunately, several disadvantages of tumor markers may preclude their use alone. For example:
• by the time the tumor cell marker level is elevated, the disease may be too far advanced to treat
• most tumor cell markers are not specific enough to identify one certain type of cancer
• some nonmalignant diseases, such as pancreatitis or ulcerative colitis, also are associated with tumor cell markers
• perhaps the worst drawback is that the absence of a tumor cell marker does not mean that a person is free of cancer.

TUMOR CLASSIFICATION

Tumors are initially classified as benign or malignant depending on their specific features. Typically, benign tumors are well differentiated; that is, their cells closely resemble those of the tissue of origin. Commonly encapsulated with well-defined borders, benign tumors grow slowly, often displacing but not infiltrating surrounding tissues, and therefore causing only slight damage. Benign tumors do not metastasize.

Conversely, most malignant tumors are undifferentiated to varying degrees, having cells that may differ considerably from those of the tissue of origin. They are seldom encapsulated and are often poorly delineated. They rapidly expand in all directions, causing extensive damage as they infiltrate surrounding tissues. Most malignant tumors metastasize through the blood or lymph to secondary sites.

Malignant tumors are further classified by tissue type, degree of differentiation (grading), and extent of the disease (staging). High-grade tumors are poorly differentiated and are more aggressive than low-grade tumors. Early-stage cancers carry a more favorable prognosis than later-stage cancers that have spread to nearby or distant sites.

TREATMENT

The number of cancer treatments is constantly increasing. They may be used alone or in combination (multimodal therapy), depending on the type, stage, localization, and responsiveness of the tumor and on limitations imposed by the patient's clinical status. Cancer treatment has four goals:
• *cure* — eradicating the cancer and promoting long-term patient survival
• *control* — arresting tumor growth
• *palliation* — alleviating symptoms when the disease is beyond control
• *prophylaxis* — providing treatment when no tumor is detectable, but the patient is known to be at high risk of tumor development or recurrence.

Cancer treatment is further categorized by type according to when it is used:
• *primary* — to eradicate the disease
• *adjuvant* — in addition to primary, to eliminate microscopic disease and promote cure or improve the patient's response
• *salvage* — to manage recurrent disease.

Any treatment regimen can cause complications. Indeed, many complications of cancer are related to the adverse effects of treatment.

Surgery, once the mainstay of cancer treatment, is now typically combined with other therapies. It may be performed to diagnose the disease, initiate primary treatment, or achieve palliation, and is occasionally done for prophylaxis.

Radiation therapy uses high-energy radiation to treat cancer. Used alone or in conjunction with other therapies, it aims to destroy dividing cancer cells while damaging normal cells as little as possible. Two types of radiation are used to treat cancer: ionizing radiation and particle beam radiation. Radiation therapy has both local and systemic adverse effects, because it affects both normal and malignant cells.

Chemotherapy includes a wide range of antineoplastic drugs, which may induce regression of a tumor and its metastasis. It's particularly useful in controlling residual disease and as an adjunct to surgery or radiation therapy. It can induce long remissions and sometimes effect cure. As a palliative treatment, chemotherapy aims to improve the patient's quality of life by temporarily relieving pain and other symptoms.

Every dose of a chemotherapeutic agent destroys only a percentage of tumor cells. Therefore, regression of the tumor requires repeated doses of drugs. The goal is to eradicate enough of the tumor so that the immune system can destroy the remaining malignant cells. Unfortunately, chemotherapy also causes numerous adverse effects.

Hormonal therapy is based on studies showing that certain hormones can inhibit the growth of certain cancers.

Immunotherapy, now commonly called biotherapy, is treatment with agents known as biologic response modifiers. Biologic agents are usually combined with chemotherapy or radiation therapy, and are most effective in the early stages of cancer. Many types of immunotherapy are still experimental; their availability may be restricted and their adverse effects are generally unpredictable. However, several approaches appear promising. Examples of immunotherapy include: bone marrow transplantation, monoclonal antibodies, and colony stimulating factors.

INFECTION

Infection is the invasion and multiplication of microorganisms in or on body tissue that cause signs, symptoms, and an immune response. Such reproduction injures the host by causing cell damage from toxins produced by the microorganisms or from intracellular multiplication, or by competing with host metabolism. Infectious diseases range from relatively mild illnesses to debilitating and lethal conditions: from the common cold through chronic hepatitis to acquired immunodeficiency syndrome (AIDS). The severity of the infection varies with the pathogenicity and number of the invading microorganisms and the strength of host defenses.

For infection to be transmitted, the following must be present: causative agent, infectious reservoir with a portal of exit, mode of transmission, a portal of entry into the host, and a susceptible host.

CAUSES

Microorganisms that are responsible for infectious diseases include viruses, bacteria, fungi, mycoplasmas, rickettsia, chlamydia, and parasites.

Viruses

Viruses are subcellular organisms made up only of a ribonucleic acid (RNA) nucleus or a deoxyribonucleic acid (DNA) nucleus covered with proteins. They're the smallest known organisms, so tiny that only an electron microscope can make them visible. Independent of the host cells, viruses can't replicate. Rather, they invade a host cell and stimulate it to participate in forming additional virus particles. Some viruses destroy surrounding tissue and release toxins. Viruses lack the genes necessary for energy production. They depend on the ribosomes and nutrients of infected host cells for protein production. The estimated 400 viruses that infect humans are classified according to their size, shape, and means of transmission (respiratory, fecal, oral, sexual).

Retroviruses are a unique type of virus that carry their genetic code in RNA rather than the more common carrier DNA. These RNA viruses contain the enzyme reverse transcriptase, which changes viral RNA into DNA. The host cell then incorporates the alien DNA into its own genetic material. The most notorious retrovirus today is human immunodeficiency virus (HIV).

Bacteria

Bacteria are simple one-celled microorganisms with a cell wall that protects them from many of the defense mechanisms of the human body. Although they lack a nucleus, bacteria possess all the other mechanisms they need to survive and rapidly reproduce.

Bacteria can be classified according to shape — spherical cocci, rod-shaped bacilli, and spiral-shaped spirilla. Bacteria can also be classified according to their need for oxygen (aerobic or anaerobic), their mobility (motile or nonmotile), and their tendency to form protective capsules (encapsulated or nonencapsulated) or spores (sporulating or nonsporulating).

Bacteria damage body tissues by interfering with essential cell function or by releasing exotoxins or endotoxins, which cause cell damage.

Fungi

Fungi have rigid walls and nuclei that are enveloped by nuclear membranes. They occur as yeast (single-cell, oval-shaped organisms) or molds (organisms with hyphae, or branching filaments). Depending on the environment, some fungi may occur in both forms. Found almost everywhere on earth, fungi live on organic matter, in water and soil, on animals and plants, and on a wide variety of unlikely materials. They can live both inside and outside their host.

Mycoplasmas

Mycoplasmas are bacterialike organisms, the smallest of the cellular microbes that can live outside a host cell, although some may be parasitic. Lacking cell walls, they can assume many different shapes ranging from coccoid to filamentous. The lack of a cell wall makes them resistant to penicillin and other antibiotics that work by inhibiting cell wall synthesis.

Rickettsia

Rickettsia are small, gram-negative, aerobic bacterialike organisms that can cause life-threatening illness. They may be coccoid, rod-shaped, or irregularly shaped. Because they're live viruses, rickettsia require a host cell for replication. They have no cell wall, and their cell membranes are leaky; thus, they must live inside another, better protected cell. Rickettsia are transmitted by the bites of arthropod carriers, such as lice, fleas, and ticks, and through exposure to their waste products. Rickettsial infections that occur in the United States include Rocky Mountain spotted fever, typhus, and Q fever.

Chlamydia

Chlamydia are smaller than rickettsia and bacteria but larger than viruses. They depend on host cells for replication and are susceptible to antibiotics. Chlamydia are transmitted by direct contact such as occurs during sexual activity.

Parasites

Parasites are unicellular or multicellular organisms that live on or within another organism and obtain nourishment from the host. They take only the nutrients they need and usually don't kill their hosts. Examples of parasites that can produce an infection if they cause cellular damage to the host include helminths, such as pinworms and tapeworms, and arthropods, such as mites, fleas, and ticks. Helminths can infect the human gut; arthropods commonly cause skin and systemic disease.

RISK FACTORS

A healthy person can usually ward off infections with the body's own built-in defense mechanisms:
- intact skin
- normal flora that inhabit the skin and various organs

- lysozymes secreted by eyes, nasal passages, glands, stomach, and genitourinary organs
- defensive structures such as the cilia that sweep foreign matter from the airways
- a healthy immune system.

However, if an imbalance develops, the potential for infection increases. Risk factors for the development of infection include weakened defense mechanisms, environmental and developmental factors, and pathogen characteristics.

Weakened defense mechanisms

The body has many defense mechanisms for resisting entry and multiplication of both exogenous and endogenous microbes. However, a weakened immune system makes it easier for these pathogens to invade the body and launch an infectious disease. This weakened state is referred to as immunodeficiency or immunocompromise.

Impaired function of white blood cells (WBCs), as well as low levels of T and B cells, characterizes immunodeficiencies. An immunodeficiency may be congenital or acquired. Acquired immunodeficiency may result from infection, malnutrition, chronic stress, or pregnancy. Diabetes, renal failure, and cirrhosis can suppress the immune response, as can drugs such as corticosteroids and chemotherapy.

Regardless of cause, the result of immunodeficiency is the same. The body's ability to recognize and fight pathogens is impaired. People who are immunodeficient are more susceptible to all infections, are more acutely ill when they become infected, and require a much longer time to heal.

Environmental factors

Other conditions that may weaken a person's immune defenses include poor hygiene, malnutrition, inadequate physical barriers, emotional and physical stressors, chronic diseases, medical and surgical treatments, and inadequate immunization.

Good hygiene promotes normal host defenses; poor hygiene increases the risk of infection. Unclean skin harbors microbes, offers an environment for them to colonize, and is more open to invasion. Frequent washing removes surface microbes and maintains an intact barrier to infection, but it may damage the skin. To maintain skin integrity, lubricants and emollients may be used to prevent cracks and breaks.

The body requires a balanced diet to provide the nutrients, vitamins, and minerals needed for an effective immune system. Protein malnutrition inhibits the production of antibodies, without which the body is unable to mount an effective attack against microbe invasion. Malnutrition has been shown to have a direct relationship to the incidence of nosocomial infections.

Dust can facilitate transportation of pathogens. For example, dustborne spores of the fungus aspergillus transmit the infection. If the inhaled spores become established in the lungs, they're notoriously difficult to expel. Fortunately, most persons with intact immune systems can resist infection with aspergillus, which is usually dangerous only in the presence of severe immunosuppression.

Developmental factors

The very young and very old are at higher risk for infection. The immune system doesn't fully develop until about age 6 months. An infant exposed to an infectious agent usually develops an infection. The most common type of infection in toddlers affects the respiratory tract. When young children put toys and other objects in their mouths, they increase their exposure to a variety of pathogens.

Exposure to communicable diseases continues throughout childhood, as children progress from daycare facilities to schools. Skin diseases, such as impetigo, and lice infestation commonly pass from one child to the next at this age. Accidents are common in childhood as well, and broken or abraded skin opens the way for bacterial invasion. Lack of immunization also contributes to incidence of childhood diseases.

Advancing age, on the other hand, is associated with a declining immune system, partly as a result of decreasing thymus function. Chronic diseases, such as diabetes and atherosclerosis, can weaken defenses by impairing blood flow and nutrient delivery to body systems.

Pathogen characteristics

A microbe must be present in sufficient quantities to cause a disease in a healthy human. The number needed to cause a disease varies from one microbe to the next and from host to host and may be affected by the mode of transmission. The severity of an infection depends on several factors, including the microbe's pathogenicity, that is, the likelihood that it will cause pathogenic changes or disease. Factors that affect pathogenicity include:

- *specificity* — the range of hosts to which a microbe is attracted. Some microbes may be attracted to a wide range of both humans and animals, while others select only human or only animal hosts.
- *invasiveness* (sometimes called *infectivity*) — ability of a microbe to invade and multiply in the host tissues. Some microbes can enter through intact skin; others can enter only if the skin or mucous membrane is broken. Some microbes produce enzymes that enhance their invasiveness.
- *quantity* — the number of microbes that succeed in invading and reproducing in the body
- *virulence* — severity of the disease a pathogen can produce. Virulence can vary depending on the host defenses; any infection can be life-threatening in an immunodeficient patient. Infection with a pathogen known to be particularly virulent requires early diagnosis and treatment.
- *toxigenicity* (related to virulence) — potential to damage host tissues by producing and releasing toxins
- *adhesiveness* — ability to attach to host tissue. Some pathogens secrete a sticky substance that helps them adhere to tissue while protecting them from the host's defense mechanisms.
- *antigenicity* — degree to which a pathogen can induce a specific immune response. Microbes that invade and localize in tissue initially stimulate a cellular response; those that disseminate quickly throughout the host's body generate an antibody response.
- *viability* — ability to survive outside its host. Most microbes can't live and multiply outside a reservoir.

STAGES OF INFECTION

Development of infection usually proceeds through four stages. (See *Stages of infection*, page 14.)

PATHOPHYSIOLOGIC CONCEPTS

Clinical expressions of infectious disease vary, depending on the pathogen involved and the body system affected. Most of

Stages of infection

Stage I

Incubation	• Duration can range from instantaneous to several years. • Pathogen is replicating and the infected person becomes contagious, thus capable of transmitting the disease.

Stage II

Prodromal stage	• Host makes vague complaints of feeling unwell. • Host is still contagious.

Stage III

Acute illness	• Microbes actively destroy host cells and affect specific host systems. • Patient recognizes which area of the body is affected. • Complaints are more specific.

Stage IV

Convalescence	• Begins when the body's defense mechanisms have contained the microbes. • Damaged tissue is healing.

the signs and symptoms result from host responses, which may be similar or very different from host to host. During the prodromal stage, a person will complain of some common, nonspecific signs and symptoms, such as fever, muscle aches, headache, and lethargy. In the acute stage, signs and symptoms that are more specific provide evidence of the microbe's target. However, some diseases remain asymptomatic and are discovered only by laboratory tests.

The inflammatory response is a major reactive defense mechanism in the battle against infective agents. Inflammation may be the result of tissue injury, infection, or allergic reaction. Acute inflammation has two stages: vascular and cellular. In the vascular stage, arterioles at or near the site of the injury briefly constrict and then dilate, causing an increase in fluid pressure in the capillaries. The consequent movement of plasma into the interstitial space causes edema. At the same time, inflammatory cells release histamine and bradykinin, which further increase capillary permeability. Red blood cells and fluid flow into the interstitial space, contributing to edema. The extra fluid arriving in the inflamed area dilutes microbial toxins.

During the cellular stage of inflammation, WBCs and platelets move toward the damaged cells, and phagocytosis of the dead cells and microorganisms begins. Platelets control any excess bleeding in the area, and mast cells arriving at the site release heparin to maintain blood flow to the area.

Signs and symptoms

Acute inflammation is the body's immediate response to cell injury or cell death. The cardinal signs of inflammation include:

• *redness (rubor)* — dilation of arterioles and increased circulation to the site; a localized blush caused by filling of previously empty or partially distended capillaries
• *heat (calor)* — local vasodilatation, fluid leakage into the interstitial spaces, and increased blood flow to the area
• *pain (dolor)* — pain receptors stimulated by swollen tissue, local pH changes, and chemicals excreted during the inflammatory process
• *edema (tumor)* — local vasodilatation, leakage of fluid into interstitial spaces, and blockage of lymphatic drainage
• *loss of function (functio laesa) of a body part* — primarily a result of edema and pain.

CLINICAL TIP
Localized infections produce a rapid inflammatory response with obvious signs and symptoms. Disseminated infections have a slow inflammatory response and take longer to identify and treat, thereby increasing morbidity and mortality.

Fever

Fever follows the introduction of an infectious agent. An elevated temperature helps fight an infection because many microorganisms are unable to survive in a hot environment. When the body temperature rises too high, body cells can be damaged, particularly those of the nervous system.

Diaphoresis (sweating) is the body's method of cooling itself and returning the temperature to "normal" for that individual. Artificial methods to reduce a slight fever can actually impede the body's defenses against infection.

Leukocytosis

The body responds to the introduction of pathogens by increasing the number and types of circulating WBCs. This process is called *leukocytosis*. In the acute or early stage, the neutrophil count increases. Bone marrow begins to release immature leukocytes, because existing neutrophils cannot meet the body's demand for defensive cells. The immature neutrophils (called "bands" in the differential WBC count) can't serve any defensive purpose.

As the acute phase comes under control and the damage is isolated, the cellular stage of the inflammatory process takes place. Neutrophils, monocytes, and macrophages begin the process of phagocytosis of dead tissue and bacteria. Neutrophils and monocytes are attracted to the site of infection by chemotaxis, and they identify the foreign antigen and attach to it. Then they engulf, kill, and degrade the microorganism that carries the antigen on its surface. Macrophages, a mature type of monocyte, arrive at the site later and remain in the area of inflammation longer than the other cells. Besides phagocytosis, macrophages play several other key roles at the site, such as preparing the area for healing and processing antigens for a cellular immune response. An elevated monocyte count is common during resolution of any injury and in chronic infections.

Chronic inflammation

An inflammatory reaction lasting longer than 2 weeks is referred to as chronic inflammation. It may or may not follow an acute process. A poorly healed wound or an unresolved infection can lead to chronic inflammation. The body may encapsulate a pathogen that it can't destroy in order to isolate it. An example of such a pathogen is mycobacteria, one of the species which cause tuberculosis; encapsulated mycobacteria appear in X-rays as identifiable spots in the lungs. With chronic inflammation, there can be permanent scarring and loss of tissue function.

DIAGNOSTIC TESTS

Accurate assessment helps identify infectious diseases, appropriate treatment, and avoidable complications. It begins with obtaining the patient's complete medical history, performing a thorough physical examination, and performing or ordering appropriate diagnostic tests. Tests that can help identify and gauge the extent of infection include laboratory studies, radiographic tests, and scans.

Most often, the first test is a WBC count and a differential. Any elevation in the overall number of WBCs is a positive result. The differential count is the relative number of each of five types of white blood cells — neutrophils, eosinophils, basophils, lymphocytes, and monocytes. This test recognizes only that something has stimulated an immune response. Bacterial infection usually causes an elevation in the counts; viruses may cause no change or a decrease in normal WBC level.

Erythrocyte sedimentation rate may be done as a general test to reveal that an inflammatory process is occurring within the body.

To determine the causative agent, a stained smear from a specific body site is obtained. Stains that may be used to visualize the microorganism include:
- *Gram stain* — identifies gram-negative or gram-positive bacteria
- *acid-fast stain* — identifies mycobacteria and nocardia
- *silver stain* — identifies fungi, legionella, and pneumocystis.

Although stains provide rapid and valuable diagnostic information, they only tentatively identify a pathogen. Confirmation requires culturing. Growth sufficient to identify the microbe may occur as quickly as 8 hours or as long as several weeks, depending on how rapidly the microbe replicates. Types of cultures that may be ordered are blood, urine, sputum, throat, nasal, wound, skin, stool, and cerebrospinal fluid, but any body substance can be cultured.

A specimen obtained for culture must not be contaminated with any other substance. For example, a urine specimen must not contain any debris from the perineum or vaginal area. If obtaining a clean urine specimen isn't possible, the patient must be catheterized to make sure that only the urine is being examined. Contaminated specimens may mislead and prolong treatment.

Additional tests that may be requested include magnetic resonance imaging to locate infection sites, chest X-rays to search the lungs for respiratory changes, and gallium scans to detect abscesses.

TREATMENTS

Treatment for infections can vary widely. Vaccines may be administered to induce a primary immune response under conditions that won't cause disease. If infection does occur, treatment is tailored to the specific causative organism. Drug therapy should be used only when it is appropriate. Supportive therapy can play an important role in fighting infections.
- Antibiotics work in a variety of ways, depending on the class of antibiotic. Their action is either bactericidal or bacteriostatic. Antibiotics may inhibit cell-wall synthesis, protein synthesis, bacterial metabolism, or nucleic acid synthesis or activity, or they may increase cell-membrane permeability.
- Antifungal drugs destroy the invading microbe by increasing cell-membrane permeability. The antifungal binds sterols in the cell membrane, resulting in leakage of intracellular contents, such as potassium, sodium, and nutrients.
- Antiviral drugs stop viral replication by interfering with DNA synthesis.

The overuse of antimicrobials has created widespread resistance to some specific drugs. Some pathogens that were once well controlled by medicines are again surfacing with increased virulence. One such pathogen is that which is known to cause tuberculosis.

Some diseases, including most viral infections, don't respond to available drugs. Supportive care is the only recourse while the host defenses repel the invader. To help the body fight an infection, the patient should:
- use universal precautions to avoid spreading the infection
- drink plenty of fluids
- get plenty of rest
- avoid people who may have other illnesses
- take only over-the-counter medications appropriate for his symptoms, with full knowledge about dosage, actions, and possible side effects or adverse reactions
- follow the doctor's orders for taking any prescription drugs and be sure to complete the medication as ordered and not share the prescription with others.

DISORDERS

The following chart describes a variety of infectious disorders, along with the causes, pathophysiologic concepts, and associated signs and symptoms. (See *Common infectious disorders*, pages 16 to 19.)

COMMON INFECTIOUS DISORDERS

DISORDER	CHARACTERISTICS
Bacterial infections	
Conjunctivitis	Bacterial or viral infection of the conjunctiva of the eye. ● Culture from the conjunctiva identifies the causative organism. ● Associated with hyperemia of the eye, discharge, tearing, pain, and photophobia.
Gonorrhea	Sexually transmitted disease caused by *Neisseria gonorrhoeae*. ● After exposure, epithelial cells at infection site become infected and disease begins to spread locally. ● Disease pattern depends on individual infected and site of infection.
Listeriosis	Infection caused by weakly hemolytic, gram-positive bacillus *Listeria monocytogenes*. ● Primary method of person-to-person transmission is neonatal infection in utero or during passage through an infected birth canal. ● Other modes of transmission include: - inhaling contaminated dust - drinking contaminated, unpasteurized milk - contact with infected animals, contaminated sewage or mud, or soil contaminated with feces containing the organism - possibly, postpartum person-to-person transmission.
Lyme disease	Infection caused by spirochete *Borrelia burgdorferi*. ● Transmitted by ixodid tick, which injects spirochete-laden saliva into bloodstream or deposits fecal matter on skin. ● After 3 to 32 days, spirochetes migrate outward, typically causing a ringlike rash. ● Spirochetes disseminate to other skin sites or organs through bloodstream or lymphatic system. ● Spirochetes may survive for years in joints, or they may die after triggering an inflammatory response in host. ● As infection progresses through three stages, neurologic symptoms and impairment worsen.
Meningitis	Meningeal inflammation caused by bacteria, viruses, protozoa, or fungi. The most common types are bacterial and viral. ● Bacterial meningitis occurs when bacteria enter the subarachnoid space and cause an inflammatory response. The organisms gain access to the subarachnoid space and the cerebrospinal fluid (CSF), where they cause irritation of the tissues bathed by the fluid. ● Viral meningitis may result from a direct infection or secondary to disease, such as mumps, herpes, measles, or leukemia.
Otitis media	Inflammation of the middle ear caused by a bacterial infection. ● Often accompanied by a viral upper respiratory infection ● Viral symptoms generally followed by ear pain.
Peritonitis	Acute or chronic inflammation of the peritoneum due to bacterial invasion. ● Onset often sudden, with severe and diffuse abdominal pain ● Pain intensifies and localizes in region of the disorder.
Pneumonia	Infection of the lung parenchyma that is bacterial, fungal, or protozoal in origin. ● The lower respiratory tract can be exposed to pathogens by inhalation, aspiration, vascular dissemination, or direct contact with contaminated equipment. Once inside, the pathogen begins to colonize and infection develops. ● Bacterial infection initially triggers alveolar inflammation and edema, which produces an area of low ventilation with normal perfusion. Capillaries become engorged with blood, causing stasis. As alveolocapillary membranes break down, alveoli fill with blood and exudate, causing atelectasis, or lung collapse.
Salmonellosis	Disease caused by a serotype of the genus *Salmonella*, a member of the *Enterobacteriaceae* family. ● Most common species of *Salmonella* include *S. typhi*, which causes typhoid fever; *S. enteritidis*, which causes enterocolitis; and *S. choleraesuis*, which causes bacteremia. ● Nontyphoidal salmonellosis usually follows ingestion of contaminated dry milk, chocolate bars, pharmaceuticals of animal origin, or contaminated or inadequately processed foods, especially eggs and poultry. ● Characteristic symptoms include abdominal pain, severe diarrhea with enterocolitis.

DISORDER	CHARACTERISTICS
Bacterial infections *(continued)*	
Shigellosis	Acute intestinal infection caused by the bacteria shigella, a short, nonmotile, gram-negative rod. ● Transmission occurs through the fecal-oral route, by direct contact with contaminated objects, or through ingestion of contaminated food or water. Occasionally, the housefly is a vector. ● After an incubation period of 1 to 4 days, shigella organisms invade the intestinal mucosa and cause inflammation.
Syphilis	Sexually transmitted infection caused by the spirochete *Treponema pallidum*. ● Prenatal transmission from an infected mother to her fetus is possible. ● Syphilis begins in the mucous membranes and quickly becomes systemic, spreading to nearby lymph nodes and the bloodstream. ● Characteristic sign of primary syphilis is chancres at the local infection site. Secondary and late complications may involve multiple organ systems.
Tetanus	Acute exotoxin-mediated infection caused by the anaerobic, spore-forming, gram-positive bacillus *Clostridium tetani*. ● Transmission occurs through a puncture wound that is contaminated by soil, dust, or animal excreta containing *C. tetani*, or by way of burns and minor wounds. ● After *C. tetani* enters the body, it causes local infection and tissue necrosis. It also produces toxins that then enter the bloodstream and lymphatics and eventually spread to central nervous system tissue. ● Characterized by marked muscle hypertonicity, hyperactive deep tendon reflexes, and painful, involuntary muscle contractions.
Toxic shock syndrome (TSS)	Acute bacterial infection caused by toxin-producing, penicillin-resistant strains of *Staphylococcus aureus*, such as TSS toxin-1 or staphylococcal enterotoxins B and C. ● Menstrual toxic shock is associated with menstruation and tampon use. ● Nonmenstrual toxic shock is associated with infections, such as abscesses, osteomyelitis, and postsurgical infections.
Tuberculosis	Infectious disease transmitted by inhaling airborne bacilli from a person infected with active tuberculosis (TB). ● Bacilli are deposited in the lungs and the immune system responds by sending leukocytes, and inflammation results. After a few days, leukocytes are replaced by macrophages. Bacilli are then ingested by the macrophages and carried off by the lymphatics to the lymph nodes. Macrophages that ingest the bacilli fuse to form epithelioid cell tubercles, tiny nodules surrounded by lymphocytes. ● Caseous necrosis develops in the lesion, and scar tissue encapsulates the tubercle. The organism may or may not be killed in the process. ● If the tubercles and inflamed nodes rupture, the infection contaminates the surrounding tissue and may spread through the blood and lymphatic circulation to distant sites.
Urinary tract infections	Infection most commonly caused by enteric gram-negative bacilli. ● Results from microorganisms entering the urethra and then ascending to the bladder.
Whooping cough (pertussis)	Highly contagious respiratory infection usually caused by the nonmotile, gram-negative coccobacillus *Bordetella pertussis* and, occasionally, by the related similar bacteria *B. parapertussis* or *B. bronchiseptica*. ● Transmitted by direct inhalation of contaminated droplets from a patient in an acute stage. It may also spread indirectly through soiled linen and other articles contaminated by respiratory secretions. ● After approximately 7 to 10 days, *B. pertussis* enters the tracheobronchial mucosa, where it produces progressively tenacious mucus. ● Known for its associated spasmodic cough, characteristically ending in a loud, crowing inspiratory whoop.
Viral infections	
Chickenpox (varicella)	Common, highly contagious, exanthem caused by the varicella-zoster virus. ● Transmitted by respiratory droplets or direct contact with vesicles.

(continued)

DISORDER	CHARACTERISTICS
Viral infections (*continued*)	
Cytomegalovirus infection	Viral infection transmitted through contact with infected secretions. • The virus spreads through the body in lymphocytes or mononuclear cells to the lungs, liver, GI tract, eyes, and central nervous system, where it commonly produces inflammatory reactions.
Herpes simplex	Herpes virus hominis causes both herpes simplex type 1 and type 2. • Type 1 is transmitted via oral and respiratory secretions; type 2 is transmitted via sexual contact. • During exposure, the virus fuses to the host cell membrane and releases proteins, turning off the host cell's protein production or synthesis. The virus then replicates and synthesizes structural proteins. The virus pushes its nucleocapsid (protein coat and nucleic acid) into the cytoplasm of the host cell and releases the viral DNA. Complete virus particles capable of surviving and infecting a living cell are transported to the cell's surface. • Characteristic painful, vesicular lesions are usually observed at the site of initial infection.
Herpes zoster	Herpes zoster is caused by a reactivation of varicella-zoster virus that has been lying dormant in the cerebral ganglia or the ganglia of posterior nerve roots. • Small, painful, red, nodular skin lesions develop on areas along nerve paths. • Lesions change to vesicles filled with pus or fluid.
Human immunodeficiency virus (HIV) infection	HIV is the virus that causes acquired immunodeficiency deficiency syndrome (AIDS). • Virus passes from one person to another through blood-to-blood and sexual contact. In addition, an infected pregnant woman can pass HIV to her baby during pregnancy or delivery as well as through breast-feeding. • Most people with HIV infection develop AIDS; however, current combination drug therapy in conjunction with treatment and prophylaxis of common opportunistic infections can delay the natural progression and prolong survival.
Infectious mononucleosis	Viral illness caused by the Epstein-Barr virus (EBV). • Most cases spread by the oropharyngeal route, but transmission by blood transfusion or during cardiac surgery is also possible. • The virus invades the B cells of the oropharyngeal lymphoid tissues and then replicates. • Dying B cells release virus into the blood, causing fever and other symptoms. During this period, antiviral antibodies appear and the virus disappears from the blood, lodging mainly in the parotid gland.
Mumps	Acute viral disease caused by a paramyxovirus. • Transmitted by droplets or by direct contact. • Characterized by enlargement and tenderness of parotid gland and swelling of other salivary glands.
Rabies	Rapidly progressive infection of the central nervous system caused by an RNA virus. • Transmitted by the bite of an infected animal through the skin or mucous membranes or, occasionally, in airborne droplets or infected tissue. • The rabies virus begins replicating in the striated muscle cells at the bite site. • The virus spreads along the nerve pathways to the spinal cord and brain, where it replicates again. • The virus moves through the nerves into other tissues, including into the salivary glands.
Respiratory syncytial virus infection	Infection of the respiratory tract from an organism belonging to a subgroup of myxoviruses. • The organism is transmitted from person to person by respiratory secretions. • Bronchiolitis or pneumonia ensues and, in severe cases, may damage the bronchiolar epithelium. • Interalveolar thickening and filling of alveolar spaces with fluid may occur.
Rubella	Viral infection transmitted through contact with the blood, urine, stool, or nasopharyngeal secretions of an infected person. It can also be transmitted transplacentally. • The virus replicates first in the respiratory tract and then spreads through the bloodstream. • Characteristic maculopapular rash usually begins on the face and then spreads rapidly.
Rubeola	Acute, highly contagious paramyxovirus infection that is spread by direct contact or by contaminated airborne respiratory droplets. • Portal of entry is the upper respiratory tract. • Characterized by Koplik's spots, a pruritic macular rash that becomes papular and erythematous.

DISORDER	CHARACTERISTICS

Viral infections *(continued)*

| Viral pneumonia | Lung infection caused by any one of a variety of viruses, transmitted through contact with an infected individual.
● The virus first attacks bronchiolar epithelial cells, causing interstitial inflammation and desquamation.
● Virus invades bronchial mucous glands and goblet cells and then spreads to the alveoli, which fill with blood and fluid. In advanced infection, a hyaline membrane may form. |

Fungal infections

| Chlamydia | Sexually transmitted disease caused by *Chlamydia trachomatis*. The pattern depends on the individual infected and the site of infection. |
| Histoplasmosis | Fungal infection caused by *Histoplasma capsulatum*.
● Transmitted through inhalation of *H. capsulatum* spores or invasion of spores after minor skin trauma.
● Initially, infected person may be asymptomatic or have symptoms of mild respiratory illness, progressing into more severe illness affecting several organ systems. |

Protozoal infections

Malaria	Acute and chronic infection with *Plasmodium falciparum, P. vivax, P. malariae,* or *P. ovale,* transmitted by the anopheles mosquito to humans. ● Plasmodium sporozoites migrate by blood circulation to parenchymal cells of the liver; there they form cystlike structures containing thousands of merozoites. ● Upon release, each merozoite invades an erythrocyte and feeds on hemoglobin. ● Eventually the erythrocyte ruptures, releasing heme (malaria pigment), cell debris, and more merozoites, which, unless destroyed by phagocytes, enter other erythrocytes.
Schistosomiasis	A slowly progressive disease caused by blood flukes of the class Trematoda: *Schistosoma mansoni* and *S. japonicum* infect the intestinal tract; *S. haematobium* infects the urinary tract. ● Modes of transmission include bathing, swimming, wading, or working in water contaminated with *Schistosoma* larvae. ● Larvae penetrate the skin or mucous membranes and eventually work their way to the liver's portal venous circulation, where they mature in 1 to 3 months. ● The adults then migrate to other parts of the body. ● The female cercariae (the final free-swimming larval stage of the organism) lay spiny eggs in blood vessels surrounding the large intestine or bladder. After penetrating the mucosa of these organs, the eggs are excreted in feces or urine.
Toxoplasmosis	Infection caused by the intracellular parasite *Toxoplasma gondii*, which affects both birds and mammals. ● Transmitted to humans by ingestion of tissue cysts in raw or undercooked meat or by fecal-oral contamination from infected cats. Direct transmission can also occur during blood transfusions or organ transplants. ● When tissue cysts are ingested, parasites are released, which quickly invade and multiply within the GI tract. The parasitic cells rupture the invaded host cell and then disseminate to the CNS, lymphatic tissue, skeletal muscle, myocardium, retina, and placenta. ● As the parasites replicate and invade adjoining cells, cell death and focal necrosis occur, surrounded by an acute inflammatory response, which are the hallmarks of this infection. ● Once the cysts reach maturity, the inflammatory process is undetectable and the cysts remain latent within the brain until they rupture. ● In the normal host, the immune response checks the infection, but this is not so with immunocompromised or fetal hosts. In these patients, focal destruction results in necrotizing encephalitis, pneumonia, myocarditis, and organ failure.
Trichinosis	Infection caused by the parasite *Trichinella spiralis* and transmitted through ingestion of uncooked or undercooked meat that contains encysted larvae. ● After gastric juices free the larva from the cyst capsule, it reaches sexual maturity in a few days. The female roundworm burrows into the intestinal mucosa and reproduces. ● Larvae then travel through the lymphatic system and the bloodstream. They become embedded as cysts in striated muscle, especially in the diaphragm, chest, arms, and legs.

GENETICS

Genetics is the study of heredity — the passing of physical, biochemical, and physiologic traits, both healthy and pathogenic, from biological parents to their children. In this transmission, mistakes or mutations can cause disability or death.

Genetic information is carried in genes, which are strung together on the deoxyribonucleic acid (DNA) double helix to form chromosomes. Every normal human cell (except reproductive cells) has 46 chromosomes, 22 paired chromosomes called autosomes, and 2 sex chromosomes (a pair of Xs in females and an X and a Y in males). A person's individual set of chromosomes is called his karyotype. The human genome has been under intense study for only about 15 years to determine the structure of each gene in the genome and its location within each of the 23 chromosomes comprising the set of human chromosomes. In June 2000, two teams of scientists announced the completion of the "rough draft" of the entire genome sequence. The sequence consists of more than 3.1 billion pairs of chemicals. Decoding the genome will enable people to know who is likely to get a specific inherited disease and enable researchers to eradicate or improve the treatment of many diseases.

For a wide variety of reasons, not every gene that might be expressed is. Genetic principles are based on studies of thousands of individuals. Those studies have led to generalities that are usually true, but exceptions occur. Genetics remains an inexact science.

GENETIC COMPONENTS

Each of the two strands of DNA in a chromosome consists of thousands of combinations of four nucleotides: adenine (A), thymine (T), cytosine (C), and guanine (G), arranged in complementary triplet pairs (called codons), each of which represents an amino acid; a specific sequence of triplets represents a gene. The strands are held together loosely by chemical bonds between adenine and thymine or cytosine and guanine. The looseness of the bonds allows the strands to separate easily during cell division. The genes carry a code for each trait a person inherits, from blood type to eye color to body shape and a myriad of other traits.

DNA ultimately controls the formation of essential substances throughout the life of every cell in the body. It does this through the genetic code, the precise sequence of AT and CG pairs on the DNA molecule. Genes not only control hereditary traits, transmitted from parents to offspring, but also cell reproduction and the daily functions of all cells. Genes control cell function by controlling the structures and chemicals that are synthesized within the cell.

TRANSMITTING TRAITS

Germ cells, or gametes, are one of two classes of cells in the body; each germ cell (ovum or sperm) contains 23 chromosomes (called the *haploid* number) in its nucleus. All the other cells in the body are somatic cells, which are *diploid*; that is, they contain 23 *pairs* of chromosomes.

When human ovum and sperm unite, the corresponding chromosomes pair up, so that the fertilized cell and every somatic cell of the new person has 23 pairs of chromosomes in its nucleus.

Germ cells

The body produces germ cells through a type of cell division called *meiosis*. Meiosis occurs only when the body is creating haploid germ cells from their diploid precursors. Each of the 23 pairs of chromosomes in the diploid precursor cell separates, so that, when the cell then divides, each new germ cell (ovum or sperm) contains one set of 23 chromosomes.

Most of the genes on one chromosome are identical or almost identical to those on its mate. The location (or locus) of a gene on a chromosome is specific and doesn't vary from person to person. This allows each of the thousands of genes on a strand of DNA in an ovum to join the corresponding gene in a sperm when the chromosomes pair up at fertilization.

Determining sex

Only one pair of the 23 pairs of chromosomes in each cell is primarily involved in determining a person's sex. These are the sex chromosomes; the other 22 chromosome pairs are called autosomes. Females have two X chromosomes and males have one X and one Y chromosome.

Each germ cell produced by a male contains either an X or a Y chromosome. When a sperm with an X chromosome fertilizes an ovum, the offspring is female (two X chromosomes); when a sperm with a Y chromosome fertilizes an ovum, the offspring is male (one X and one Y chromosome). Very rare errors in cell division can result in a germ cell that has no sex chromosome or has two X chromosomes. After fertilization, the zygote may have an XO or XXY karyotype and still survive. Most other errors in sex chromosome division are incompatible with life.

Mitosis

The fertilized ovum — now called a zygote, undergoes a kind of cell division called *mitosis*. Before a cell divides, its chromosomes replicate. During this process, the double helix of DNA separates into two chains; each chain serves as a template for constructing a new chain. Individual DNA nucleotides are linked into new strands with bases complementary to those in the originals. In this way, two identical double helices are formed, each containing one of the original strands and a newly formed complementary strand. These double helices are duplicates of the original DNA chain.

Mitotic cell division occurs in five phases: *interphase, prophase, metaphase, anaphase,* and *telophase.* The result of every mitotic cell division is two new daughter cells, each genetically identical to the original and to each other. Then, each of the two resulting cells divides, and so on, eventually forming a many-celled human embryo. Thus, each cell in a person's body (except ovum or sperm) contains an identical set of 46 chromosomes that are unique to that person.

TRAIT PREDOMINANCE

Each parent contributes one set of chromosomes (and therefore one set of genes) so that every offspring has two genes for every locus on the autosomes. Some characteristics, or traits, such as eye color, are determined by one gene that may have many variants (alleles). Others, called *polygenic* traits, require the interaction of two or more genes. In addition, environmental factors may affect how genes are expressed, although the environmental factors do not affect the genetic structure.

Variations in a particular gene — such as brown, blue, or green eye color — are called alleles. A person who has identical genes on each member of the chromosome pair is *homozygous* for that gene; if the alleles are different, the person is said to be *heterozygous.*

Autosomal inheritance

For unknown reasons, on autosomes, one allele may be more influential than another in determining a specific trait. The more powerful, or *dominant,* gene is more likely to be expressed in the offspring than the less influential, or *recessive,* gene. Offspring will express a dominant allele when one or both chromosomes in a pair carry it. A recessive allele won't be expressed unless both chromosomes carry identical copies of the allele. For example, a child may receive a gene for brown eyes from one parent and a gene for blue eyes from the other parent. The gene for brown eyes is dominant, and the gene for blue eyes is recessive. Because the dominant gene is more likely to be expressed, the child is more likely to have brown eyes.

Sex-linked inheritance

The X and Y chromosomes are not literally a pair because the X chromosome is much larger than the Y, with more genetic material. The male has only one copy of the genes on the X chromosome. Inheritance of those genes is called *X-linked.* A man will transmit one copy of each X-linked gene to his daughters and none to his sons. A woman will transmit one copy to each child, whether male or female.

Inheritance of genes on the X chromosomes is different in another way. Some recessive genes on the X chromosomes act like dominants in females. For reasons that are not yet clear, one recessive allele will be expressed in some somatic cells and another in other somatic cells.

Multifactorial inheritance

Environmental factors can affect the expression of some genes; this is called multifactorial inheritance. Some diseases have genetic predisposition but multifactorial inheritance, that is, the gene for the disease is expressed only under certain environmental conditions. Environmental factors that may contribute to multifactorial inheritance include:
● maternal age
● use of drugs, alcohol, or hormones by either parent
● maternal infection during pregnancy or existing diseases in the mother
● maternal or paternal exposure to radiation
● nutritional factors
● general maternal or paternal health
● other factors, including high altitude, maternal smoking, maternal-fetal blood incompatibility, and inadequate prenatal care.

PATHOPHYSIOLOGIC CONCEPTS

Autosomal disorders, sex-linked disorders, and multifactorial disorders result from changes to genes or chromosomes. Some defects arise spontaneously, and others may be caused by environmental teratogens.

Environmental teratogens

Teratogens are environmental agents (infectious toxins, maternal systemic diseases, drugs, chemicals, and physical agents) that can harm the developing fetus by causing congenital structural or functional defects. Teratogens may also cause spontaneous abortion, complications during labor and delivery, hidden defects in later development (such as cognitive or behavioral problems), or neoplastic transformations.

Gene errors

A permanent change in genetic material is a *mutation,* which may occur spontaneously or after exposure of a cell to radiation, certain chemicals, or viruses. Mutations can occur anywhere in the genome.

Every cell has built-in defenses against genetic damage. However, if a mutation isn't identified or repaired, the mutation may produce a trait different from the original trait and will be transmitted to offspring. Mutations may have no effect; some may change expression of a trait, and others change the way a cell functions. Some mutations cause serious or deadly defects, such as congenital anomalies or cancer.

Autosomal disorders

In single-gene disorders, an error occurs at a single gene site on the DNA strand. A mistake may occur in the copying and transcribing of a single codon through additions, deletions, or excessive repetitions.

Single-gene disorders are inherited in clearly identifiable patterns that are the same as those seen in inheritance of normal traits. Because every person has 22 pairs of autosomes and only 1 pair of sex chromosomes, most hereditary disorders are caused by autosomal defects.

Autosomal dominant transmission usually affects male and female offspring equally. Children of an affected parent have a 50% chance of being affected. Autosomal recessive inheritance also usually affects male and female offspring equally. If both parents are affected, all their offspring will be affected. If both parents are unaffected but are heterozygous for the trait (carriers of the defective gene), each child has a 25% chance of being affected. If only one parent is affected, none of the offspring will be affected, but all will carry the defective gene. If one parent is affected and the other is a carrier, 50% of their children will be affected. Autosomal recessive disorders may occur when there is no family history of the disease.

Sex-linked disorders

Genetic disorders caused by genes located on the sex chromosomes are termed sex-linked disorders. Most sex-linked disorders are controlled by genes located on the X chromosome, usually as recessive traits. Because males have only one X chromosome, a single X-linked recessive gene can cause disease to be exhibited in a male. Females receive two X chromosomes, so they can be homozygous for a disease allele, homozygous for a normal allele, or heterozygous.

(Text continues on page 24.)

COMMON GENETIC DISORDERS

DISORDER	PATHOPHYSIOLOGY	SIGNS AND SYMPTOMS
Autosomal recessive disorders		
Cystic fibrosis (CF) Inborn error in a cell-membrane transport protein. Dysfunction of the exocrine glands affects multiple organ systems. The disease affects males and females. It is the most common fatal genetic disease in white children.	Most cases arise from the mutation that affects the genetic coding for a single amino acid, resulting in a protein (cystic fibrosis transmembrane regulator [CFTR]) that doesn't function properly. The CFTR resembles other transmembrane transport proteins, but it lacks the phenylalanine in the protein produced by normal genes. This regulator interferes with cAMP-regulated chloride channels and transport of other ions by preventing adenosine triphosphate from binding to the protein or by interfering with activation by protein kinase. The mutation affects volume-absorbing epithelia in the airways and intestines, salt-absorbing epithelia in sweat ducts, and volume-secretory epithelia in the pancreas. Lack of phenylalanine leads to dehydration, which increases the viscosity of mucus-gland secretions and consequently obstructs glandular ducts. CF has varying effects on electrolyte and water transport.	• Chronic airway infections leading to bronchiectasis • Bronchiolectasis • Exocrine pancreatic insufficiency • Intestinal dysfunction • Abnormal sweat-gland function • Reproductive dysfunction
Phenylketonuria (PKU) Inborn error in metabolism of the amino acid phenylalanine. PKU has a low incidence among Blacks and Ashkenazic Jews and a high incidence among people of Irish and Scottish descent.	Patients with classic PKU have almost no activity of phenylalanine hydroxylase, an enzyme that helps convert phenylalanine to tyrosine. As a result, phenylalanine accumulates in the blood and urine, and tyrosine levels are low.	• By age 4 months, signs of arrested brain development, including mental retardation • Personality disturbances • Seizures • Decreased IQ • Macrocephaly • Eczematous skin lesions or dry, rough skin • Hyperactivity • Irritability • Purposeless, repetitive motions • Awkward gait • Musty odor from skin and urine excretion of phenylacetic acid
Sickle cell anemia Congenital hemolytic anemia resulting from defective hemoglobin molecules. In the United States, sickle cell anemia occurs primarily in persons of African and Mediterranean descent. It also affects populations in Puerto Rico, Turkey, India, the Middle East, and the Mediterranean.	Abnormal hemoglobin S in red blood cells becomes insoluble during hypoxia. As a result, these cells become rigid, rough, and elongated, forming a crescent or sickle shape. The sickling produces hemolysis. The altered cells also pile up in the capillaries and smaller blood vessels, making the blood more viscous. Normal circulation is impaired, causing pain, tissue infarctions, and swelling. Each patient with sickle cell anemia has a different hypoxic threshold and different factors that trigger a sickle cell crisis. Illness, exposure to cold, stress, acidotic states, or a pathophysiologic process that pulls water out of the sickle cells precipitates a crisis in most patients. The blockages then cause anoxic changes that lead to further sickling and obstruction.	• Symptoms of sickle cell anemia don't develop until after the age of 6 months because fetal hemoglobin protects infants for the first few months after birth. • Chronic fatigue • Unexplained dyspnea on exertion • Joint swelling • Aching bones • Severe localized and generalized pain • Leg ulcers • Frequent infections • Priapism in males *In sickle cell crisis:* • Severe pain • Hematuria • Lethargy
Tay-Sachs disease Also known as GM$_2$ gangliosidosis, the most common lipid-storage disease. Tay-Sachs affects Ashkenazic Jews about 100 times more often than the general population.	The enzyme hexosaminidase A is absent or deficient. This enzyme is necessary to metabolize gangliosides, water-soluble glycolipids found primarily in the central nervous system (CNS). Without hexosaminidase A, lipid molecules accumulate, progressively destroying and demyelinating CNS cells.	• Exaggerated Moro (startle) reflex at birth and apathy (response only to loud sounds) by age 3 to 6 months • Inability to sit up, lift head, or grasp objects; difficulty turning over; progressive vision loss • Deafness, blindness, seizures, paralysis, spasticity, and continued neurologic deterioration (by 18 months of age) • Recurrent bronchopneumonia

DISORDER	PATHOPHYSIOLOGY	SIGNS AND SYMPTOMS
Autosomal dominant disorders		
Marfan syndrome Rare degenerative, generalized disease of the connective tissue that results from elastin and collagen defects. The syndrome occurs in 1 of 20,000 individuals, affecting males and females equally.	The syndrome is caused by mutation in a single gene on chromosome 15, the gene that codes for fibrillin, a glycoprotein component of connective tissue. These small fibers are abundant in large blood vessels and the suspensory ligaments of the ocular lenses. The effect on connective tissue is variable and includes excessive bone growth, ocular disorders, and cardiac defects.	• Increased height, long extremities, and arachnodactyly (long, spiderlike fingers) • Defects of sternum (funnel chest or pigeon breast, for example), chest asymmetry, scoliosis, or kyphosis • Hypermobile joints • Myopia • Lens displacement • Valvular abnormalities (redundancy of leaflets, stretching of chordae tendineae, or dilation of valvulae annulus) • Mitral valve prolapse • Aortic regurgitation
X-linked recessive disorders		
Hemophilia Bleeding disorder; severity and prognosis vary with the degree of deficiency, or nonfunction, and the site of bleeding. Hemophilia occurs in 20 of 100,000 male births. Hemophilia A, or classic hemophilia, is a deficiency of clotting factor VIII; it's more common than type B, affecting more than 80% of all hemophiliacs. Hemophilia B, or Christmas disease, affects 15% of all hemophiliacs and results from a deficiency of factor IX. There's no relationship between factor VIII and factor IX inherited defects.	Abnormal bleeding occurs because of specific clotting factor malfunction. Factors VIII and IX are components of the intrinsic clotting pathway; factor IX is an essential factor and factor VIII is a critical cofactor. Factor VIII accelerates the activation of factor X by several thousandfold. Excessive bleeding occurs when these clotting factors are reduced by more than 75%. Hemophilia may be severe, moderate, or mild, depending on the degree of activation of clotting factors. A person with hemophilia forms a platelet plug at a bleeding site, but clotting factor deficiency impairs the ability to form a stable fibrin clot. Delayed bleeding is more common than immediate hemorrhage.	• Spontaneous bleeding in severe hemophilia • Excessive or continued bleeding or bruising • Large subcutaneous and deep intramuscular hematomas • Prolonged bleeding in mild hemophilia after major trauma or surgery, but no spontaneous bleeding after minor trauma • Pain, swelling, and tenderness in joints • Internal bleeding, often manifested as abdominal, chest, or flank pain • Hematuria • Hematemesis or tarry stools
Polygenic (multifactorial) disorders		
Cleft lip and cleft palate May occur separately or together. Cleft lip with or without cleft palate occurs twice as often in males as in females. Cleft palate without cleft lip is more common in females. Cleft lip deformities can occur unilaterally, bilaterally, or, rarely, in the midline. Only the lip may be involved, or the defect may extend into the upper jaw or nasal cavity. Incidence is highest in children with a family history of cleft defects.	During the second month of pregnancy, the front and sides of the face and the palatine shelves develop. Because of a chromosomal abnormality, exposure to teratogens, genetic abnormality, or environmental factors, the lip or palate fuses imperfectly. The deformity may range from a simple notch to a complete cleft. A cleft palate may be partial or complete. A complete cleft includes the soft palate, the bones of the maxilla, and the alveolus on one or both sides of the premaxilla. A double cleft is the most severe of the deformities. The cleft runs from the soft palate forward to either side of the nose. A double cleft separates the maxilla and premaxilla into freely moving segments. The tongue and other muscles can displace the segments, enlarging the cleft.	• Obvious cleft lip or cleft palate • Feeding difficulties due to incomplete fusion of the palate

(continued)

DISORDER	PATHOPHYSIOLOGY	SIGNS AND SYMPTOMS
Polygenic (multifactorial) disorders *(continued)*		
Spina bifida Incomplete fusion of one or more vertebrae, resulting in dimpling of the area (spina bifida occulta) or protrusion of the spinal tissue (spina bifida cystica). Spina bifida occulta occurs in as many as 25% of births, and spina bifida cystica occurs in 1 in 1,000 births in the United States. Incidence varies greatly with countries and regions.	Neural tube closure normally occurs at 24 days' gestation in the cranial region and continues distally, with closure of the lumbar regions by 26 days. As the nervous system develops and differentiates, it's vulnerable to teratogenic effects. The specific cause of spina bifida, incomplete fusion of the vertebrae in the developing nervous system of the embryo, is unknown, but neural tube defects have been associated with such noninfectious maternal disorders as folic acid deficiency. Spina bifida occulta rarely affects the structure or function of the cord and peripheral nerve roots. Spina bifida cystica can occur as a meningocele, in which the meninges protrude in a cerebrospinal fluid-filled sac, or as a myelomeningocele, in which peripheral nerves, root segments, or the spinal cord also protrude. Varying degrees of sensory and motor dysfunction below the level of the lesion are present.	• Weak feet • Bowel and bladder disturbances • Dimple, tuft of hair, soft fatty deposits, port wine nevi, or combination over spine (spina bifida occulta) • Saclike protrusion over the spine due to meningocele or myelomeningocele (spina bifida cystica) • Possible permanent neurologic dysfunction due to meningocele or myelomeningocele (spina bifida cystica)
Disorders of chromosome number		
Down's syndrome (trisomy 21) Spontaneous chromosome abnormality that causes characteristic facial features, other distinctive physical abnormalities (cardiac defects in 60% of affected persons), and mental retardation. It occurs in 1 of 650 to 700 live births.	Nearly all cases of Down's syndrome result from trisomy 21 (3 copies of chromosome 21). The result is a karyotype of 47 chromosomes instead of the usual 46. In 4% of patients, Down's syndrome results from an unbalanced translocation or chromosomal rearrangement in which the long arm of chromosome 21 breaks and attaches to another chromosome. Some affected persons and some asymptomatic parents may have chromosomal mosaicism, a mixture of two cell types, some with the normal 46 and some with an extra chromosome 21.	• Distinctive facial features (low nasal bridge, epicanthic folds, protruding tongue, and low-set ears); small open mouth and disproportionately large tongue • Single transverse crease on the palm (Simian crease) • Small white spots on the iris (Brushfield's spots) • Mental retardation (estimated IQ of 20 to 50) • Developmental delay • Congenital heart disease, mainly septal defects and especially of the endocardial cushion • Impaired reflexes

Most people who express X-linked *recessive* traits are males with unaffected parents. In rare cases, the father is affected and the mother is a carrier. All daughters of an affected male will be carriers. Sons of an affected male will be unaffected, and the unaffected sons aren't carriers. Unaffected male children of a female carrier don't transmit the disorder.

Characteristics of X-linked *dominant* inheritance include evidence of the inherited trait in the family history. A person with the abnormal trait must have one affected parent. If the father has an X-linked dominant disorder, all his daughters and none of his sons will be affected. If a mother has an X-linked dominant disorder, each of her children has a 50% chance of being affected.

Multifactorial disorders

Most multifactorial disorders result from the effects of several different genes and an environmental component. In polygenic inheritance, each gene has a small additive effect, and the effect of a combination of genetic errors in a person is unpredictable. Multifactorial disorders can result from a less-than-optimum expression of many different genes, not from a specific error.

Some multifactorial disorders are apparent at birth, such as cleft lip, cleft palate, congenital heart disease, anencephaly, clubfoot, and myelomeningocele. Others don't become apparent until later, such as type II diabetes mellitus, hypertension, hyperlipidemia, most autoimmune diseases, and many cancers. Multifactorial disorders that develop during adulthood are often believed to be strongly related to environmental factors, not only in incidence but also in the degree of expression.

Chromosome defects

Aberrations in chromosome structure or number cause a class of disorders called congenital anomalies, or birth defects. The aberration may be loss, addition, or rearrangement of genetic material. If the remaining genetic material is sufficient to maintain life, an endless variety of clinical manifestations may occur. Most clinically significant chromosome aberrations arise during meiosis. Meiosis is an incredibly complex process that can go wrong in many ways. Potential contributing factors include maternal age, radiation, and use of some therapeutic or recreational drugs.

Translocation, the relocation of a segment of a chromosome to a nonhomologous chromosome, occurs when chromosomes split apart and rejoin in an abnormal arrangement. The cells still have a normal amount of genetic material, so often there are no visible abnormalities. However, the children of parents with translocated chromosomes may have serious genetic defects, such as monosomies or trisomies.

During both meiosis and mitosis, chromosomes normally separate in a process called *disjunction*. Failure to separate, called nondisjunction, causes an unequal distribution of chromosomes between the two resulting cells. If nondisjunction occurs during mitosis soon after fertilization, it may affect all the resulting cells. Gain or loss of chromosomes usually is caused by nondisjunction of autosomes or sex chromosomes during meiosis. The incidence of nondisjunction increases with parental age.

The presence of one chromosome less than the normal number is called *monosomy*; an autosomal monosomy is nonviable. The presence of an extra chromosome is called a *trisomy*. A mixture of both trisomic and normal cells results in *mosaicism*, which is the presence of two or more cell lines in the same person. The effect of mosaicism depends on the proportion and anatomic location of abnormal cells.

GENETIC DISORDERS

Genetic disorders are commonly classified by pattern of inheritance, as shown in the accompanying chart. (See *Common genetic disorders*, pages 22 to 24.)

FLUIDS AND ELECTROLYTES

The body is mostly liquid — various electrolytes dissolved in water. Electrolytes are ions (electrically charged versions) of essential elements — predominantly sodium (Na^+), chloride (Cl^-), oxygen (O_2^-), hydrogen (H^+), bicarbonate (HCO_3^-), calcium (Ca^{2+}), potassium (K^+), sulfate (SO_4^{2-}), and phosphate (PO_4^{3-}). Only ionic forms of elements can dissolve or combine with other elements. Electrolyte balance must remain in a narrow range for the body to function. The kidneys maintain chemical balance throughout the body by producing and eliminating urine. They regulate the volume, electrolyte concentration, and acid-base balance of body fluids; detoxify and eliminate wastes; and regulate blood pressure by regulating fluid volume. The skin and lungs also play a role in fluid and electrolyte balance. Sweating results in loss of sodium and water, and every breath contains water vapor.

FLUID BALANCE

The kidneys maintain fluid balance in the body by regulating the amount and components of fluid inside and around the cells.

Intracellular fluid

The fluid inside each cell is called the intracellular fluid (ICF). Each cell has its own mixture of components in the intracellular fluid, but the amounts of these substances are similar in every cell. ICF contains large amounts of potassium, magnesium, and phosphate ions.

Extracellular fluid

The fluid in the spaces outside the cells, called extracellular fluid (ECF), is constantly moving. Normally, ECF includes blood plasma and interstitial fluid. In some pathologic states, it accumulates in a so-called third space, the space around organs in the chest or abdomen.

ECF is rapidly transported through the body by circulating blood and between blood and tissue fluids by fluid and electrolyte exchange across the capillary walls. ECF contains large amounts of sodium, chloride, and bicarbonate ions, plus such cell nutrients as oxygen, glucose, fatty acids, and amino acids. It also contains carbon dioxide (CO_2), transported from the cells to the lungs for excretion, and other cellular products, transported from the cells to the kidneys for excretion.

The kidneys maintain the volume and composition of ECF and, to a lesser extent, ICF by continually exchanging water and ionic solutes, such as hydrogen, sodium, potassium, chloride, bicarbonate, sulfate, and phosphate ions, across the cell membranes of the renal tubules.

Fluid exchange

Four forces act to equalize concentrations of fluids, electrolytes, and proteins on both sides of the capillary wall by moving fluid between the vessels and the interstitial fluid. Forces that move fluid out of vessels are:
- hydrostatic pressure of blood
- osmotic pressure of tissue fluid.
  Forces that move fluid into vessels are:
- oncotic pressure of plasma proteins
- hydrostatic pressure of interstitial fluid.

Hydrostatic pressure is higher at the arteriolar end of the capillary bed than at the venular end. Oncotic pressure of plasma increases slightly at the venular end as fluid escapes. When the endothelial barrier (capillary wall) is normal and intact, fluid escapes at the arteriolar end of the capillary bed and is returned at the venular end. The small amount of fluid lost from the capillaries into the interstitial tissue spaces is drained off

ALTERATIONS OF TONICITY

ALTERATIONS	PATHOPHYSIOLOGY	CAUSES
Isotonic	• Intracellular fluids (ICF) and extracellular fluids (ECF) have equal osmotic pressure, but there's a dramatic change in total-body fluid volume. • No cellular swelling or shrinkage because osmosis does not occur.	• Blood loss from penetrating trauma • Expansion of fluid volume if a patient receives too much normal saline
Hypertonic	• ECF is more concentrated than ICF. • Water flows out of the cell through the semipermeable cell membrane, causing cell shrinkage.	• Administration of hypertonic (>0.9%) saline • Hypernatremia from severe dehydration • Sodium retention from renal disease
Hypotonic	• Osmotic pressure forces some ECF into the cells, causing them to swell. • In extreme hypotonicity, cells may swell until they burst and die.	• Overhydration

MAJOR ELECTROLYTES

ELECTROLYTE	CHARACTERISTICS
Sodium	• Major extracellular fluid (ECF) cation • Maintains tonicity of ECF • Regulates acid-base balance by renal reabsorption of sodium ion (base) and excretion of hydrogen ion (acid) • Facilitates nerve conduction and neuromuscular function • Facilitates glandular secretion • Maintains water balance
Potassium	• Major intracellular fluid (ICF) cation • Maintains cell electrical neutrality • Facilitates cardiac muscle contraction and electrical conductivity • Facilitates neuromuscular transmission of nerve impulses • Maintains acid-base balance
Chloride	• Mainly an ECF anion • Accounts for two-thirds of all serum anions • Secreted by the stomach mucosa as hydrochloric acid, providing an acid medium for digestion and enzyme activation • Helps maintain acid-base and water balances • Influences tonicity of ECF • Facilitates exchange of oxygen and carbon dioxide in red blood cells • Helps activate salivary amylase, which triggers the digestive process
Calcium	• Indispensable to cell permeability, bone and teeth formation, blood coagulation, nerve impulse transmission, and normal muscle contraction • *Hypo*calcemia can cause tetany and seizures • *Hyper*calcemia can cause cardiac arrhythmias and coma
Magnesium	• Present in small quantities, but physiologically as significant as the other major electrolytes • Enhances neuromuscular communication • Stimulates parathyroid hormone secretion, which regulates intracellular calcium • Activates many enzymes in carbohydrate and protein metabolism • Facilitates cell metabolism • Facilitates sodium, potassium, and calcium transport across cell membranes • Facilitates protein transport
Phosphate	• Involved in cellular metabolism as well as neuromuscular regulation and hematologic function • Phosphate reabsorption in the renal tubules inversely related to calcium levels: an increase in urinary phosphorous triggers calcium reabsorption and vice versa

through the lymphatic system and returned to the bloodstream.

Acid-base balance

Regulation of the ECF environment involves the ratio of acid to base, measured clinically as pH. In physiology, all positively charged ions are acids and all negatively charged ions are bases. To regulate acid-base balance, the kidneys secrete hydrogen ions (acid), reabsorb sodium (acid) and bicarbonate ions (base), acidify phosphate salts, and produce ammonium ions (acid). This keeps the blood at its normal pH of 7.37 to 7.43. The following are important pH boundaries:

<6.8	incompatible with life
<7.2	cell function seriously impaired
<7.35	acidosis
7.37 to 7.43	normal
>7.45	alkalosis
>7.55	cell function seriously impaired
>7.8	incompatible with life.

PATHOPHYSIOLOGIC CONCEPTS

The regulation of intracellular and extracellular electrolyte concentrations depends on the following:
• balance between intake of substances containing electrolytes and output of electrolytes in urine, feces, and sweat
• transport of fluid and electrolytes between ECF and ICF.

Fluid imbalance occurs when regulatory mechanisms can't compensate for abnormal intake and output at any level from the cell to the organism. Fluid and electrolyte imbalances include edema, isotonic alterations, hypertonic alterations, hypotonic alterations, and electrolyte imbalances. Disorders of fluid volume or osmolarity result. Many conditions also affect capillary exchange, resulting in fluid shifts.

Edema

Despite almost constant interchange through the endothelial barrier, the body maintains a steady state of extracellular water balance between the plasma and interstitial fluid. Increased fluid volume in the interstitial spaces is called edema. It's clas-

DISORDERS OF FLUID BALANCE: HYPOVOLEMIA

CAUSES	PATHOPHYSIOLOGY	SIGNS/SYMPTOMS	DIAGNOSIS	TREATMENT
Hypovolemia is an isotonic disorder. Fluid volume deficit decreases capillary hydrostatic pressure and fluid transport. Cells are deprived of normal nutrients that serve as substrates for energy production, metabolism, and other cellular functions. It results from the following causes: *Fluid loss:* • Hemorrhage • Excessive perspiration • Renal failure with polyuria • Abdominal surgery • Vomiting or diarrhea • Nasogastric drainage • Diabetes mellitus with polyuria or diabetes insipidus • Fistulas • Excessive use of laxatives, diuretic therapy • Fever *Reduced fluid intake:* • Dysphagia • Coma • Environmental conditions preventing fluid intake • Psychiatric illness *Fluid shift from extracellular fluid (ECF):* • Burns (during the initial phase) • Acute intestinal obstruction • Acute peritonitis • Pancreatitis • Crushing injury • Pleural effusion • Hip fracture	Decreased renal blood flow triggers the renin-angiotensin system to increase sodium and water reabsorption. The cardiovascular system compensates by increasing heart rate, cardiac contractility, venous constriction, and systemic vascular resistance, thus increasing cardiac output and mean arterial pressure. Hypovolemia also triggers the thirst response, releasing more antidiuretic hormone and producing more aldosterone. When compensation fails, hypovolemic shock occurs in the following sequence: • decreased intravascular fluid volume • diminished venous return, which reduces preload and decreases stroke volume • reduced cardiac output • decreased mean arterial presure • impaired tissue perfusion • decreased oxygen and nutrient delivery to cells • multisystem organ failure.	• Orthostatic hypotension • Tachycardia • Thirst • Flattened neck veins • Sunken eyeballs • Dry mucous membranes • Diminished skin turgor • Rapid weight loss • Decreased urine output • Prolonged capillary refill time	• Increased blood urea nitrogen • Elevated serum creatinine level • Increased serum protein, hemoglobin, and hematocrit (unless caused by hemorrhage, when loss of blood elements causes subnormal values) • Rising blood glucose • Elevated serum osmolality (except in hyponatremia, where serum osmolality is low) • Serum electrolyte and arterial blood gas (ABG) analysis may reflect associated clinical problems due to underlying cause of hypovolemia or treatment regimen • Urine specific gravity > 1.030 • Increased urine osmolality • Urine sodium level < 50 mEq/L	• Oral fluids • Parenteral fluids • Fluid resuscitation by rapid I.V. administration • Blood or blood products (with hemorrhage) • Antidiarrheals as needed • Antiemetics as needed • I.V. dopamine (Intropin) or norepinephrine (Levophed) to increase cardiac contractility and renal perfusion (if patient remains symptomatic after fluid replacement) • Autotransfusion (for some patients with hypovolemia caused by trauma)

sified as localized or systemic. Obstruction of the veins or lymphatic system or increased vascular permeability usually causes localized edema in the affected area, such as the swelling around an injury. Systemic, or generalized edema, may be due to heart failure or renal disease. Massive systemic edema is called *anasarca*.

Edema results from abnormal expansion of the interstitial fluid or the accumulation of fluid in a third space, such as the peritoneum (ascites), pleural cavity (hydrothorax), or pericardial sac (pericardial effusion).

Tonicity

Many fluid and electrolyte disorders are classified according to how they affect osmotic pressure, or tonicity. Tonicity describes the relative concentrations of electrolytes (osmotic pressure) on both sides of a semipermeable membrane (the cell wall or the capillary wall). The word *normal* in this context refers to the usual electrolyte concentration of physiologic fluids. Normal saline has a sodium chloride concentration of 0.9%.

• *Isotonic* solutions have the same electrolyte concentration and therefore the same osmotic pressure as ECF.

DISORDERS OF FLUID BALANCE: HYPERVOLEMIA

CAUSES	PATHOPHYSIOLOGY	SIGNS/SYMPTOMS	DIAGNOSIS	TREATMENT
Hypervolemia is an abnormal increase in the volume of circulating fluid (plasma) in the body. It results from the following causes: *Increased risk for sodium and water retention:* ● Heart failure ● Hepatic cirrhosis ● Nephrotic syndrome ● Corticosteroid therapy ● Low dietary protein intake ● Renal failure *Excessive sodium and water intake:* ● Parenteral fluid replacement with normal saline or lactated Ringer's solution ● Blood or plasma replacement ● Dietary intake of water, sodium chloride, or other salts *Fluid shift to ECF:* ● Remobilization of fluid after burn treatment ● Intake of hypertonic fluids ● Intake of colloid oncotic fluids	Increased ECF volume causes the following sequence of events: ● circulatory overload ● increased cardiac contractility and mean arterial pressure ● increased capillary hydrostatic pressure ● shift of fluid to the interstitial space ● edema. Elevated mean arterial pressure inhibits secretion of antidiuretic hormone and aldosterone and consequent increased urinary elimination of water and sodium. These compensatory mechanisms usually restore normal intravascular volume. If hypervolemia is severe or prolonged or the patient has a history of cardiovascular dysfunction, compensatory mechanisms may fail, and heart failure and pulmonary edema may ensue.	● Rapid breathing ● Dyspnea ● Crackles ● Rapid, bounding pulse ● Hypertension ● Distended neck veins ● Moist skin ● Acute weight gain ● Edema ● S_3 gallop	● Decreased serum potassium and blood urea nitrogen ● Decreased hematocrit due to hemodilution ● Normal serum sodium ● Low urine sodium excretion ● Increased hemodynamic values	● Treatment of underlying condition ● Oxygen administration ● Use of thromboembolic disease support hose to help mobilize edematous fluid ● Bed rest ● Restricted sodium and water intake ● Preload reduction agents and afterload reduction agents ● Hemodialysis or peritoneal dialysis ● Continuous arteriovenous hemofiltration ● Continuous venovenous hemofiltration

● *Hypertonic* solutions have a greater than normal concentration of some essential electrolyte, usually sodium.
● *Hypotonic* solutions have a lower than normal concentration of some essential electrolyte, also usually sodium. (See *Alterations of tonicity*, page 26.)

Electrolyte balance

The major electrolytes are the cations sodium, potassium, calcium, and magnesium and the anions chloride, phosphate, and bicarbonate. The body continuously attempts to maintain intracellular and extracellular equilibrium of electrolytes. Too much or too little of any electrolyte will affect most body systems. (See *Major electrolytes*, page 27.)

Electrolyte imbalances can affect all body systems. Too much or too little potassium or too little calcium or magnesium can increase the excitability of the cardiac muscle, causing arrhythmias. Multiple neurologic symptoms may result from electrolyte imbalance, ranging from disorientation or confusion to a completely depressed central nervous system. Too much or too little sodium or too much potassium can

cause oliguria. Blood pressure may be increased or decreased. The GI tract is particularly susceptible to electrolyte imbalance:
● too much potassium — leads to abdominal cramps, nausea, and diarrhea
● too little potassium — leads to paralytic ileus
● too much magnesium — leads to nausea, vomiting, and diarrhea
● too much calcium — leads to nausea, vomiting, and constipation.

Acid-base imbalance

Acid-base balance is essential to life. Concepts related to imbalance include:
● *acidemia* — arterial pH less than 7.35, which reflects a relative excess of acid in the blood. The hydrogen ion content in ECF increases, and the hydrogen ions move to the ICF. To keep the ICF electrically neutral, an equal amount of potassium leaves the cell, creating a relative hyperkalemia.
● *alkalemia* — arterial blood pH greater than 7.45, which reflects a relative excess of base in the blood. In alkalemia, an excess of hydrogen ions in the ICF forces them into the ECF. To

DISORDERS OF ELECTROLYTE BALANCE

ELECTROLYTE IMBALANCE	SIGNS AND SYMPTOMS	DIAGNOSTIC TEST RESULTS
Hyponatremia	• Muscle twitching and weakness • Lethargy, confusion, seizures, and coma • Hypotension and tachycardia • Nausea, vomiting, and abdominal cramps • Oliguria or anuria	• Serum sodium < 135 mEq/L • Decreased urine specific gravity • Decreased serum osmolality • Urine sodium > 100 mEq/24 hours • Increased red blood cell count
Hypernatremia	• Agitation, restlessness, fever, and decreased level of consciousness • Hypertension, tachycardia, pitting edema, and excessive weight gain • Thirst, increased viscosity of saliva, rough tongue • Dyspnea, respiratory arrest, and death	• Serum sodium > 145 mEq/L • Urine sodium < 40 mEq/24 hours • High serum osmolality
Hypokalemia	• Dizziness, hypotension, arrhythmias, electrocardiogram (ECG) changes, and cardiac arrest • Nausea, vomiting, anorexia, diarrhea, decreased peristalsis, and abdominal distention • Muscle weakness, fatigue, and leg cramps	• Serum potassium < 3.5 mEq/L • Coexisting low serum calcium and magnesium levels not responsive to treatment for hypokalemia usually suggest hypomagnesemia • Metabolic alkalosis • ECG changes, including flattened T waves, elevated U waves, depressed ST segment
Hyperkalemia	• Tachycardia changing to bradycardia, ECG changes, and cardiac arrest • Nausea, diarrhea, and abdominal cramps • Muscle weakness and flaccid paralysis	• Serum potassium > 5 mEq/L • Metabolic acidosis • ECG changes, including tented and elevated T waves, widened QRS complex, prolonged PR interval, flattened or absent P waves, depressed ST segment
Hypochloremia	• Muscle hypertonicity and tetany • Shallow, depressed breathing • Usually associated with hyponatremia and its characteristic symptoms, such as muscle weakness and twitching	• Serum chloride < 98 mEq/L • Serum pH > 7.45 (supportive value) • Serum CO_2 > 32 mEq/L (supportive value)
Hyperchloremia	• Deep, rapid breathing • Weakness • Diminished cognitive ability, possibly leading to coma	• Serum chloride > 108 mEq/L • Serum pH < 7.35, serum CO_2 < 22 mEq/L (supportive values)
Hypocalcemia	• Anxiety, irritability, twitching around the mouth, laryngospasm, seizures, positive Chvostek's and Trousseau's signs • Hypotension and arrhythmias due to decreased calcium influx	• Serum calcium < 8.5 mg/dl • Low platelet count • ECG changes: lengthened QT interval, prolonged ST segment, arrhythmias • Possible changes in serum protein levels
Hypercalcemia	• Drowsiness, lethargy, headaches, irritability, confusion, depression, or apathy • Weakness and muscle flaccidity • Bone pain and pathological fractures • Heart block • Anorexia, nausea, vomiting, constipation, and dehydration • Flank pain	• Serum calcium > 10.5 mg/dl • ECG changes: signs of heart block and shortened QT interval • Azotemia • Decreased parathyroid hormone level • Sulkowitch urine test results: increased calcium precipitation
Hypomagnesemia	• Nearly always coexists with hypokalemia and hypocalcemia • Hyperirritability, tetany, leg and foot cramps, positive Chvostek's and Trousseau's signs, confusion, delusions, and seizures • Arrhythmias, vasodilation, and hypotension	• Serum magnesium < 1.5 mEq/L • Coexisting low serum potassium and calcium levels

ELECTROLYTE IMBALANCE	SIGNS AND SYMPTOMS	DIAGNOSTIC TEST RESULTS
Hypermagnesemia	• Uncommon, caused by decreased renal excretion (renal failure) or increased intake of magnesium • Diminished reflexes, muscle weakness to flaccid paralysis • Respiratory distress • Heart block, bradycardia • Hypotension	• Serum magnesium > 2.5 mEq/L • Coexisting elevated potassium and calcium levels
Hypophosphatemia	• Muscle weakness, tremor, and paresthesia • Peripheral hypoxia	• Serum phosphate < 2.5 mg/dl • Urine phosphate > 1.3 g/24 hours
Hyperphosphatemia	• Usually asymptomatic unless leading to hypocalcemia, then evidenced by tetany and seizures	• Serum phosphate > 4.5 mg/dl • Serum calcium < 9 mg/dl • Urine phosphorus < 0.9 g/24 hours

keep the ICF electrically neutral, potassium moves from the ECF to the ICF, creating a relative hypokalemia.

• *acidosis* — a systemic increase in hydrogen ion concentration. If the lungs fail to eliminate CO_2 or if volatile (carbonic) or nonvolatile (lactic) acid products of metabolism accumulate, hydrogen ion concentration rises. Acidosis can also occur if persistent diarrhea causes loss of basic bicarbonate anions or the kidneys fail to reabsorb bicarbonate or secrete hydrogen ions.

• *alkalosis* — a bodywide decrease in hydrogen ion concentration. An excessive loss of CO_2 during hyperventilation, loss of nonvolatile acids during vomiting, or excessive ingestion of base may decrease hydrogen ion concentration.

• *compensation* — the lungs and kidneys, along with a number of chemical buffer systems in the intracellular and extracellular compartments, work together to maintain plasma pH in the range of 7.35 to 7.45.

Buffer systems

A buffer system consists of a weak acid (one that doesn't readily release free hydrogen ions) and a corresponding base, such as sodium bicarbonate. These buffers resist or minimize a change in pH when an acid or base is added to the buffered solution. Buffers work in seconds.

The four major buffers or buffer systems are:
• carbonic acid-bicarbonate system
• hemoglobin-oxyhemoglobin system
• other protein buffers
• phosphate system.

When primary disease processes alter either the acid or base component of the ratio, the lungs or kidneys (whichever is not affected by the disease process) act to restore the ratio and normalize pH. Because the body's mechanisms that regulate pH occur in stepwise fashion over time, the body tolerates gradual changes in pH better than abrupt ones.

Renal mechanisms

If a respiratory disorder causes acidosis or alkalosis, the kidneys respond by altering the processing of hydrogen and bicarbonate ions to return the pH to normal. Renal compensation begins hours to days after a respiratory alteration in pH. Despite this delay, renal compensation is powerful.

• *Acidemia* — Kidneys excrete excess hydrogen ions, which may combine with phosphate or ammonia to form titratable acids in the urine. The net effect is to *raise* the concentration of bicarbonate ions in the ECF and restore acid–base balance.

• *Alkalemia* — Kidneys excrete excess bicarbonate ions, usually with sodium ions. The net effect is to *reduce* the concentration of bicarbonate ions in the ECF and restore acid-base balance.

Pulmonary mechanisms

If acidosis or alkalosis results from a metabolic or renal disorder, the respiratory system regulates the respiratory rate to return the pH to normal. The partial pressure of CO_2 in arterial blood (Pa_{CO_2}) reflects CO_2 levels proportionate to blood pH. As the concentration of the gas increases, so does its partial pressure. Within minutes after the slightest change in Pa_{CO_2}, central chemoreceptors in the medulla that regulate the rate and depth of ventilation detect the change and respond as follows:

• *acidemia* — increased respiratory rate and depth to eliminate CO_2

• *alkalemia* — decreased respiratory rate and depth to retain CO_2.

DISORDERS

Fluid and electrolyte balance is essential for health. Many factors, such as illness, injury, surgery, and treatments, can disrupt fluid and electrolyte balances. (See *Disorders of fluid balance*, pages 28 and 29, and *Disorders of electrolyte balance*, pages 30 and 31.)

Acid-base disturbances can cause respiratory acidosis or alkalosis or metabolic acidosis or alkalosis. (See *Disorders of acid-base balance*, pages 32 and 33.)

DISORDERS OF ACID-BASE BALANCE

DISORDER/CAUSES	PATHOPHYSIOLOGY	SIGNS/SYMPTOMS	DIAGNOSIS	TREATMENT
Respiratory acidosis				
• Airway obstruction or parenchymal lung disease • Mechanical ventilation • Chronic metabolic alkalosis as respiratory compensatory mechanisms try to normalize pH • Chronic bronchitis • Extensive pneumonia • Large pneumothorax • Pulmonary edema • Asthma • Chronic obstructive pulmonary disorder (COPD) • Drugs • Cardiac arrest • Central nervous system (CNS) trauma • Neuromuscular diseases • Sleep apnea	When pulmonary ventilation decreases, partial pressure of carbon dioxide in arterial blood (Pa_{CO_2}) increases and CO_2 level rises. Retained CO_2 combines with water (H_2O) to form carbonic acid (H_2CO_3), which dissociates to release free hydrogen (H^+) and bicarbonate (HCO_3^-) ions. Increased Pa_{CO_2} and free H^+ ions stimulate the medulla to increase respiratory drive and expel CO_2. As pH falls, 2,3-diphosphoglycerate (2,3-DPG) accumulates in red blood cells, where it alters hemoglobin (hgb) to release oxygen. The hgb picks up H^+ ions and CO_2 and removes them from the serum. As respiratory mechanisms fail, rising Pa_{CO_2} stimulates kidneys to retain HCO_3^- and sodium (Na^+) ions and excrete H^+ ions. . As the H^+ ion concentration overwhelms compensatory mechanisms, H^+ ions move into cells and potassium (K^+) ions move out. Without enough oxygen, anaerobic metabolism produces lactic acid.	• Restlessness • Confusion • Apprehension • Somnolence • Asterixis • Headaches • Dyspnea and tachypnea • Papilledema • Depressed reflexes • Hypoxemia • Tachycardia • Hypertension/hypotension • Atrial and ventricular arrhythmias • Coma	• ABG analysis: Pa_{CO_2} > 45 mm Hg; pH < 7.35 to 7.45; and normal HCO_3^- in the acute stage and elevated HCO_3^- in the chronic stage	*For pulmonary causes:* • Removal of foreign body obstructing the airway • Mechanical ventilation • Bronchodilators • Antibiotics for pneumonia • Chest tubes for pneumothorax • Thrombolytics or anticoagulants for pulmonary emboli • Bronchoscopy to remove excess secretions *For COPD:* • Bronchodilators • Oxygen at low flow rates • Corticosteroids *For other causes:* • Drug therapy • Dialysis or activated charcoal to remove toxins • Correction of metabolic alkalosis • I.V. sodium bicarbonate
Respiratory alkalosis				
• Acute hypoxemia, pneumonia, interstitial lung disease, pulmonary vascular disease, or acute asthma • Anxiety • Hypermetabolic states such as fever and sepsis • Excessive mechanical ventilation • Salicylate toxicity • Metabolic acidosis • Hepatic failure • Pregnancy	As pulmonary ventilation increases, excessive CO_2 is exhaled. Resulting hypocapnia leads to reduction of H_2CO_3, excretion of H^+ and HCO_3^- ions, and rising serum pH. Against rising pH, the hydrogen–potassium buffer system pulls H^+ ions out of cells and into blood in exchange for K^+ ions. H^+ ions entering blood combine with HCO_3^- ions to form H_2CO_3, and pH falls. Hypocapnia causes an increase in heart rate, cerebral vasoconstriction, and decreased cerebral blood flow. After 6 hours, kidneys secrete more HCO_3^- and less H^+. Continued low Pa_{CO_2} and vasoconstriction increases cerebral and peripheral hypoxia. Severe alkalosis inhibits calcium (Ca^+) ionization; increasing nerve/muscle excitability.	• Deep, rapid breathing • Light-headedness or dizziness • Agitation • Circumoral and peripheral paresthesias • Carpopedal spasms, twitching, and muscle weakness	ABG analysis showing Pa_{CO_2} <35 mm Hg; elevated pH in proportion to decrease in Pa_{CO_2} in the acute stage but decreasing toward normal in the chronic stage; normal HCO_3^- in the acute stage but less than normal in the chronic stage	• Removal of ingested toxins, such as salicylates, by inducing emesis or using gastic lavage4 • Treatment of fever or sepsis • Oxygen for acute hypoxemia • Treatment of CNS disease • Having patient breathe into paper bag • Adjustments to mechanical ventilation to decrease minute ventilation

DISORDER/CAUSES	PATHOPHYSIOLOGY	SIGNS/SYMPTOMS	DIAGNOSIS	TREATMENT
Metabolic acidosis				
• Excessive acid accumulation • Deficient HCO_3^- stores • Decreased acid excretion by the kidneys • Diabetic ketoacidosis • Chronic alcoholism • Malnutrition or a low-carbohydrate, high-fat diet • Anaerobic carbohydrate metabolism • Underexcretion of metabolized acids or inability to conserve base • Diarrhea, intestinal malabsorption, or loss of sodium bicarbonate from the intestines • Salicylate intoxication, exogenous poisoning, or less frequently, Addison's disease • Inhibited secretion of acid	As H^+ ions begin accumulating in the body, chemical buffers (plasma HCO_3^- and proteins) in cells and ECF bind them. Excess H^+ ions decrease blood pH and stimulate chemoreceptors in the medulla to increase respiration. Consequent fall of partial pressure of $PaCO_2$ frees H^+ ions to bind with HCO_3^- ions. Respiratory compensation occurs but isn't sufficient to correct acidosis. Healthy kidneys compensate, excreting excess H^+ ions, buffered by phosphate or ammonia. For each H^+ ion excreted, renal tubules reabsorb and return to blood one Na^+ ion and one HCO_3^- ion. Excess H^+ ions in ECF passively diffuse into cells. To maintain balance of charge across cell membrane, cells release K^+ ions. Excess H^+ ions change the normal balance of K^+, Na^+, and Ca^+ ions, impairing neural excitability.	• Headache and lethargy progressing to drowsiness, CNS depression, Kussmaul's respirations, hypotension, stupor, and coma and death • Associated GI distress leading to anorexia, nausea, vomiting, diarrhea, and possibly dehydration • Warm, flushed skin • Fruity-smelling breath	• Arterial pH < 7.35; $PaCO_2$ normal or < 34 mm Hg as respiratory compensatory mechanisms take hold; HCO_3^- may be < 22 mEq/L • Urine pH < 4.5 in the absence of renal disease • Elevated plasma lactic acid in lactic acidosis • Anion gap > 14 mEq/L in high-anion gap metabolic acidosis, lactic acidosis, ketoacidosis, aspirin overdose, alcohol poisoning, renal failure, or other disorder characterized by accumulation of organic acids, sulfates, or phosphates • Anion gap 12 mEq/L or less in normal anion gap metabolic acidosis from HCO_3^- loss, GI or renal loss, increased acid load, rapid I.V. saline administration, or other disorders characterized by HCO_3^- loss	• Sodium bicarbonate I.V. for severe high anion gap • I.V. lactated Ringer's solution • Evaluation and correction of electrolyte imbalances • Correction of underlying cause • Mechanical ventilation to maintain respiratory compensation, if needed • Antibiotic therapy to treat infection • Dialysis for patients with renal failure or certain drug toxicities • Antidiarrheal agents for diarrhea-induced HCO_3^- loss • Position patient to prevent aspiration • Seizure precautions
Metabolic alkalosis				
• Chronic vomiting • Nasogastric tube drainage or lavage without adequate electrolyte replacement • Fistulas • Use of steroids and certain diuretics (furosemide [Lasix], thiazides, and ethacrynic acid [Edecrin]) • Massive blood transfusions • Cushing's disease, primary hyperaldosteronism, and Bartter's syndrome • Excessive intake of bicarbonate of soda, other antacids, or absorbable alkali • Excessive amounts of I.V. fluids, high serum concentrations of bicarbonate or lactate • Respiratory insufficiency • Low serum chloride • Low serum potassium	Chemical buffers in ECF and ICF bind HCO_3^- in the body. Excess unbound HCO_3^- raises blood pH, depressing chemoreceptors in the medulla, inhibiting respiration and raising $PaCO_2$. CO_2 combines with H_2O to form H_2CO_3. Low oxygen limits respiratory compensation. When blood HCO_3^- rises to 28 mEq/L, the amount filtered by renal glomeruli exceeds reabsorptive capacity of the renal tubules. Excess HCO_3^- is excreted in urine, and H^+ ions are retained. To maintain electrochemical balance, Na^+ ions and water are excreted with HCO_3^- ions. When H^+ ion levels in ECF are low, H^+ ions diffuse passively out of cells and extracellular K^+ ions move into cells. As intracellular H^+ ion levels fall, calcium ionization decreases, and nerve cells become permeable to Na^+ ions. Na^+ ions moving into cells trigger neural impulses in PNS and in CNS.	• Irritability, picking at bedclothes (carphology), twitching, and confusion • Nausea, vomiting, and diarrhea • Cardiovascular abnormalities due to hypokalemia • Respiratory disturbances (such as cyanosis and apnea) and slow, shallow respirations • Possible carpopedal spasm in the hand, due to diminished peripheral blood flow during repeated blood pressure checks	• Blood pH > 7.45; HCO_3^- > 29 mEq/L • Low potassium (< 3.5 mEq/L), calcium (< 8.9 mg/dl), and chloride (< 98 mEq/L)	• Cautious use of ammonium chloride I.V. (rarely) or HCl to restore ECF hydrogen and chloride levels • KCl and normal saline solution • Discontinuation of diuretics and supplementary KCl • Oral or I.V. acetazolamide

PART II

DISORDERS

AORTIC ANEURYSM

A thoracic aortic aneurysm is an abnormal widening of the ascending, transverse, or descending part of the aorta. Aneurysm of the ascending aorta is the most common type and has the highest mortality. An abdominal aneurysm generally occurs in the aorta between the renal arteries and iliac branches.

Causes

Aneurysms commonly result from atherosclerosis, which weakens the aortic wall and gradually distends the lumen. Other causes include:
• fungal infection (mycotic aneurysms) of the aortic arch and descending segments
• congenital disorders, such as coarctation of the aorta or Marfan syndrome
• trauma
• syphilis
• hypertension (in dissecting aneurysm).

AGE ALERT
Ascending aortic aneurysms, the most common type, are usually seen in hypertensive men under age 60.
   Descending aortic aneurysms, usually found just below the origin of the subclavian artery, are most common in elderly hypertensive men. They may also occur in younger patients after traumatic chest injury or, less often, infection.

Pathophysiology

First, degenerative changes create a focal weakness in the muscular layer of the aorta (tunica media), allowing the inner layer (tunica intima) and outer layer (tunica adventitia) to stretch outward. The outward bulge is the aneurysm. The pressure of blood pulsing through the aorta progressively weakens the vessel walls and enlarges the aneurysm. As the vessel dilates, wall tension increases. This increases arterial pressure and dilates the aneurysm further.

Aneurysms may be *dissecting*, a hemorrhagic separation in the aortic wall, usually within the medial layer; *saccular*, an outpouching of the arterial wall; or *fusiform*, a spindle-shaped enlargement encompassing the entire aortic circumference.

A false aneurysm occurs when the entire wall is injured, with blood contained in surrounding tissue. A sac eventually forms and communicates with an artery or the heart.

Signs and symptoms

Ascending aneurysm:
• Pain, the most common symptom of thoracic aortic aneurysm

• Bradycardia
• Aortic insufficiency
• Pericardial friction rub (caused by a hemopericardium)
• Unequal intensities of the right carotid and left radial pulses
• Difference in blood pressure between the right and left arms.
   Descending aneurysm:
• Pain, usually starting suddenly between the shoulder blades; may radiate to chest
• Hoarseness
• Dyspnea
• Dysphagia
• Dry cough.
   Abdominal aneurysm:
Although abdominal aneurysms usually don't produce symptoms, most are evident as a pulsating mass in the periumbilical area. Other signs include:
• systolic bruit over the aorta
• tenderness on deep palpation
• lumbar pain that radiates to the flank and groin.

CLINICAL TIP
Pain caused by a dissecting aortic aneurysm:
   • feeling of "ripping" or "tearing"
   • radiation to anterior chest, neck, back, or abdomen
   • abrupt onset.

Diagnostic tests
• Aortography
• Electrocardiography
• Echocardiography
• Hemoglobin levels
• Computed tomography scan
• Magnetic resonance imaging
• Transesophageal echocardiography
• Serial ultrasound (sonography)
• Anteroposterior and lateral X-rays.

Treatment
A dissecting aortic aneurysm is an emergency that requires prompt surgery and stabilizing measures. Treatment includes:
• antihypertensives, such as nitroprusside
• negative inotropic agents to decrease force of contractility
• oxygen for respiratory distress
• narcotics for pain
• I.V. fluids
• possibly, whole blood transfusions.

TYPES OF AORTIC ANEURYSMS

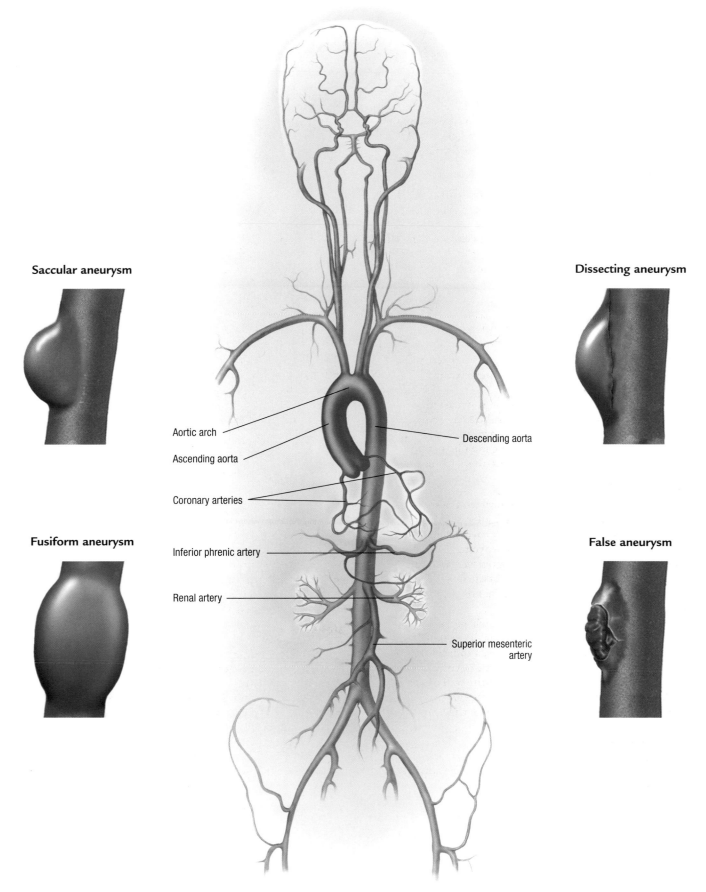

Saccular aneurysm

Dissecting aneurysm

Fusiform aneurysm

False aneurysm

Aortic arch

Ascending aorta

Coronary arteries

Inferior phrenic artery

Renal artery

Descending aorta

Superior mesenteric artery

CARDIAC ARRHYTHMIAS

Abnormal electrical conduction or automaticity changes heart rate and rhythm. Arrhythmias vary in severity — from mild, asymptomatic, and requiring no treatment (such as sinus arrhythmia, in which heart rate increases and decreases with respiration) to catastrophic ventricular fibrillation, which mandates immediate resuscitation. Arrhythmias are generally classified according to their origin (ventricular or supraventricular). Their effect on cardiac output and blood pressure, partially influenced by the site of origin, determines their clinical significance. (See *Types of cardiac arrhythmias,* see Appendix.)

Causes

Each arrhythmia may have its own specific causes. Common causes include:
- congenital defects
- myocardial ischemia or infarction
- organic heart disease
- drug toxicity
- degeneration or obstruction of conductive tissue
- connective tissue disorders
- electrolyte imbalances
- hypertrophy of heart muscle
- acid-base imbalances
- emotional stress.

AGE ALERT
Electrocardiogram changes that occur with age include:
- longer PR, QRS, and QT intervals
- lower amplitude of QRS complex
- leftward shift of QRS axis.

Pathophysiology

Altered automaticity, reentry, or conduction disturbances may cause cardiac arrhythmias. Enhanced automaticity is the result of partial depolarization, which may increase the intrinsic rate of the SA node or latent pacemakers, or may induce ectopic pacemakers to reach threshold and depolarize.

Ischemia or deformation causes an abnormal circuit to develop within conductive fibers. Although current flow is blocked in one direction within the circuit, the descending impulse can travel in the other direction. By the time the impulse completes the circuit, the previously depolarized tissue within the circuit is no longer refractory to stimulation; therefore, arrhythmias occur.

Conduction disturbances occur when impulses are conducted too quickly or too slowly.

Signs and symptoms

Signs and symptoms of arrhythmias result from reduced cardiac output and altered perfusion to the organs and may include:
- asymptomatic
- dyspnea
- hypotension
- dizziness, syncope, and weakness
- chest pain
- cool, clammy skin
- altered level of consciousness
- reduced urinary output
- palpitations.

Diagnostic tests
- Electrocardiography
- Laboratory testing
- 24-hour Holter monitoring
- Exercise testing
- Electrophysiologic testing.

Treatment

Follow the specific treatment guidelines or protocols for each arrhythmia. Treatment generally focuses on the underlying problem and may include:
- antiarrhythmic medications
- electrolyte correction
- oxygen
- correction of acid-base balance
- cardioversion
- pacemaker
- cardiopulmonary resuscitation.

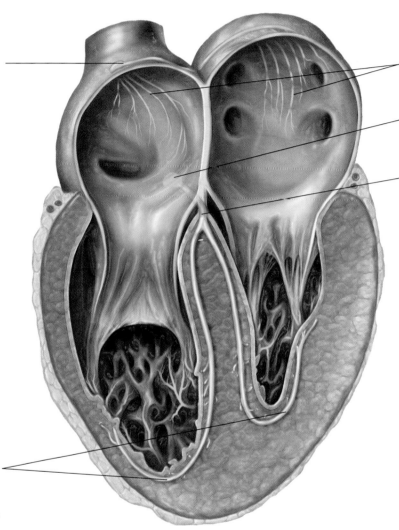

Sinus node arrhythmias
- Sino-atrial block
- Sinus bradycardia
- Sinus tachycardia

Atrial arrhythmias
- Premature atrial contractions
- Atrial fibrillation
- Atrial flutter

Atrioventricular (AV) blocks
- First-degree AV block
- Second-degree AV block
- Third-degree AV block

Junctional arrhythmias
- AV junctional rhythm

Ventricular arrhythmias
- Premature ventricular contractions
- Ventricular fibrillation
- Ventricular tachycardia

Cardiac arrhythmias   **39**

CARDIOMYOPATHY

Cardiomyopathy is classified as dilated, hypertrophic, or restrictive.

Dilated cardiomyopathy results from damage to cardiac muscle fibers; loss of muscle tone grossly dilates all four chambers of the heart, giving the heart a globular shape.

Hypertrophic cardiomyopathy, also called idiopathic hypertrophic subaortic stenosis, is characterized by disproportionate, asymmetrical thickening of the interventricular septum and left ventricular hypertrophy.

Restrictive cardiomyopathy is characterized by restricted ventricular filling (the result of left ventricular hypertrophy) and endocardial fibrosis and thickening. If severe, it is irreversible.

Causes

Most patients with cardiomyopathy have idiopathic disease, but some cases are secondary to the following possible causes:

Dilated cardiomyopathy:
- Viral or bacterial infection
- Hypertension
- Peripartum syndrome (related to toxemia)
- Ischemic heart disease or valvular disease
- Drug hypersensitivity or chemotherapy
- Cardiotoxic effects of drugs or alcohol.

Hypertrophic cardiomyopathy:
- Autosomal dominant inheritance
- Hypertension
- Obstructive valvular disease
- Thyroid disease.

Restrictive cardiomyopathy:
- Amyloidosis or sarcoidosis
- Hemochromatosis
- Infiltrative neoplastic disease.

Pathophysiology

In *dilated cardiomyopathy*, extensive damage to cardiac muscle fibers reduces contractility in the left ventricle. As systolic function declines, stroke volume, ejection fraction, and cardiac output fall.

In *hypertrophic cardiomyopathy,* hypertrophy of the left ventricle and interventricular septum obstruct left ventricular outflow. The heart compensates for the decreased cardiac output (due to obstructed outflow) by increasing the rate and force of contractions. The hypertrophied ventricle becomes stiff and unable to relax and fill during diastole. As left ventricular volume diminishes and filling pressure rises, pulmonary venous pressure also rises, leading to venous congestion and dyspnea.

In *restrictive cardiomyopathy*, left ventricular hypertrophy and endocardial fibrosis limit myocardial contraction and emptying during systole as well as ventricular relaxation and filling during diastole. As a result, cardiac output falls.

Signs and symptoms

Dilated cardiomyopathy:
- Shortness of breath, orthopnea, dyspnea on exertion, paroxysmal nocturnal dyspnea, fatigue, and dry cough at night
- Peripheral edema, hepatomegaly, jugular venous distention, and weight gain
- Peripheral cyanosis
- Tachycardia
- Pansystolic murmur or S_3 and S_4 gallop rhythms
- Irregular pulse if atrial fibrillation is present.

Hypertrophic cardiomyopathy:
- Angina, syncope, dyspnea, or fatigue
- Systolic ejection murmur along the left sternal border and at the apex
- Pulsus biferiens or abrupt arterial pulse
- Irregular pulse if atrial fibrillation is present.

Restrictive cardiomyopathy:
- Fatigue, dyspnea, orthopnea, chest pain, edema, liver engorgement
- Peripheral cyanosis, pallor
- S_3 or S_4 gallop rhythms, systolic murmurs.

Diagnostic tests
- Electrocardiography
- Radionuclide studies
- Chest X-ray
- Echocardiography
- Cardiac catheterization.

Treatment

Dilated cardiomyopathy:
- Treatment of underlying cause
- Angiotensin-converting enzyme (ACE) inhibitors, diuretics, digoxin, hydralazine, isosorbide dinitrate, beta-adrenergic blockers, antiarrythmics such as amiodarone
- Cardioversion or pacemaker insertion
- Anticoagulants
- Revascularization
- Valve repair or replacement
- Heart transplantation
- Lifestyle modifications, such as smoking cessation.

Hypertrophic cardiomyopathy:
- Beta-adrenergic blockers, antiarrhythmic drugs, anticoagulants, verapamil, diltiazem
- Cardioversion
- Ablation of atrioventricular node and implantation of a dual-chamber pacemaker
- Implantation of cardioverter-defibrillator
- Ventricular myotomy or myectomy
- Mitral valve replacement
- Heart transplantation.

Restrictive cardiomyopathy:
- Treatment of underlying cause
- Digoxin, diuretics, and restricted-sodium diet may ease symptoms of heart failure
- Oral vasodilators.

TYPES OF CARDIOMYOPATHY

Dilated

Hypertrophic

Restrictive

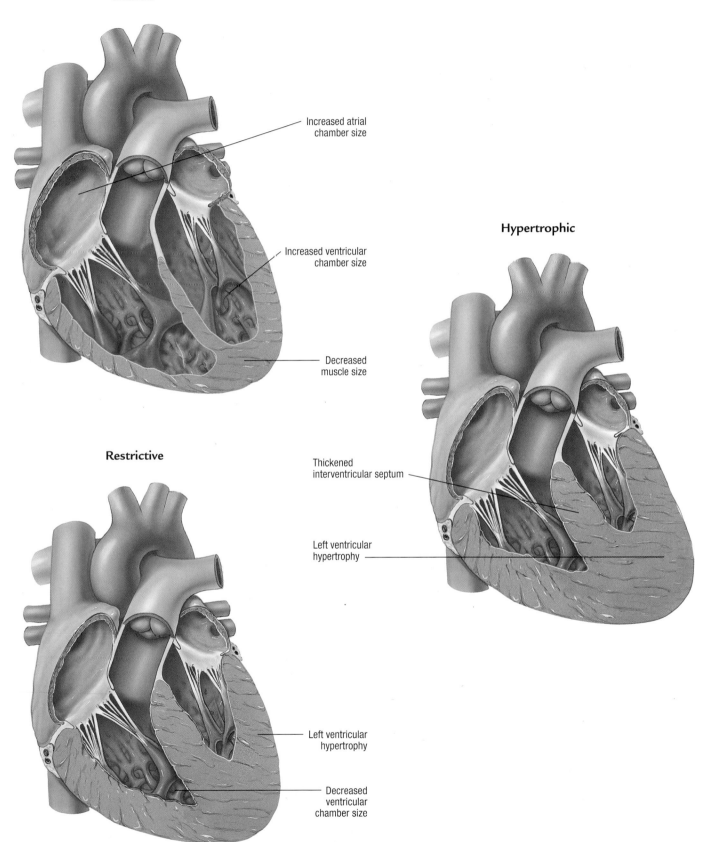

Increased atrial chamber size

Increased ventricular chamber size

Decreased muscle size

Thickened interventricular septum

Left ventricular hypertrophy

Left ventricular hypertrophy

Decreased ventricular chamber size

CONGENITAL DEFECTS

The most common congenital defects of the heart are atrial-septal defect (ASD), coarctation of the aorta, patent ductus arteriosus (PDA), tetralogy of Fallot, transposition of the great arteries, and ventricular septal defect (VSD). Causes of all six conditions remain unknown, although some have specific clinical associations. Pathophysiology and presentation are specific to each disorder, but diagnostic tests and available treatment modalities are applicable to the entire group (see page 44).

ATRIAL SEPTAL DEFECT

An opening between the left and right atria permits blood flow from left atrium to right atrium rather than left atrium to left ventricle.

Clinical association

Down's syndrome.

Pathophysiology

Blood shunts from the left atrium to the right atrium because the left atrial pressure is normally slightly higher than the right atrial pressure. In some adults, irreversible pulmonary hypertension develops and causes a right-to-left shunt, which results in unoxygenated blood entering the systemic circulation.

Signs and symptoms

- Fatigue
- Early to midsystolic murmur, low-pitched diastolic murmur
- Fixed, widely split S_2
- Systolic click or late systolic murmur at the apex
- Clubbing of nails and cyanosis, if right-to-left shunt develops.

COARCTATION OF THE AORTA

Coarctation is a narrowing of the aorta.

Clinical association

Turner's syndrome.

Pathophysiology

Obstruction causes hypertension in the aortic branches above the constriction and diminished pressure in the vessel below the constriction.

Signs and symptoms

- Heart failure
- Claudication (absence of pain or discomfort due to reduced blood flow to the legs), hypertension
- Headache, vertigo, and epistaxis (hemorrhage from the nose)
- Blood pressure greater in upper than in lower extremities
- Pink upper extremities and cyanotic lower extremities
- Absent or diminished femoral pulses
- Continuous midsystolic murmur
- Chest and arms may be more developed than legs.

PATENT DUCTUS ARTERIOSUS

The lumen of the duct between the aorta and pulmonary artery remains open after birth.

Clinical associations

- Premature birth
- Rubella syndrome
- Coarctation of the aorta
- Ventricular septal defect
- Pulmonary and aortic stenosis
- Living at high altitude, long-term exposure to low-blood oxygen tension.

Pathophysiology

Aortic pressure shunts oxygenated blood from the aorta through the ductus arteriosus to the pulmonary artery. The blood returns to the left side of the heart and is again pumped into the aorta. The result is systemic hypoxia.

Signs and symptoms

- Respiratory distress with signs of heart failure in infants
- Gibson murmur
- Thrill palpated at left sternal border
- Prominent left ventricular impulse
- Corrigan's pulse
- Wide pulse pressure
- Slow motor development, failure to thrive.

(Text continues on page 44.)

CONGENITAL HEART DEFECTS

Atrial septal defect

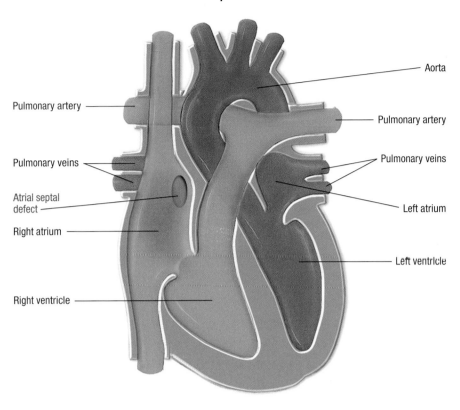

Aorta

Pulmonary artery

Pulmonary artery

Pulmonary veins

Pulmonary veins

Atrial septal defect

Left atrium

Right atrium

Left ventricle

Right ventricle

Coarctation of the aorta

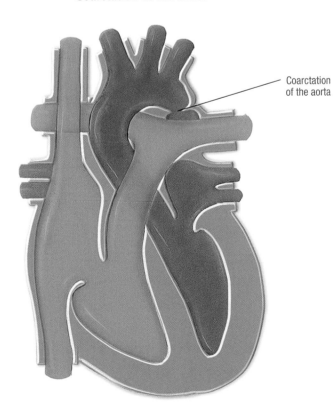

Coarctation of the aorta

Patent ductus arteriosus

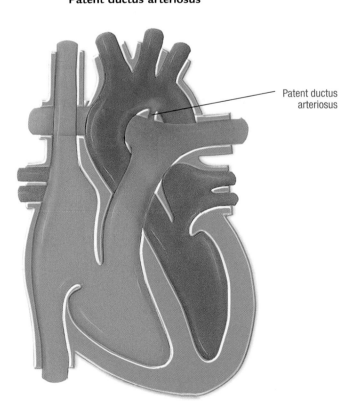

Patent ductus arteriosus

TETRALOGY OF FALLOT

Tetralogy of Fallot is a combination of four cardiac defects: VSD, right ventricular outflow tract obstruction, right ventricular hypertrophy, and an aorta positioned above the VSD (overriding aorta).

Clinical associations
- Fetal alcohol syndrome
- Thalidomide use during pregnancy.

Pathophysiology

Unoxygenated venous blood entering the right side of the heart may pass through the VSD to the left ventricle, bypassing the lungs, or it may enter the pulmonary artery, depending on the extent of the pulmonic stenosis.

Signs and symptoms
- Cyanosis
- Cyanotic or "blue" spells (Tet spells)
- Clubbing of digits, diminished exercise tolerance, increasing dyspnea on exertion, growth retardation, and eating difficulties
- Squatting to reduce shortness of breath
- Loud systolic murmur, continuous murmur of the ductus
- Thrill at left sternal border
- Right ventricular impulse and prominent inferior sternum.

TRANSPOSITION OF GREAT ARTERIES

The aorta rises from the right ventricle and the pulmonary artery from the left ventricle, producing two noncommunicating circulatory systems.

Pathophysiology

The transposed pulmonary artery carries oxygenated blood back to the lungs, rather than to the left side of the heart. The transposed aorta returns unoxygenated blood to the systemic circulation rather than to the lungs. Communication between the pulmonary and systemic circulation is necessary for survival.

Signs and symptoms
- Cyanosis and tachypnea
- Gallop rhythm, tachycardia, dyspnea, hepatomegaly, and cardiomegaly
- Murmurs of ASD, VSD, or PDA, loud S_2
- Diminished exercise tolerance, fatigue, and clubbing.

VENTRICULAR SEPTAL DEFECT

VSD is an opening in the septum between the ventricles that allows blood to shunt between the left and right ventricles.

Clinical associations
- Down's syndrome, other autosomal trisomies
- Renal anomalies, prematurity, fetal alcohol syndrome
- PDA, coarctation of the aorta.

Pathophysiology

As the pulmonary vasculature gradually relaxes, between 4 and 8 weeks after birth, right ventricular pressure decreases, allowing blood to shunt from the left to the right ventricle. Initially, large VSD shunts cause left atrial and left ventricular hypertrophy. Later, an uncorrected VSD causes right ventricular hypertrophy due to increasing pulmonary resistance. Eventually, biventricular heart failure occurs.

Signs and symptoms
- Failure to thrive
- Loud, harsh systolic murmur (along the left sternal border at the third or fourth intercostal space), palpable thrill
- Loud, widely split pulmonic component of S_2
- Displacement of point of maximal impulse to left
- Prominent anterior chest
- Liver, heart, and spleen enlargement
- Diaphoresis, tachycardia, and rapid, grunting respirations.

Diagnostic tests
- Chest X-ray
- Electrocardiography
- Echocardiography
- Cardiac catheterization
- Laboratory tests.

Treatment
- Surgery
- Medication
- Oxygen therapy
- Treatment of complications.

Tetralogy of Fallot

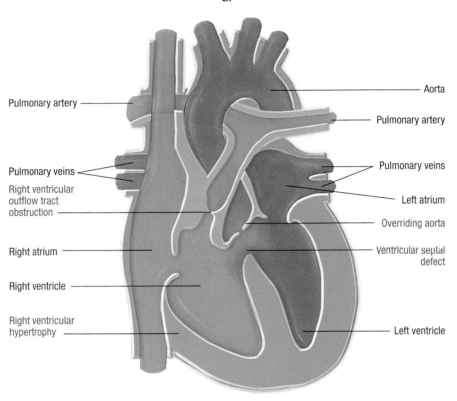

Pulmonary artery

Aorta

Pulmonary artery

Pulmonary veins

Right ventricular outflow tract obstruction

Pulmonary veins

Left atrium

Overriding aorta

Right atrium

Ventricular septal defect

Right ventricle

Right ventricular hypertrophy

Left ventricle

Transposition of great arteries

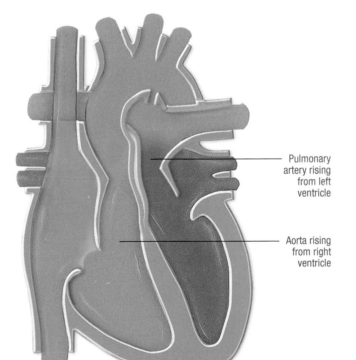

Pulmonary artery rising from left ventricle

Aorta rising from right ventricle

Ventricular septal defect

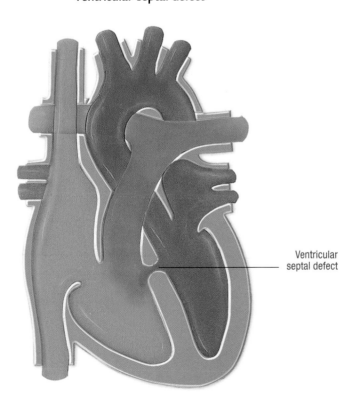

Ventricular septal defect

CORONARY ARTERY DISEASE

Coronary artery disease (CAD) results as atherosclerotic plaque fills the lumens of the coronary arteries and obstructs blood flow. The primary effect of CAD is a diminished supply of oxygen and nutrients to myocardial tissue.

AGE ALERT
As the population ages, the prevalence of CAD is rising. Approximately 11 million Americans have CAD, and it is most common among males, whites, and the middle-aged and elderly.

Causes
- Atherosclerosis, most common
- Dissecting aneurysm
- Infectious vasculitis
- Syphilis
- Congenital abnormalities.

Pathophysiology
Fatty, fibrous plaques progressively occlude the coronary arteries, reducing the volume of blood that can flow through them and leading to myocardial ischemia.

As atherosclerosis progresses, the diseased artery undergoes changes that impair its ability to dilate and thereby compensate for the obstruction. The consequent precarious balance between myocardial oxygen supply and demand threatens the myocardium distal to the lesion. When oxygen demand exceeds what the diseased vessel can supply, the result is localized myocardial ischemia.

Myocardial cells become ischemic within 10 seconds after coronary artery occlusion. Transient ischemia causes reversible changes at the cellular and tissue levels, depressing myocardial function. Within several minutes, oxygen deprivation forces the myocardium to shift from aerobic to anaerobic metabolism, leading to accumulation of lactic acid and reduction of cellular pH. Without intervention, this sequence of events can lead to tissue injury or necrosis.

The combination of hypoxia, reduced energy availability, and acidosis rapidly impairs left ventricular function. As the fibers become unable to shorten normally, the force of contractions and velocity of blood flow in the affected myocardial region become inadequate. Moreover, wall motion in the ischemic area becomes abnormal and each contraction ejects less blood from the heart . Restoring blood flow through the coronary arteries restores aerobic metabolism and contractility. Failure to do so results in myocardial infarction.

Signs and symptoms
- Angina
- Nausea and vomiting
- Cool extremities
- Diaphoresis due to sympathetic stimulation
- Xanthelasma (fat deposits on the eyelids).

AGE ALERT
CAD may be asymptomatic in the older adult because the sympathetic response to ischemia is impaired. Dyspnea and fatigue are two key signals of ischemia in an active older adult.

Diagnostic tests
- Electrocardiography
- Exercise testing
- Pharmacological stress testing
- Coronary angiography
- Myocardial perfusion imaging with thallium-201
- Stress echocardiography
- Lipid profile, thyroid function tests.

CLINICAL TIP
The lipid profile consists of the following components:
- Low-density lipoprotein (LDL): "bad" lipoprotein, carries most of the cholesterol molecules
- High-density lipoprotein (HDL): "good" lipoprotein, removes lipids from cells
- Apolipoprotein B: major component of LDL
- Apolipoprotein A-1: major component of HDL
- Lipoprotein a: one of the most atherogenic lipoproteins.

Treatment
- Drug therapy: nitrates, beta-adrenergic or calcium-channel blockers; antiplatelet, antilipemic, antihypertensive drugs
- Coronary artery bypass graft (CABG) surgery
- "Keyhole" or minimally invasive surgery, an alternative to traditional CABG
- Angioplasty
- Atherectomy
- Stent placement to maintain patency of reopened artery
- Lifestyle modifications to limit progression of CAD: smoking cessation, regular exercise, maintaining ideal body weight, and low-fat, low-sodium diet.

CORONARY ARTERIES

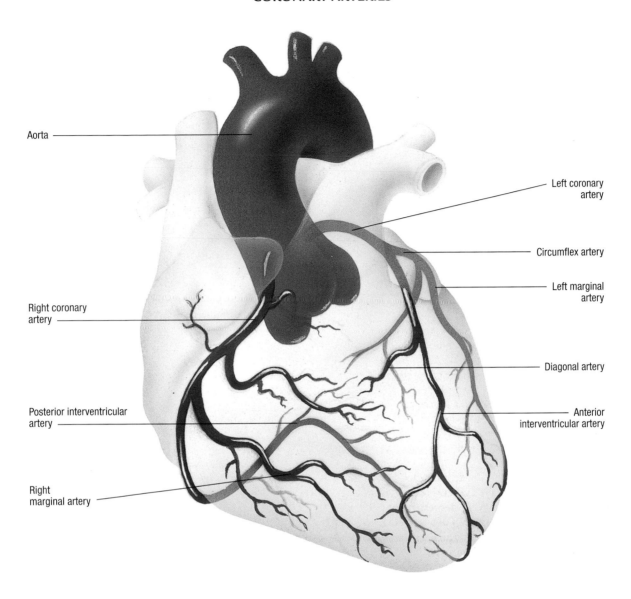

Aorta

Left coronary artery

Circumflex artery

Left marginal artery

Right coronary artery

Diagonal artery

Posterior interventricular artery

Anterior interventricular artery

Right marginal artery

CORONARY ARTERY AND ATHEROSCLEROSIS

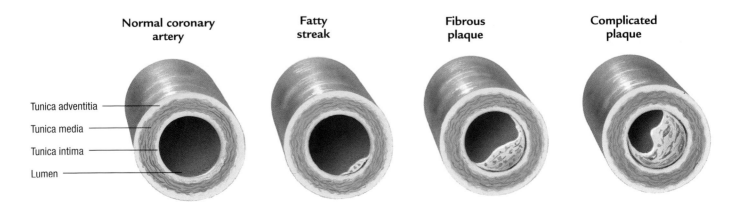

Normal coronary artery

Fatty streak

Fibrous plaque

Complicated plaque

Tunica adventitia

Tunica media

Tunica intima

Lumen

DEEP VEIN THROMBOSIS

An acute condition characterized by inflammation and thrombus formation, deep vein thrombosis (DVT) mainly refers to thrombosis in the deep veins of the legs. This disorder is typically progressive and can lead to potentially lethal pulmonary embolism. DVT often begins with localized inflammation alone (phlebitis), which rapidly provokes thrombus formation. Rarely, venous thrombosis develops without associated inflammation of the vein.

Causes
- Idiopathic
- Endothelial damage
- Accelerated blood clotting
- Reduced blood flow.
  Predisposing factors:
- Prolonged bed rest
- Trauma
- Surgery
- Childbirth
- Oral contraceptives, such as estrogens.

Pathophysiology
A thrombus forms when an alteration in the epithelial lining causes platelet aggregation and consequent fibrin entrapment of red and white blood cells and additional platelets. Thrombus formation is more rapid in areas where blood flow is slower, because contact between platelets increases and thrombin accumulates. The rapidly expanding thrombus initiates a chemical inflammatory process in the vessel epithelium, which leads to fibrosis (narrowing of the blood vessel). The enlarging clot may occlude the vessel lumen partially or totally, or it may detach and embolize to lodge elsewhere in the systemic circulation.

Signs and symptoms
- Vary with site and length of the affected vein (may be asymptomatic)
- Severe pain
- Fever, chills
- Malaise
- Edema and cyanosis of the affected arm or leg
- Redness and warmth over affected area
- Palpable vein
- Lymphadenitis.

 CLINICAL TIP
Some patients may display signs of inflammation and, possibly, a positive Homans' sign (pain on dorsiflexion of the foot) during physical examination.

Diagnostic tests
- Duplex Doppler ultrasonography
- Impedance plethysmography
- Phlebography.

Treatment
The goals of treatment are to control thrombus development, prevent complications, relieve pain, and prevent recurrence of the disorder. Treatment includes:
- bed rest with elevation of affected arm or leg
- warm, moist soaks over affected area
- analgesics
- antiembolism stockings
- anticoagulants (initially, heparin; later, warfarin)
- streptokinase
- simple ligation to vein plication, or clipping
- embolectomy and insertion of a vena caval umbrella or filter.

DEEP VEINS OF LEG

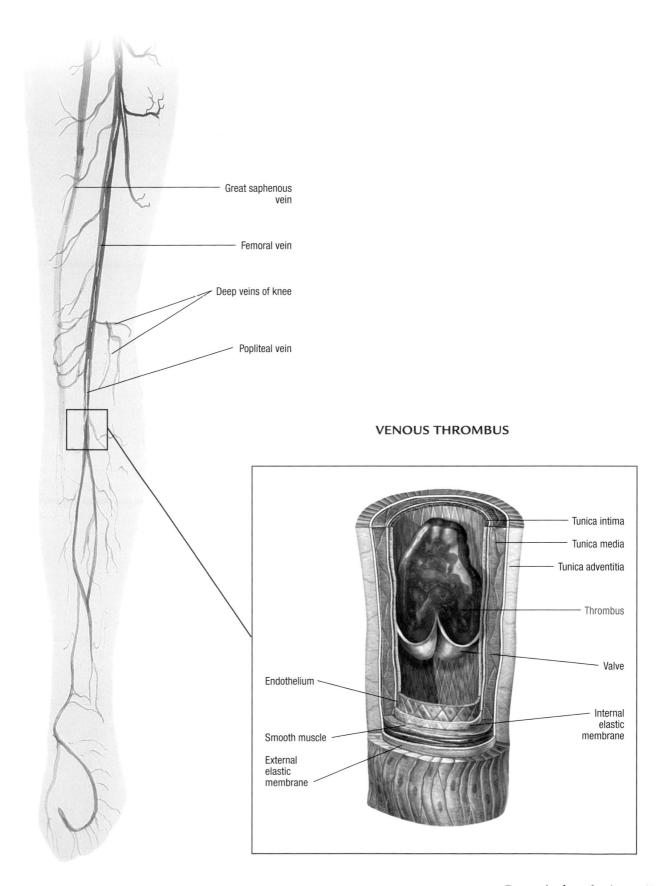

Great saphenous vein

Femoral vein

Deep veins of knee

Popliteal vein

VENOUS THROMBUS

Tunica intima

Tunica media

Tunica adventitia

Thrombus

Valve

Endothelium

Internal elastic membrane

Smooth muscle

External elastic membrane

ENDOCARDITIS

Endocarditis (also known as infective or bacterial endocarditis) is an infection of the endocardium, heart valves, or cardiac prosthesis resulting from bacterial or fungal invasion.

Causes
- I.V. drug abuse
- Prosthetic heart valves
- Mitral valve prolapse
- Rheumatic heart disease.
  Other predisposing conditions:
- Congenital abnormalities — coarctation of aorta, tetralogy of Fallot
- Subaortic and valvular aortic stenosis
- Ventricular septal defects
- Pulmonary stenosis
- Marfan syndrome
- Degenerative heart disease
- Syphilis.

Pathophysiology
Infection causes fibrin and platelets to aggregate on the valve tissue and engulf circulating bacteria or fungi. They form friable verrucous (wart-like) vegetative growths on the heart valves, endocardial lining of a heart chamber, or endothelium of a blood vessel. Such vegetations may cover the valve surfaces, causing ulceration and necrosis; they may also extend to the chordae tendineae. Ultimately, they may embolize to the spleen, kidneys, central nervous system, and lungs.

Signs and symptoms
- Malaise, weakness, fatigue
- Weight loss, anorexia
- Arthralgia
- Intermittent fever, night sweats, chills
- Valvular insufficiency
- Loud, regurgitant murmur
- Suddenly changing murmur or new murmur in the presence of fever

- Splenic infarction — left upper quadrant pain radiating to left shoulder, abdominal rigidity
- Renal infarction — hematuria, pyuria, flank pain, decreased urine output
- Cerebral infarction — hemiparesis, aphasia, other neurologic deficits
- Pulmonary infarction — cough, pleuritic pain, pleural friction rub, dyspnea, and hemoptysis
- Peripheral vascular occlusion — numbness and tingling in an arm, leg, finger, or toe.

Diagnostic tests
- Positive blood cultures

 CLINICAL TIP
Three or more blood cultures in a 24- to 48-hour period (each from a separate venipuncture) identify the causative organism in up to 90% of patients. Blood cultures should be drawn from three different sites with at least 1 to 3 hours between each draw.

- Normal or elevated white blood cell count
- Abnormal macrophages
- Elevated erythrocyte sedimentation rate
- Normocytic, normochromic anemia
- Proteinuria and microscopic hematuria
- Positive serum rheumatoid factor
- Echocardiography (particularly, transesophageal).

Treatment
- Penicillin and an aminoglycoside, usually gentamicin
- Bed rest
- Aspirin for fever and aches, or acetaminophen
- Sufficient fluid intake
- Corrective surgery if refractory heart failure develops
- Replacement of an infected prosthetic valve.

Normal heart wall

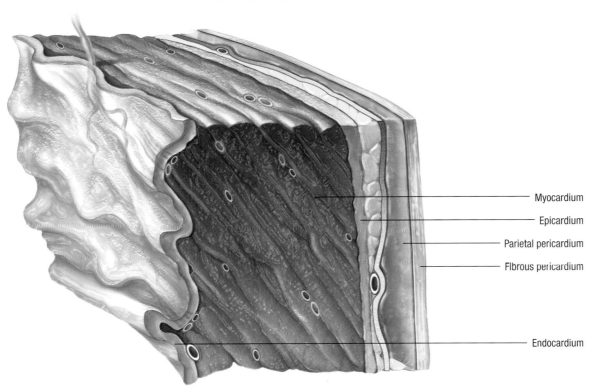

- Myocardium
- Epicardium
- Parietal pericardium
- Fibrous pericardium
- Endocardium

Endocarditis

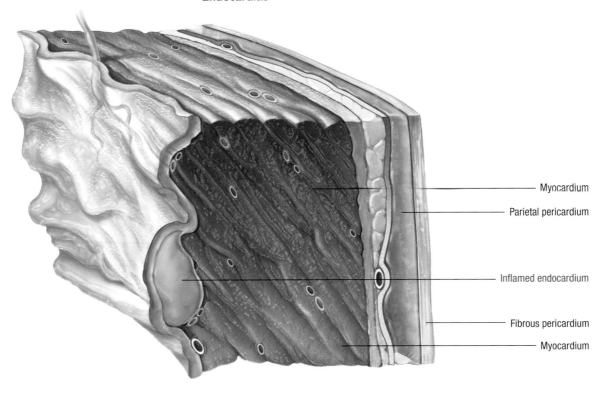

- Myocardium
- Parietal pericardium
- Inflamed endocardium
- Fibrous pericardium
- Myocardium

HEART FAILURE

A syndrome rather than a disease, heart failure occurs when the heart can't pump enough blood to meet the metabolic needs of the body. Heart failure results in intravascular and interstitial volume overload and poor tissue perfusion.

Causes
- *Left-sided heart failure*: left ventricular infarction, hypertension, aortic or mitral valve stenosis
- *Right-sided heart failure:* backward flow due to left-sided heart failure
- *Systolic dysfunction*: myocardial infarction or dilated cardiomyopathy
- *Diastolic dysfunction:* left ventricular hypertrophy, hypertension, or restrictive cardiomyopathy.

Pathophysiology
Heart failure may be classified according to the side of the heart affected or by the cardiac cycle involved.
- *Left-sided heart failure*: ineffective left ventricular contractile function. Cardiac output falls, and blood that would have been pumped into the systemic circulation backs up into the left atrium and then into the lungs.
- *Right-sided heart failure:* ineffective right ventricular contractile function. Blood not pumped effectively through the right ventricle to the lungs backs up into the right atrium and into the peripheral circulation.
- *Systolic dysfunction:* left ventricle can't pump enough blood out to the systemic circulation during systole and the ejection fraction falls. Consequently, blood backs up into the pulmonary circulation and pressure rises in the pulmonary venous system. Cardiac output falls.
- *Diastolic dysfunction*: left ventricle can't relax and fill during diastole and the stroke volume falls. Therefore, larger ventricular volumes are needed to maintain cardiac output.

All causes of heart failure eventually reduce cardiac output and trigger compensatory mechanisms. These mechanisms improve cardiac output at the expense of increased ventricular work, as described below.
- Increased sympathetic activity enhances peripheral vascular resistance, contractility, heart rate, and venous return. It also restricts blood flow to the kidneys, causing them to secrete renin which, in turn, converts angiotensinogen to angiotensin I, which then becomes angiotensin II — a potent vasoconstrictor.
- Angiotensin causes the adrenal cortex to release aldosterone, leading to sodium and water retention and an increase in circulating blood volume. This renal mechanism is helpful; however, if it persists unchecked, it can aggravate heart failure as the heart struggles to pump against the increased volume.
- The increase in end-diastolic ventricular volume (preload) causes increased stroke work and stroke volume during contraction, stretching cardiac muscle fibers so that the ventricle can accept the increased intravascular volume. Eventually, the muscle becomes stretched beyond optimum limits and contractility declines.

In heart failure, the body produces counterregulatory substances (prostaglandins and atrial natriuretic factor) to try to reduce the negative effects of the volume overload and vasoconstriction caused by the compensatory mechanisms.

When blood flow increases in the ventricles, the heart makes the following compensations:
- *Short-term:* As the end-diastolic fiber length increases, the ventricular muscle responds by dilating and increasing the force of contraction (Frank-Starling curve.)
- *Long-term:* Ventricular hypertrophy increases the heart muscles' ability to contract and push its volume of blood into the circulation.

Compensation may occur for long periods of time before signs and symptoms develop.

Signs and symptoms
Left-sided heart failure:
- Dyspnea, orthopnea, paroxysmal nocturnal dyspnea
- Fatigue
- Nonproductive cough, crackles
- Hemoptysis
- Point of maximal impulse displaced toward left anterior axillary line
- Tachycardia; S_3 and S_4 heart sounds
- Cool, pale skin.
  Right-sided heart failure:
- Jugular venous distention
- Hepatojugular reflux and hepatomegaly
- Right upper quadrant pain
- Anorexia, fullness, and nausea
- Nocturia
- Weight gain
- Edema, ascites or anasarca.

Diagnostic tests
- Chest X-ray
- Electrocardiography
- Abnormal liver function tests and elevated blood urea nitrogen and creatinine levels
- Echocardiography
- Hemodynamic monitoring using a pulmonary artery (Swan-Ganz) catheter
- Radionuclide ventriculography.

Treatment
- Treatment of the underlying cause, if known
- Angiotensin-converting enzyme (ACE) inhibitors to patients with left ventricle dysfunction
- Digoxin
- Beta-adrenergic blockers
- Diuretics, nitrates, morphine, oxygen
- Lifestyle modifications to reduce risk factors
- Coronary artery bypass surgery or angioplasty
- Heart transplantation.

 AGE ALERT
Incidence of heart failure rises with age. Approximately 1% of people older than age 50 and 10% of people older than age 80 experience heart failure.

TYPES OF HEART FAILURE

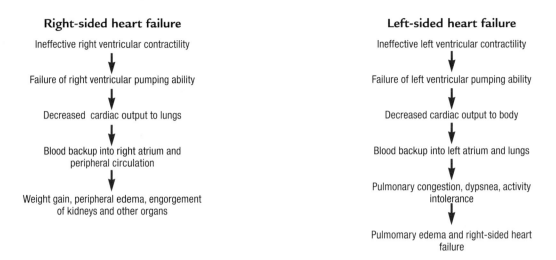

Right-sided heart failure

Ineffective right ventricular contractility

↓

Failure of right ventricular pumping ability

↓

Decreased cardiac output to lungs

↓

Blood backup into right atrium and peripheral circulation

↓

Weight gain, peripheral edema, engorgement of kidneys and other organs

Left-sided heart failure

Ineffective left ventricular contractility

↓

Failure of left ventricular pumping ability

↓

Decreased cardiac output to body

↓

Blood backup into left atrium and lungs

↓

Pulmonary congestion, dypsnea, activity intolerance

↓

Pulmomary edema and right-sided heart failure

Normal cardiac circulation

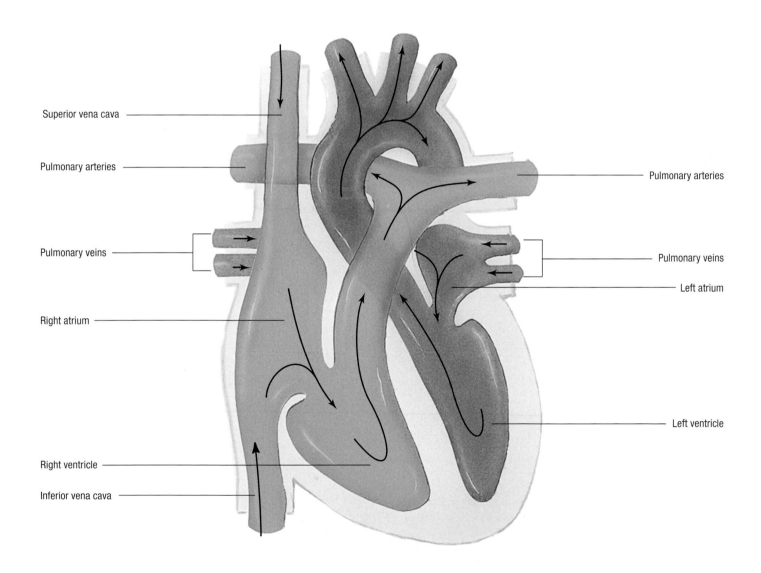

Superior vena cava

Pulmonary arteries

Pulmonary veins

Right atrium

Right ventricle

Inferior vena cava

Pulmonary arteries

Pulmonary veins

Left atrium

Left ventricle

HYPERTENSION

Hypertension, an elevation in diastolic or systolic blood pressure, occurs as two major types: primary (essential), which is the most common; and secondary, which results from renal disease or another identifiable cause. Malignant hypertension is a severe, fulminant form of either type. Hypertension is a major cause of cerebrovascular accident, cardiac disease, and renal failure.

Causes

Risk factors for primary hypertension:
- Family history
- Advancing age
- Race (most common in blacks)
- Obesity
- Tobacco use
- High intake of sodium or saturated fat
- Excessive alcohol consumption
- Sedentary lifestyle, stress.
  Causes of secondary hypertension:
- Excess renin
- Mineral deficiencies (calcium, potassium, and magnesium)
- Diabetes mellitus
- Coarctation of the aorta
- Renal artery stenosis or parenchymal disease
- Brain tumor, quadriplegia, head injury
- Pheochromocytoma, Cushing's syndrome, hyperaldosteronism
- Thyroid, pituitary, or parathyroid dysfunction
- Oral contraceptives, cocaine, epoetin alfa, sympathetic stimulants, monoamine oxidase inhibitors taken with tyramine, estrogen replacement therapy, nonsteroidal anti-inflammatory drugs
- Pregnancy.

Pathophysiology

Arterial blood pressure is a product of total peripheral resistance and cardiac output. Cardiac output is increased by conditions that increase heart rate or stroke volume, or both. Peripheral resistance is increased by factors that increase blood viscosity or reduce the lumen size of vessels.

Several mechanisms may lead to hypertension, such as:
- changes in the arteriolar bed causing increased peripheral vascular resistance
- abnormally increased tone in the sympathetic nervous system that originates in the vasomotor system centers, causing increased peripheral vascular resistance
- increased blood volume resulting from renal or hormonal dysfunction
- arteriolar thickening caused by genetic factors, leading to increased peripheral vascular resistance
- abnormal renin release, resulting in the formation of angiotensin II, which constricts the arteriole and increases blood volume.

Prolonged hypertension increases the workload of the heart as resistance to left ventricular ejection increases. To increase contractile force, the left ventricle hypertrophies, raising the oxygen demand and workload of the heart. Cardiac dilation

and failure may occur when hypertrophy can no longer maintain sufficient cardiac output. Because hypertension promotes coronary atherosclerosis, the heart may be further compromised by reduced blood flow to the myocardium, resulting in angina or myocardial infarction (MI). Hypertension also causes vascular damage, leading to accelerated atherosclerosis and target organ damage.

The pathophysiology of secondary hypertension is related to the underlying disease.

Signs and symptoms
- Generally asymptomatic
- Elevated blood pressure readings on at least two consecutive occasions after initial screening
- Occipital headache
- Epistaxis possibly due to vascular involvement
- Bruits
- Dizziness, confusion, fatigue
- Blurry vision
- Nocturia
- Edema.

CLINICAL TIP
Many older adults have a wide auscultatory gap, that is, the hiatus between the first Korotkoff sound and the next sound. Failure to inflate the blood pressure cuff high enough can lead to missing the first Korotkoff sound and underestimating the systolic blood pressure. To avoid missing the first Korotkoff sound, palpate the radial artery and inflate the cuff approximately 20 mm beyond disappearance of the pulse beat.

Diagnostic tests
- Serial blood pressure measurements.
  To detect primary causes:
- Blood urea nitrogen, creatinine, and potassium levels; complete blood count; urinalysis
- Excretory urography
- Electrocardiography
- Chest X-ray
- Echocardiography.

Treatment
- Diuretics
- Calcium channel blockers
- Angiotensin-converting enzyme (ACE) inhibitors
- Alpha-receptor blockers
- Alpha-receptor agonists
- Beta blockers
- Treatment of underlying cause
- Nitroprusside or an adrenergic inhibitor, such as propranolol
- Lifestyle modifications to reduce risk factors
- Calcium, magnesium, potassium supplementation as needed.

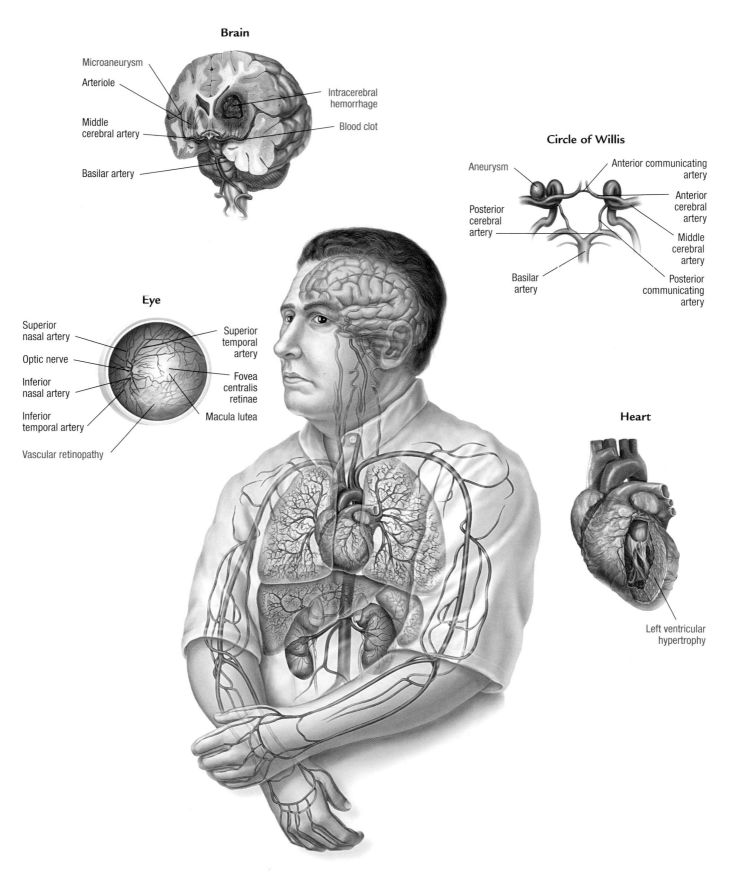

Brain

Microaneurysm

Arteriole

Middle
cerebral artery

Basilar artery

Intracerebral
hemorrhage

Blood clot

Circle of Willis

Aneurysm

Posterior
cerebral
artery

Basilar
artery

Anterior communicating
artery

Anterior
cerebral
artery

Middle
cerebral
artery

Posterior
communicating
artery

Eye

Superior
nasal artery

Optic nerve

Inferior
nasal artery

Inferior
temporal artery

Vascular retinopathy

Superior
temporal
artery

Fovea
centralis
retinae

Macula lutea

Heart

Left ventricular
hypertrophy

Mitral valve prolapse

Mitral valve prolapse is also called systolic click-murmur syndrome and floppy mitral valve syndrome. It is probably a congenital abnormality.

Causes
- Autosomal dominant inheritance
- Inherited connective tissue disorders such as Marfan syndrome, Ehlers-Danlos syndrome, and osteogenesis imperfecta
- Genetic or environmental interruption of valve development during week 5 or 6 of gestation.

Pathophysiology
The cusps of the mitral valve are enlarged, thickened, and scalloped, possible secondary to collagen abnormalities. The chordae tendineae may be longer than usual, allowing the cusps to stretch upward. Mitral regurgitation occurs when the valve permits blood to leak into the atrium.

Signs and symptoms
- Often asymptomatic
- Regurgitant murmur
- Midsystolic click
- Palpitations, arrhythmias, tachycardia
- Light-headedness or syncope
- Fatigue, especially in the morning; lethargy; weakness
- Dyspnea, hyperventilation
- Chest tightness, atypical chest pain
- Anxiety, panic attacks, depression.

CLINICAL TIP

The high incidence of mitral valve prolapse (3% to 8% of adults) suggests that it may be a normal variant. It occurs more often in women than in men. Although severe sequelae may occur (such as ruptured chordae tendineae, ventricular failure, emboli, bacterial endocarditis, and sudden death), mortality and morbidity are low. Most affected persons experience no physical limitations. The psychologic effects of the diagnosis may be more disabling than the disease process itself.

Diagnostic tests
- Two-dimensional echocardiography
- Electrocardiography (resting and exercise)
- Doppler studies
- Cardiac angiography.

Treatment
- Corresponds to degree of mitral regurgitation
- In presence of regurgitation, antibiotic prophylaxis before any invasive procedure to prevent infective endocarditis
- Beta blockers
- Measures to prevent hypovolemia, such as drinking at least 64 oz (1,893 ml) of water or noncaffeinated beverages per day, because hypovolemia can decrease ventricular volume, thereby increasing stress on the prolapsed mitral valve
- Surgical repair or valve replacement.

Cross section of left ventricle

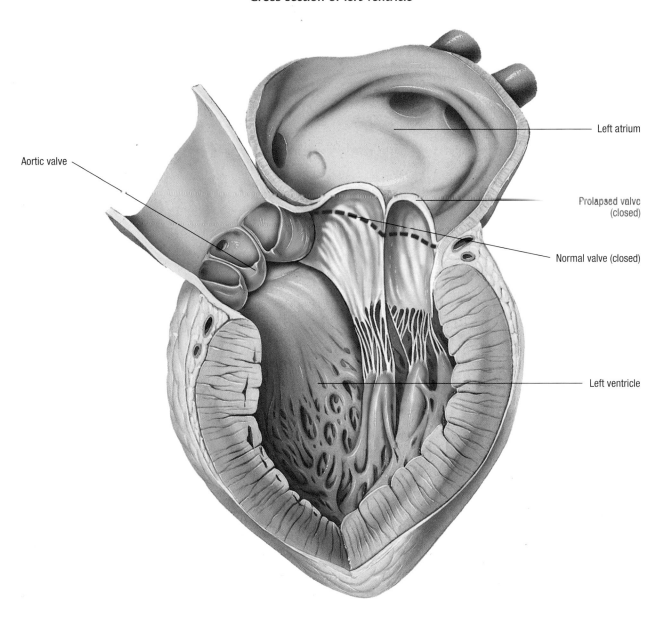

Aortic valve

Left atrium

Prolapsed valve
(closed)

Normal valve (closed)

Left ventricle

MYOCARDIAL INFARCTION

In myocardial infarction (MI), reduced blood flow through one or more of the coronary arteries initiates myocardial ischemia and necrosis. (See also "Coronary artery disease," page 46.)

Causes
- Thrombosis
- Coronary artery stenosis or spasm.
  Predisposing risk factors include:
- family history of heart disease
- atherosclerosis
- hypertension
- tobacco smoking
- elevated serum triglyceride, total cholesterol, and low-density lipoprotein levels
- diabetes mellitus
- obesity
- excessive intake of saturated fats, carbohydrates, or salt
- sedentary lifestyle
- stress or type A personality
- drug use, especially cocaine and amphetamines
- gender and age (most common in men and postmenopausal women).

Pathophysiology
If coronary artery occlusion causes prolonged ischemia, lasting longer than 30 to 45 minutes, irreversible myocardial cell damage and muscle death occur.

The site of the MI depends on the vessels involved. Occlusion of the circumflex branch of the left coronary artery causes a lateral wall infarction; occlusion of the anterior descending branch of the left coronary artery, an anterior wall infarction. True posterior or inferior wall infarctions generally result from occlusion of the right coronary artery or one of its branches.

Right ventricular infarctions can also result from right coronary artery occlusion, can accompany inferior infarctions, and may cause right-sided heart failure. In Q-wave (transmural) MI, tissue damage extends through all myocardial layers; in non–Q-wave (subendocardial) MI, damage occurs only in the innermost and possibly the middle layers.

All infarcts have a central area of necrosis (infarction) surrounded by an area of potentially viable hypoxic injury, which may be salvaged if circulation is restored, or may progress to necrosis. The zone of injury, in turn, is surrounded by viable ischemic tissue.

The infarcted myocardial cells release cardiac enzymes and proteins. Within 24 hours, the infarcted muscle becomes edematous and cyanotic. During the next several days, leukocytes infiltrate the necrotic area and begin to remove necrotic cells, thinning the ventricular wall. Scar formation begins by the third week after MI, and by the sixth week, scar tissue is well established.

The scar tissue that forms on the necrotic area inhibits contractility. Compensatory mechanisms (vascular constriction, increased heart rate, and renal retention of sodium and water) try to maintain cardiac output. Ventricular dilation may also occur in a process called remodeling. Functionally, MI may cause reduced contractility with abnormal wall motion, altered left ventricular compliance, reduced stroke volume, reduced ejection fraction, and elevated left ventricular end-diastolic pressure.

Signs and symptoms
- Persistent, crushing substernal chest pain that may radiate to the left arm, jaw, neck, or shoulder blades
- Cool extremities, perspiration, anxiety, and restlessness due to release of catecholamines
- Blood pressure and pulse initially elevated as a result of sympathetic nervous system activation
- Shortness of breath and crackles, reflecting heart failure
- Fatigue and weakness
- Nausea and vomiting
- Jugular venous distention
- S_3 and S_4 heart sounds, loud holosystolic murmur in apex
- Reduced urine output.

 AGE ALERT
Many older adults with MI do not have chest pain. Instead they may experience atypical symptoms such as fatigue, dyspnea, falls, tingling of the extremities, nausea, vomiting, weakness, syncope, and confusion.

Diagnostic tests
- Serial 12-lead electrocardiography
- Serial cardiac enzymes and the proteins troponin T and I
- Elevated white blood cell count and erythrocyte sedimentation rate
- Echocardiography
- Nuclear imaging with thallium-201 or technetium 99m
- Cardiac catheterization.

Treatment
The American College of Cardiology/American Heart Association Task Force on Practice Guidelines for treatment of MI include:
- assessment of patients with chest pain in the Emergency Department within 10 minutes of symptom onset
- oxygen
- nitroglycerin
- morphine or meperidine (Demerol)
- aspirin
- continuous cardiac monitoring to detect arrhythmias and ischemia
- I.V. thrombolytic therapy within 6 hours of symptom onset
- I.V. heparin
- percutaneous transluminal coronary angioplasty (PTCA)
- limitation of physical activity for the first 12 hours
- atropine, lidocaine, transcutaneous pacing patches or a transvenous pacemaker, a defibrillator, and epinephrine
- beta blockers
- angiotensin-converting enzyme (ACE) inhibitors
- magnesium sulfate.

TISSUE DESTRUCTION IN MYOCARDIAL INFARCTION

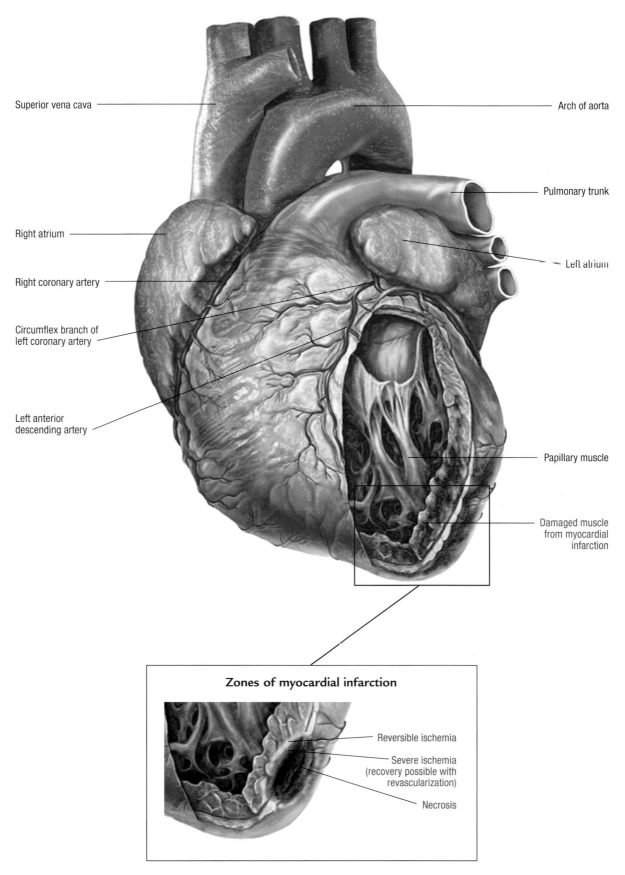

Superior vena cava

Arch of aorta

Right atrium

Pulmonary trunk

Right coronary artery

Left atrium

Circumflex branch of
left coronary artery

Left anterior
descending artery

Papillary muscle

Damaged muscle
from myocardial
infarction

Zones of myocardial infarction

Reversible ischemia

Severe ischemia
(recovery possible with
revascularization)

Necrosis

MYOCARDITIS

Myocarditis is focal or diffuse inflammation of the cardiac muscle (myocardium). It may be acute or chronic and can occur at any age. In many cases, myocarditis causes neither specific cardiovascular symptoms nor electrocardiogram abnormalities, and recovery is usually spontaneous without residual defects. Occasionally, myocarditis is complicated by heart failure; in rare cases, it leads to cardiomyopathy.

Causes
- Infections: viral, bacterial, parasitic-protozoan, fungal, or metazoal (a class of multicellular organisms) infections such as echinoccosis and trichinosis
- Hypersensitive immune reactions, such as acute rheumatic fever or postcardiotomy syndrome
- Radiation therapy
- Toxins, such as lead, chemicals, or cocaine
- Chronic alcoholism.

Pathophysiology
Damage to the myocardium occurs when an infectious organism triggers an autoimmune, cellular, or humoral reaction; noninfectious causes can lead to toxic inflammation. In either case, the resulting inflammation may lead to hypertrophy, fibrosis, and inflammatory changes of the myocardium and conduction system. The heart muscle weakens and contractility is reduced. The heart muscle becomes flabby and dilated and pinpoint hemorrhages may develop.

Signs and symptoms
- Fatigue, dyspnea, palpitations
- Fever
- Mild, continuous pressure or soreness in the chest
- Tachycardia, S_3 and S_4 gallops
- Murmur of mitral insufficiency, pericardial friction rub
- Right-sided and left-sided heart failure (neck vein distention, dyspnea, edema, pulmonary congestion, persistent fever with resting or exertional tachycardia disproportionate to the degree of fever, and supraventricular and ventricular arrhythmias).

CLINICAL TIP
To auscultate for a pericardial friction rub, have the patient sit upright, lean forward, and exhale. Listen over the third intercostal space on the left side of the chest. A pericardial rub has a scratchy, rubbing quality. If you suspect a rub and have trouble hearing one, have the patient hold his breath.

Diagnostic tests
- Elevated creatine kinase (CK), creatine kinase isoform CK-MB, aspartate aminotransferase, and lactate dehydrogenase
- White blood cell count and erythrocyte sedimentation rate
- Antibody titers
- Electrocardiography
- Chest X-ray
- Echocardiography
- Radionuclide scanning
- Cultures of stool, throat, and body fluids
- Endomyocardial biopsy.

Treatment
- No treatment for benign self-limiting disease
- Antibiotics
- Antipyretics
- Restricted activity
- Supplemental oxygen therapy
- Sodium restriction and diuretics
- Angiotensin-converting enzyme (ACE) inhibitors
- Digoxin
- Antiarrhythmic drugs, such as quinidine or procainamide
- Temporary pacemaker
- Anticoagulation to prevent thromboembolism
- Corticosteroids and immunosuppressants
- Cardiac assist devices or transplantation.

TISSUE CHANGES IN MYOCARDITIS

Normal heart wall

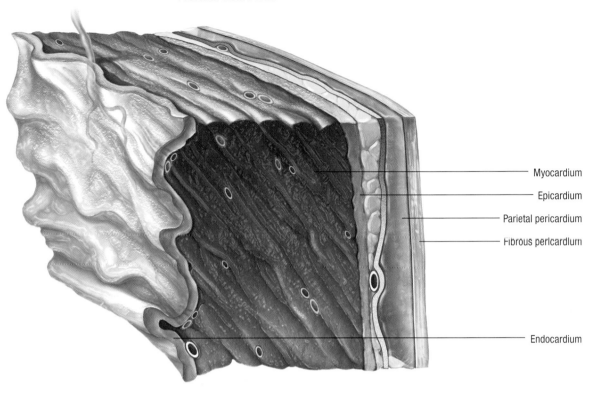

Myocardium

Epicardium

Parietal pericardium

Fibrous pericardium

Endocardium

Myocarditis

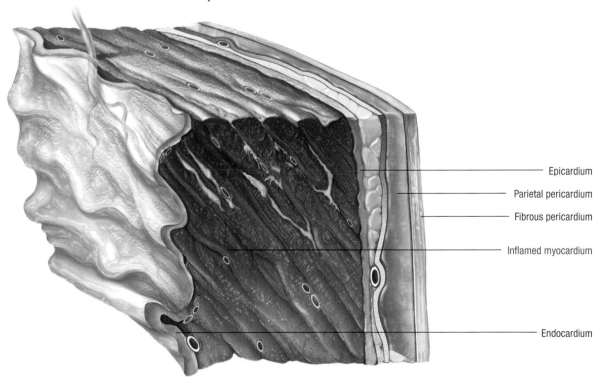

Epicardium

Parietal pericardium

Fibrous pericardium

Inflamed myocardium

Endocardium

Pericardial effusion and cardiac tamponade

Cardiac tamponade is a rapid, unchecked rise in pressure in the pericardial sac that compresses the heart, impairs diastolic filling, and limits cardiac output. The rise in pressure usually results from blood or fluid accumulation in the pericardial sac (pericardial effusion). Even a small amount of fluid (50 to 100 ml) can cause a serious tamponade if it accumulates rapidly.

Causes
- Idiopathic
- Effusion (due to cancer, bacterial infections, tuberculosis or, rarely, acute rheumatic fever)
- Traumatic or nontraumatic hemorrhage
- Viral or postirradiation pericarditis
- Chronic renal failure requiring dialysis
- Drug reaction (procainamide, hydralazine, minoxidil, isoniazid, penicillin, methysergide maleate, daunorubicin)
- Heparin- or warfarin-induced tamponade
- Connective tissue disorders
- Acute myocardial infarction.

Pathophysiology
In cardiac tamponade, the progressive accumulation of fluid in the pericardial sac causes compression of the heart chambers. This compression obstructs blood flow into the ventricles and reduces the amount of blood that can be pumped out of the heart with each contraction.

Each time the ventricles contract, more fluid accumulates in the pericardial sac. This further limits the amount of blood that can fill the ventricular chambers, especially the left ventricle, during the next cardiac cycle.

The amount of fluid necessary to cause cardiac tamponade varies greatly; it may be as little as 50 to 100 ml when the fluid accumulates rapidly or more than 2,000 ml if the fluid accumulates slowly and the pericardium stretches to adapt. Prognosis is inversely proportional to the amount of fluid accumulated.

Signs and symptoms
- Elevated central venous pressure (CVP) with neck vein distention
- Muffled heart sounds
- Pulsus paradoxus
- Diaphoresis and cool, clammy skin
- Anxiety, restlessness, syncope
- Cyanosis
- Weak, rapid pulse
- Cough, dyspnea, orthopnea, tachypnea.

CLINICAL TIP
Cardiac tamponade has three classic features known as Beck's triad:
- elevated CVP with neck vein distention
- muffled heart sounds
- pulsus paradoxus.

Diagnostic tests
- Chest X-ray
- Electrocardiography (ECG)
- Pulmonary artery catheterization
- Echocardiography.

Treatment
- Supplemental oxygen
- Continuous ECG and hemodynamic monitoring
- Pericardiocentesis
- Pericardectomy
- Resection of a portion or all of the pericardium
- Trial volume loading with crystalloids
- Inotropic drugs
- Posttraumatic injury: blood transfusion, thoracotomy to drain reaccumulating fluid, or repair of bleeding sites may be necessary
- Heparin-induced tamponade: heparin antagonist protamine sulfate to stop bleeding
- Warfarin-induced tamponade: vitamin K to stop bleeding.

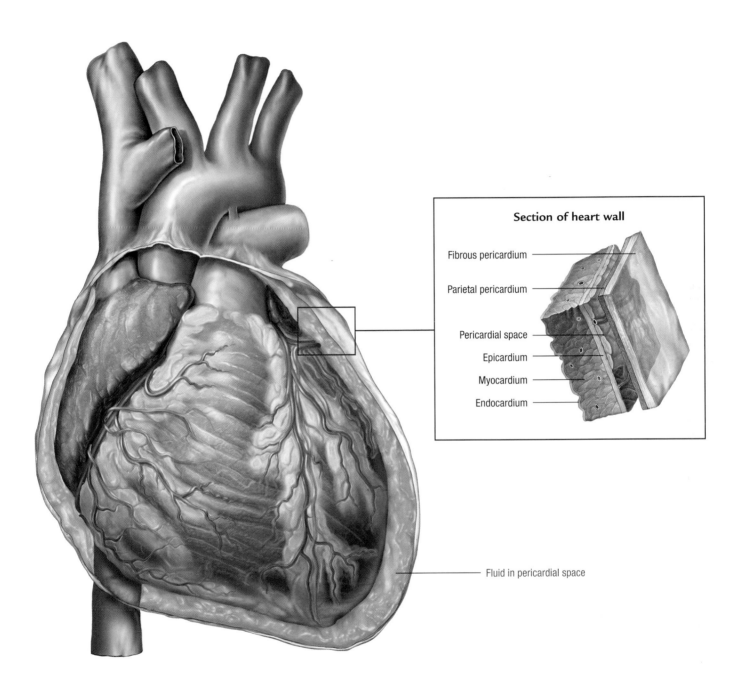

Section of heart wall

Fibrous pericardium

Parietal pericardium

Pericardial space

Epicardium

Myocardium

Endocardium

Fluid in pericardial space

PERICARDITIS

Pericarditis is inflammation of the pericardium — the fibroserous sac that envelops, supports, and protects the heart. Acute pericarditis can be fibrinous or effusive, with purulent, serous, or hemorrhagic exudate. Chronic constrictive pericarditis is characterized by dense fibrous pericardial thickening. The prognosis depends on the underlying cause but is generally good in acute pericarditis, unless constriction occurs.

Causes

- Bacterial, fungal, or viral infection
- Neoplasm
- High-dose radiation to the chest
- Uremia
- Hypersensitivity or autoimmune disease
- Previous cardiac injury, such as myocardial infarction, trauma, or surgery
- Drugs, such as hydralazine or procainamide
- Idiopathic factors
- Aortic aneurysm
- Myxedema.

AGE ALERT
The most common cause of pericarditis in children is acute rheumatic fever.

Pathophysiology

Pericardial tissue damaged by bacteria or other substances releases chemical mediators of inflammation (prostaglandins, histamines, bradykinins, and serotonin) into the surrounding tissue, thereby initiating the inflammatory process. Friction occurs as the inflamed pericardial layers rub against each other. Histamines and other chemical mediators dilate vessels and increase vessel permeability. Vessel walls then leak fluids and protein (including fibrinogen) into tissues, causing extracellular edema. Macrophages already present in the tissue begin to phagocytize the invading bacteria and are joined by neutrophils and monocytes. After several days, the area fills with an exudate composed of necrotic tissue and dead and dying bacteria, neutrophils, and macrophages. If the cause of pericarditis is not infection, the exudate may be serous (as with autoimmune disease) or hemorrhagic (seen with trauma or surgery). Eventually, the contents of the cavity autolyze and are gradually reabsorbed into healthy tissue.

Chronic constrictive pericarditis develops if the chronic or recurrent pericarditis makes the pericardium thick and stiff, encasing the heart in a stiff shell and preventing proper filling during diastole. Consequently, left and right-side filling pressures rise as stroke volume and cardiac output fall.

Signs and symptoms

- Pericardial friction rub
- Sharp and often sudden pain, usually starting over the sternum and radiating to the neck, shoulders, back, and arms
- Shallow, rapid respirations
- Mild fever
- Dyspnea, orthopnea, tachycardia
- Heart failure
- Muffled, distant heart sounds
- Pallor, clammy skin, hypotension, pulsus paradoxus, neck vein distention
- Eventually, cardiovascular collapse
- Fluid retention, ascites, hepatomegaly, jugular venous distention
- Pericardial knock in early diastole along the left sternal border produced by restricted ventricular filling
- Kussmaul's sign (increased jugular vein distention on inspiration due to restricted right-sided filling).

CLINICAL TIP
The pain in pericarditis is often pleuritic, increasing with deep inspiration and decreasing when the patient sits up and leans forward, pulling the heart away from the diaphragmatic pleurae of the lungs.

Diagnostic tests

To diagnose the condition:
- Electrocardiography
- Echocardiography
- Chest X-ray.
  To identify the underlying cause:
- Erythrocyte sedimentation rate, white blood cell count, blood urea nitrogen
- Blood cultures
- Antistreptolysin-O titers
- Purified protein derivative skin test.

Treatment

- Bed rest as long as fever and pain persist
- Treatment of the underlying cause, if it can be identified
- Nonsteroidal anti-inflammatory drugs, corticosteroids
- Antibacterial, antifungal, or antiviral therapy
- Partial or total pericardectomy.

Normal heart wall

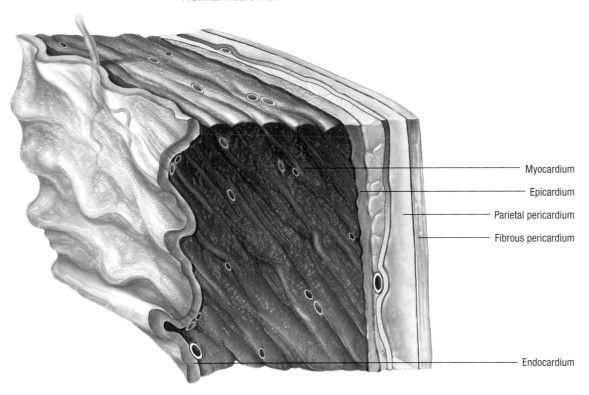

Myocardium

Epicardium

Parietal pericardium

Fibrous pericardium

Endocardium

Pericarditis

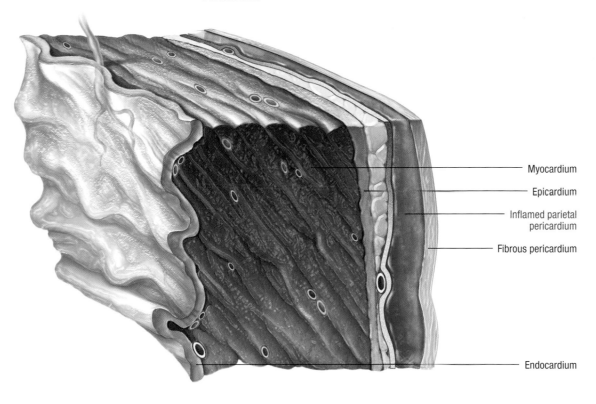

Myocardium

Epicardium

Inflamed parietal pericardium

Fibrous pericardium

Endocardium

Raynaud's disease

Raynaud's *disease* is one of several primary disorders characterized by episodic spasms of the small peripheral arteries and arterioles, precipitated by exposure to cold or stress. This condition occurs bilaterally and usually affects the hands or, less often, the feet. It is benign, requires no specific treatment, and has no serious sequelae. Raynaud's *phenomenon*, however, is secondary to any of several connective disorders — such as scleroderma, systemic lupus erythematosus, or polymyositis — and progresses to ischemia, gangrene, and amputation. Distinguishing between the two disorders is difficult because some patients experience mild symptoms of Raynaud's disease for several years and then develop overt connective tissue disease, especially scleroderma.

 AGE ALERT
Raynaud's disease is most prevalent in females, particularly between puberty and age 40.

Causes

Raynaud's disease:
- Unknown; family history is a risk factor.
  Raynaud's phenomenon:
- Connective tissue disorders, such as scleroderma, rheumatoid arthritis, systemic lupus erythematosus, or polymyositis
- Pulmonary hypertension
- Thoracic outlet syndrome
- Arterio-occlusive disease
- Myxedema
- Trauma
- Serum sickness
- Exposure to heavy metals
- Long-term exposure to cold, vibrating machinery (such as operating a jackhammer), or pressure to the fingertips (as in typists and pianists).

Pathophysiology

Raynaud's disease is a syndrome of episodic constriction of the arterioles and arteries of the extremities, resulting in pallor and cyanosis of the fingers and toes. Several mechanisms may account for the reduced digital blood flow, including:
- intrinsic vascular wall hyperactivity to cold
- increased vasomotor tone due to sympathetic stimulation

- antigen-antibody immune response (most likely because abnormal immunologic test results accompany Raynaud's phenomenon).

Signs and symptoms

- Bilateral blanching (pallor) of the fingers after exposure to cold or stress:
- vasoconstriction or vasospasm reduces blood flow.
- cyanosis due to increased oxygen extraction resulting from sluggish blood flow
- spasm resolves, and fingers turn red (rubor) as blood rushes back into the arterioles
- Cold and numbness
- Throbbing, aching pain, swelling, and tingling
- Trophic changes (as a result of ischemia), such as sclerodactyly, ulcerations, or chronic paronychia.

Diagnostic tests

- Clinical criteria:
- skin color changes induced by cold or stress
- bilateral involvement
- absence of gangrene or, if present, minimal cutaneous gangrene
- normal arterial pulses
- history of symptoms for at least 2 years
- Antinuclear antibody titer
- Arteriography
- Doppler ultrasonography.

Treatment

- Avoiding triggers such as cold, and mechanical or chemical injury
- Stopping smoking and avoiding decongestants and caffeine to reduce vasoconstriction
- Calcium channel blockers
- Alpha-adrenergic blockers
- Biofeedback and relaxation exercises to reduce stress and improve circulation
- Sympathectomy or amputation.

PROGRESSIVE VASCULAR CHANGES

Pallor due to decreased or absent blood flow

Cyanosis due to capillary dilatation

Rubor due to excessive hyperemia resulting from reactive vasodilation

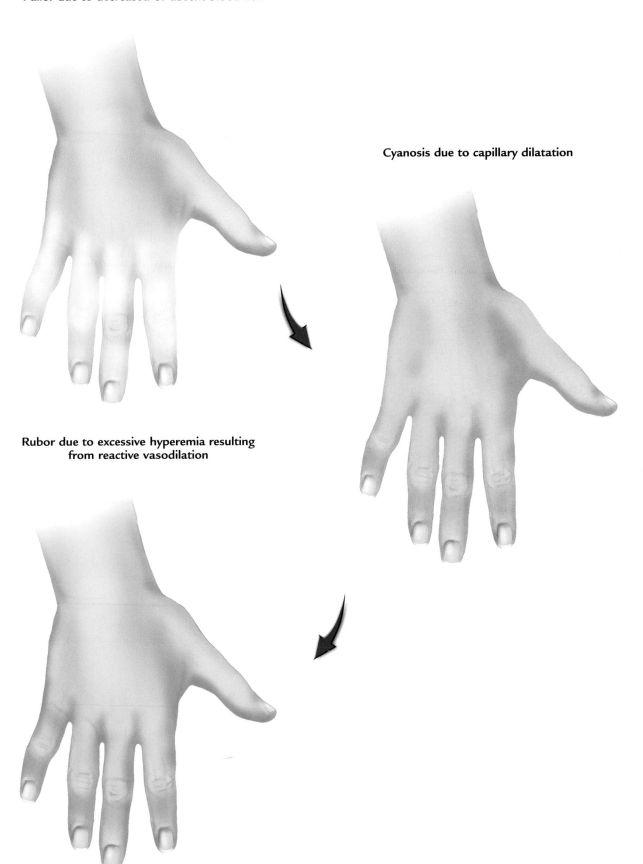

RHEUMATIC HEART DISEASE

A systemic inflammatory disease of childhood, acute rheumatic fever develops after infection of the upper respiratory tract with group A beta-hemolytic streptococci. It mainly involves the heart, joints, central nervous system, skin, and subcutaneous tissues, and often recurs. Rheumatic heart disease refers to the cardiac manifestations of rheumatic fever and includes pancarditis during the early acute phase and chronic valvular disease later. Cardiac involvement develops in up to 50% of patients.

Rheumatic fever tends to run in families, lending support to the existence of genetic predisposition. Environmental factors also seem to be significant in the development of the disorder.

 AGE ALERT
In lower socioeconomic groups, the incidence is highest in children between ages 5 and 15, probably due to malnutrition and crowded living conditions.

Causes

Rheumatic fever is caused by group A beta-hemolytic streptococcal pharyngitis.

Pathophysiology

Rheumatic fever appears to be a hypersensitivity reaction to a group A beta-hemolytic streptococcal infection. Because very few persons (3%) with streptococcal infections contract rheumatic fever, altered host resistance must be involved in its development or recurrence. The antigens of group A streptococci bind to receptors in the heart, muscle, brain, and synovial joints, causing an autoimmune response. Because the antigens of the streptococcus are similar to some antigens of the body's own cells, antibodies may attack healthy body cells.

Carditis may affect the endocardium, myocardium, or pericardium during the early acute phase. Later, heart-valve damage may cause chronic valvular disease.

Signs and symptoms

- Streptococcal infection a few days to 6 weeks before onset of symptoms
- New or worsening mitral or aortic murmur
- Pericardial friction rub
- Chest pain, often pleuritic
- Dyspnea, tachypnea, nonproductive cough, bibasilar crackles, edema.

Diagnostic tests

- White blood cell count, erythrocyte sedimentation rate
- Hemoglobin, hematocrit

- C-reactive protein
- Cardiac enzymes
- Antistreptolysin-O titer
- Throat cultures
- Electrocardiography
- Chest X-rays
- Echocardiography
- Cardiac catheterization.

 CLINICAL TIP
Jones Criteria for diagnosis require either two major criteria or one major criterion and two minor plus evidence of a previous group A streptococcal infection.
Major criteria:
- Carditis
- Migratory joint pain
- Sydenham's chorea
- Subcutaneous nodules, usually near tendons or bony prominences of joints, especially the elbows, knuckles, wrists, and knees
- Erythema marginatum.
Minor criteria:
- Fever
- Arthralgia
- Elevated acute phase reactants
- Prolonged PR interval.

Treatment

- Prompt treatment of all group A beta-hemolytic streptococcal pharyngitis with oral penicillin V or I.M. benzathine penicillin G; erythromycin for patients with penicillin hypersensitivity
- Salicylates
- Corticosteroids
- Strict bed rest for about 5 weeks
- Sodium restriction, angiotensin-converting enzyme (ACE) inhibitors, digoxin, and diuretics
- Corrective surgery, such as commissurotomy, valvuloplasty, or valve replacement for severe mitral or aortic valvular dysfunction that causes persistent heart failure
- Secondary prevention of rheumatic fever, which begins after the acute phase subsides:
– monthly I.M. injections of penicillin G benzathine or daily doses of oral penicillin V or sulfadiazine
– continued treatment, usually for at least 5 years or until age 21, whichever is longer
- Prophylactic antibiotics for dental work and other invasive or surgical procedures.

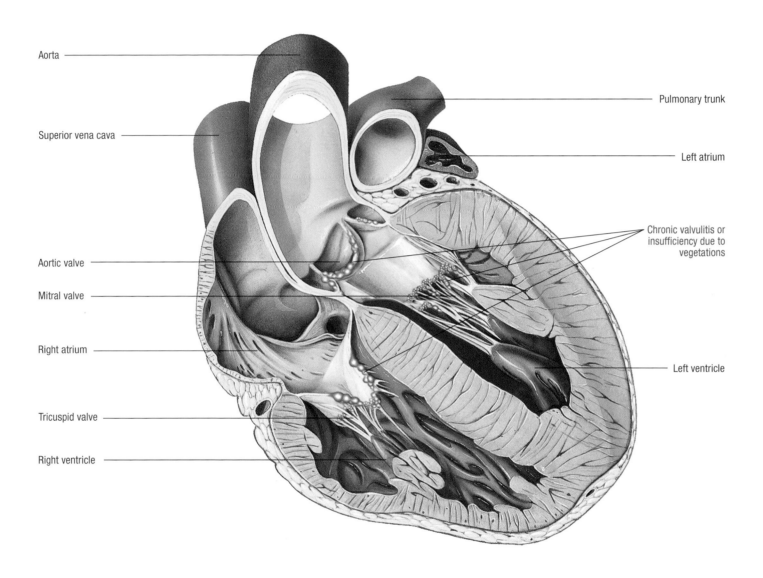

Aorta

Superior vena cava

Aortic valve

Mitral valve

Right atrium

Tricuspid valve

Right ventricle

Pulmonary trunk

Left atrium

Chronic valvulitis or insufficiency due to vegetations

Left ventricle

SHOCK

Shock is a clinical syndrome that leads to reduced perfusion of tissues and organs and organ failure. Shock can be classified into three categories: distributive (neurogenic, septic, and anaphylactic); cardiogenic; and hypovolemic.

Causes

Neurogenic shock:
- Spinal cord injury, spinal anesthesia
- Vasomotor center depression
- Severe pain
- Medications
- Hypoglycemia.
  Septic shock:
- Gram-negative bacteria, gram-positive bacteria
- Viruses, fungi, rickettsiae, parasites, yeast, protozoa, or mycobacteria.
  Anaphylactic shock:
- Medications, vaccines, contrast media
- Venom
- Foods
- ABO-incompatible blood.
  Cardiogenic shock:
- Myocardial infarction (most common cause)
- Heart failure, cardiomyopathy
- Pericardial tamponade
- Tension pneumothorax
- Pulmonary embolism.
  Hypovolemic shock:
- Blood loss (most common cause)
- GI fluid loss, renal loss, fluid shifts
- Burns
- Ascites, peritonitis
- Hemothorax.

Pathophysiology

Each type of shock has three stages.

Compensatory stage: When arterial pressure and tissue perfusion fall, compensatory mechanisms are activated to maintain cardiac output and perfusion to the heart and brain. As the baroreceptors in the carotid sinus and aortic arch sense a drop in blood pressure, epinephrine and norepinephrine are secreted to increase peripheral resistance, blood pressure, and myocardial contractility. Reduced blood flow to the kidney activates the renin-angiotensin-aldosterone system, causing vasoconstriction and sodium and water retention and thereby increasing blood volume and venous return.

Progressive stage: When compensatory mechanisms cannot maintain cardiac output, tissues become hypoxic because perfusion is inadequate. Cells switch to anaerobic metabolism and lactic acid accumulates, producing metabolic acidosis (depressing myocardial function). Tissue hypoxia promotes the release of endothelial mediators, causing vasodilation and endothelial abnormalities, leading to venous pooling and increased capillary permeability. Sluggish blood flow increases the risk of disseminated intravascular coagulation.

Irreversible (refractory) stage: Inadequate perfusion damages cell membranes, lysosomal enzymes are released, and energy stores are depleted, leading to cell death. Lactic acid continues to accumulate, increasing capillary permeability and the movement of fluid out of the vascular space. This loss of intravascular fluid further contributes to hypotension. Perfusion to the coronary arteries is reduced, causing myocardial depression and a further reduction in cardiac output. Circulatory and respiratory failure occur.

Signs and symptoms

Compensatory stage:
- Tachycardia and bounding pulse
- Restlessness and irritability
- Tachypnea
- Reduced urinary output
- Cool, pale skin (or warm, dry skin in septic shock).
  Progressive stage:
- Hypotension
- Narrowed pulse pressure; weak, rapid, thready pulse
- Shallow respirations
- Cold, clammy skin; cyanosis.
  Irreversible stage:
- Unconsciousness and absent reflexes
- Rapidly falling blood pressure; weak pulse
- Slow, shallow or Cheyne-Stokes respirations
- Anuria.

Diagnostic tests

- Hematocrit
- Blood, urine, and sputum cultures
- Coagulation studies
- White blood cell count and erythrocyte sedimentation rate
- Blood urea nitrogen, creatinine, and serum glucose levels
- Cardiac enzymes and proteins
- Arterial blood gas analysis
- Chest X-ray
- Hemodynamic monitoring
- Electrocardiography
- Echocardiography.

Treatment

- Identification and treatment of the underlying cause
- Maintaining a patent airway; oxygen
- Continuous cardiac monitoring
- I.V. fluids, crystalloids, colloids, or blood products
- *For neurogenic shock:* vasopressor drugs
- *For septic shock:*
- antibiotic therapy
- inotropic and vasopressor drugs
- *For cardiogenic shock:*
- inotropic drugs, vasodilators,diuretics
- intra-aortic balloon pump therapy
- thrombolytic therapy or coronary artery revascularization
- ventricular assist device
- heart transplantation
- *For hypovolemic shock:* pneumatic antishock garment.

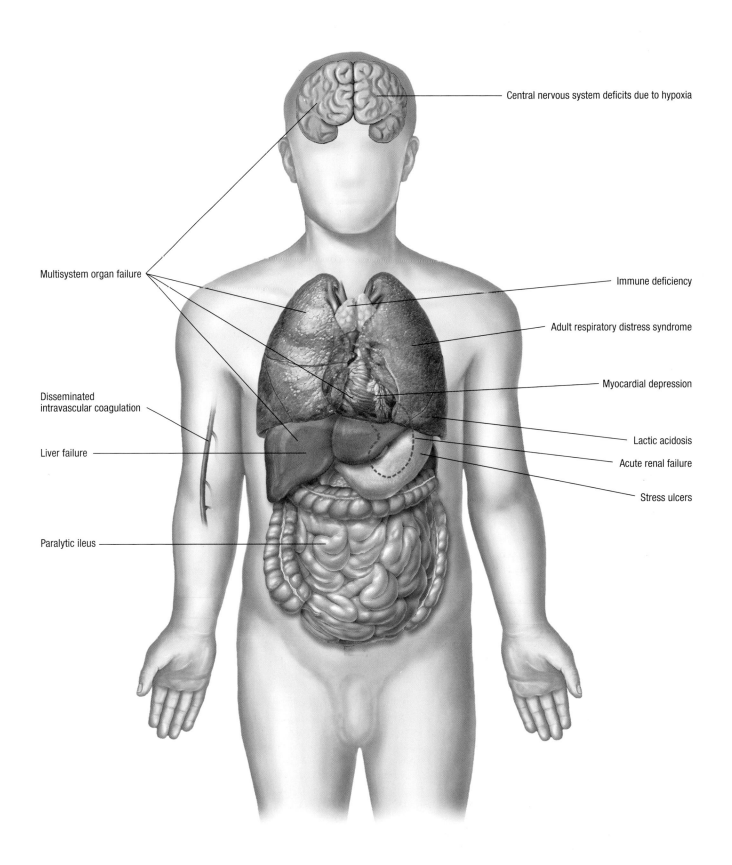

Central nervous system deficits due to hypoxia

Multisystem organ failure

Immune deficiency

Adult respiratory distress syndrome

Disseminated intravascular coagulation

Myocardial depression

Liver failure

Lactic acidosis

Acute renal failure

Stress ulcers

Paralytic ileus

VALVULAR HEART DISEASE

In valvular heart disease, three types of mechanical disruptions can occur: stenosis, or narrowing, of the valve opening; incomplete closure of the valve; or prolapse of the valve.

Causes
The causes of valvular heart disease are varied and are different for each type of valve disorder.

Mitral stenosis:
- Rheumatic fever
- Congenital anomalies.

Mitral insufficiency:
- Rheumatic fever
- Mitral valve prolapse
- Myocardial infarction
- Severe left ventricular failure
- Ruptured chordae tendinae.

Aortic insufficiency:
- Rheumatic fever
- Syphilis
- Hypertension
- Endocarditis
- Marfan syndrome.

Aortic stenosis:
- Congenital
- Rheumatic fever
- Atherosclerosis.

Pulmonic stenosis:
- Congenital
- Rheumatic fever.

Pathophysiology
Pathophysiology of valvular heart disease varies according to the valve and the disorder.

Mitral insufficiency: Any abnormality of the mitral leaflets, mitral annulus, chordae tendineae, papillary muscles, left atrium, or left ventricle can lead to mitral regurgitation. Blood from the left ventricle flows back into the left atrium during systole, and the atrium enlarges to accommodate the backflow. The left ventricle also dilates to accommodate the increased volume of blood from the atrium and to compensate for diminishing cardiac output. Ventricular hypertrophy and increased end-diastolic pressure raise pulmonary artery pressure, eventually leading to left-sided and right-sided heart failure.

Mitral stenosis: Structural abnormality, fibrosis, or calcification obstructs blood flow from the left atrium to the left ventricle. Left atrial volume and pressure rise and the chamber dilates. Greater resistance to blood flow causes pulmonary hypertension, right ventricular hypertrophy, and right-sided heart failure. Inadequate filling of the left ventricle causes low cardiac output.

Aortic insufficiency: Blood flows back into the left ventricle during diastole, causing fluid overload in the ventricle, which dilates and hypertrophies. The excess volume causes fluid overload in the left atrium and, finally, the pulmonary system. Left-sided heart failure and pulmonary edema result.

Aortic stenosis: Left ventricular pressure rises to overcome the resistance of the narrowed valvular opening. The added work-load increases the demand for oxygen, and diminished cardiac output causes poor coronary artery perfusion, ischemia of the left ventricle, and left-sided heart failure.

Pulmonic stenosis: Obstructed right ventricular outflow causes right ventricular hypertrophy, resulting in right-sided heart failure.

Signs and symptoms
The clinical manifestations vary according to valvular defects and the severity of the defect. Patient may be asymptomatic.

Common to all valvular disorders:
- Dyspnea, weakness and fatigue.

Mitral stenosis:
- Orthopnea
- Palpitations, right-sided heart failure, crackles
- Atrial fibrillation
- Diastolic thrill, loud S_1, opening snap-diastolic murmur.

Mitral insufficiency:
- Palpitations, angina, tachycardia
- Right-sided heart failure, pulmonary edema, crackles
- Split S_2; S_3; holosystolic murmur at apex
- Apical thrill.

Aortic insufficiency:
- Palpitations, angina, syncope
- Cough
- Pulmonary congestion, left-sided heart failure
- Quincke's sign
- Pulsus biferiens, visible apical pulse
- S_3 and blowing diastolic murmur at left sternal border.

Aortic stenosis:
- Palpitations, angina, arrhythmias
- Syncope
- Pulmonary congestion, left-sided heart failure
- Diminished carotid pulses, systolic thrill (carotid)
- Decreased cardiac output
- Systolic murmur at base of carotids, S_4.

Pulmonic stenosis:
- Syncope, chest pain, right-sided heart failure
- Systolic murmur at left sternal border, S_2 split.

Diagnostic tests
- Cardiac catheterization
- Chest X-ray
- Echocardiography
- Electrocardiography.

Treatment
- Digoxin, anticoagulants, nitroglycerin, beta blockers, diuretics, vasodilators, angiotensin-converting enzyme (ACE) inhibitors
- Low-sodium diet
- Oxygen
- Prophylactic antibiotics before and after invasive procedures
- Cardioversion
- Open or closed commissurotomy
- Annuloplasty or valvuloplasty
- Prosthetic valve for mitral or aortic valve disease.

HEART VALVES

Normal

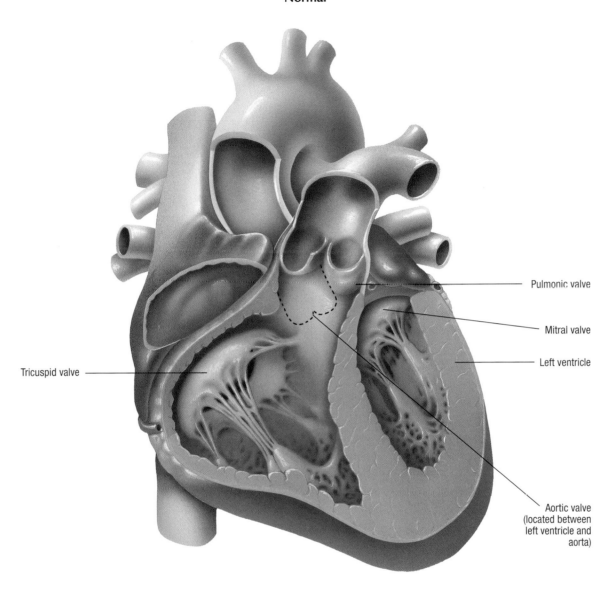

Tricuspid valve

Pulmonic valve

Mitral valve

Left ventricle

Aortic valve
(located between
left ventricle and
aorta)

Superior view of the heart

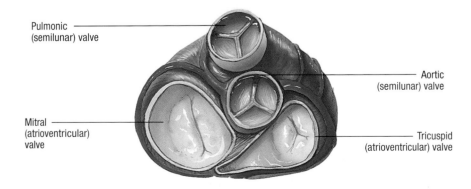

Pulmonic
(semilunar) valve

Mitral
(atrioventricular)
valve

Aortic
(semilunar) valve

Tricuspid
(atrioventricular) valve

Normal atrioventricular valve

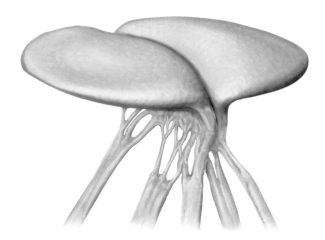

Stenotic atrioventricular valve

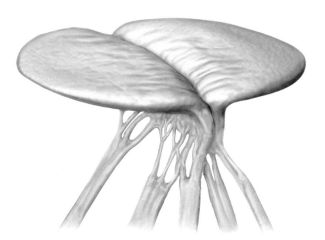

Insufficient atrioventricular valve

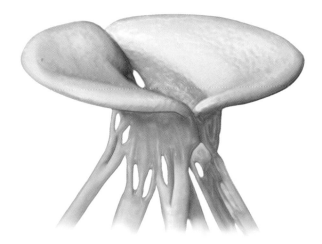

Normal semilunar valve

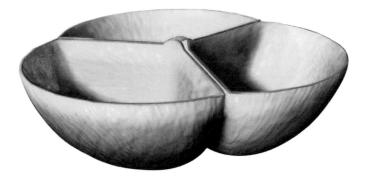

Stenotic semilunar valve

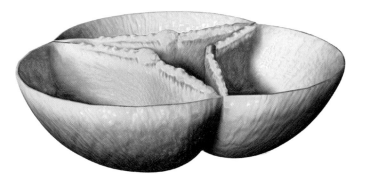

Insufficient semilunar valve

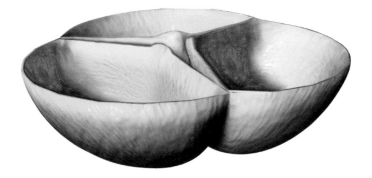

VARICOSE VEINS

Varicose veins are dilated, tortuous veins, engorged with blood and resulting from poor venous valve function. They can be primary, originating in the superficial veins, or secondary, occurring in the deep veins.

Causes

Primary varicose veins:
- Congenital weakness of valves or vein wall
- Prolonged venous stasis or increased intra-abdominal pressure, as in pregnancy, obesity, constipation, or wearing tight clothes
- Standing for an extended period of time
- Family tendency.
  Secondary varicose veins:
- Deep vein thrombosis
- Venous malformation
- Arteriovenous fistulas
- Venous trauma
- Occlusion.

Pathophysiology

Veins are thin-walled, distensible vessels with valves that keep blood flowing in one direction. Any condition that weakens, destroys, or distends these valves allows the backflow of blood to the previous valve. If a valve cannot hold the pooling blood, it can become incompetent, allowing even more blood to flow backward. The increasing volume of blood in the vein raises pressure and distends the vein. As the veins are stretched, their walls weaken and lose their elasticity, and the veins become lumpy and tortuous. Rising hydrostatic pressure forces plasma into the surrounding tissues, resulting in edema.

Signs and symptoms

- Dilated, tortuous, purplish, ropelike veins, particularly in the calves
- Edema of the calves and ankles
- Leg heaviness that worsens in the evening and in warm weather
- Dull aching in the legs after prolonged standing or walking
- Aching during menses.

AGE ALERT
As a person ages, veins dilate and stretch, increasing susceptibility to varicose veins and chronic venous insufficiency. Because the skin becomes friable and can easily break down, ulcers caused by chronic venous insufficiency may take longer to heal.

Diagnostic tests

CLINICAL TIP
Manual compression test detects a palpable impulse when the vein is firmly occluded at least 8" above the point of palpation, indicating incompetent valves in the vein.

Trendelenburg's test (retrograde filling test) detects incompetent valves when the vein is occluded with the patient in the supine position and the leg elevated 90°. When the person stands (still with the vein occluded) the saphenous veins should fill slowly from below in approximately 30 seconds.

- Photoplethysmography
- Doppler ultrasonography
- Venous outflow and reflux plethysmography
- Ascending and descending venography.

Treatment

- Treatment of underlying cause (if possible), such as abdominal tumor or obesity
- Antiembolism stockings or elastic bandages
- Regular exercise
- Injection of a sclerosing agent into small to medium-sized varicosities
- Surgical stripping and ligation of severe varicose veins
- Phlebectomy (removing the varicose vein through small incisions in the skin).

VASCULAR CHANGES IN VARICOSE VEINS

Normal
Varicose veins
Incompetent valve
Reverse blood flow
Varicose veins
Normal blood flow

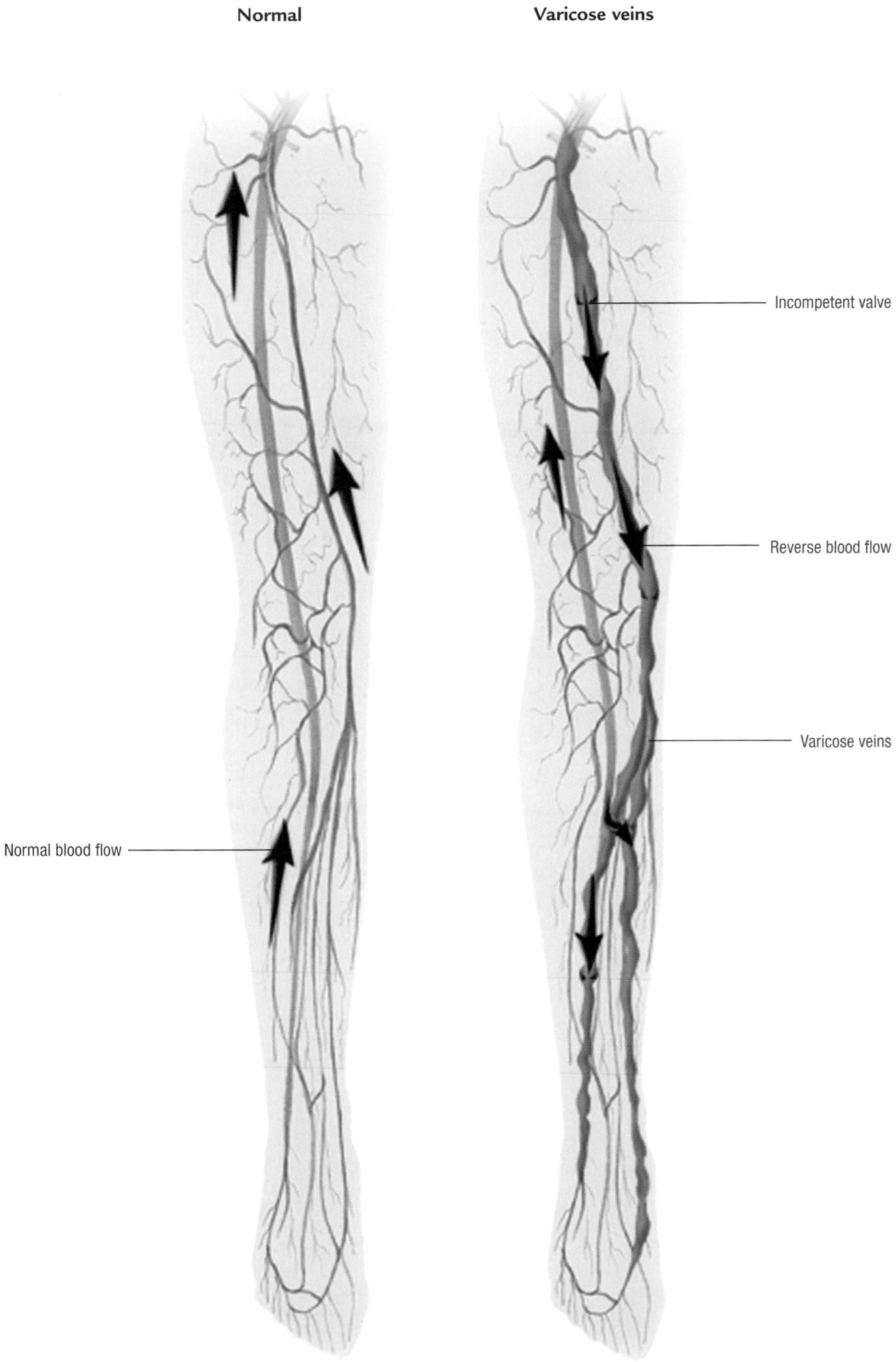

ADULT RESPIRATORY DISTRESS SYNDROME

Adult respiratory distress syndrome (ARDS) is a form of pulmonary edema that can quickly lead to acute respiratory failure. Also known as shock lung, stiff lung, white lung, wet lung, or Da Nang lung, ARDS may follow direct or indirect injury to the lung. However, diagnosis is difficult; death can occur within 48 hours of onset if ARDS is not promptly diagnosed and treated.

Causes

- Injury to the lung from trauma
- Trauma-related factors, such as fat emboli, sepsis, shock, pulmonary contusions, and multiple transfusions
- Anaphylaxis
- Aspiration of gastric contents or diffuse pneumonia, especially viral pneumonia
- Drug overdose
- Idiosyncratic drug reaction to ampicillin or hydrochlorothiazide
- Inhalation of noxious gases, such as nitrous oxide, ammonia, or chlorine
- Near drowning
- Oxygen toxicity
- Sepsis
- Coronary artery bypass grafting
- Hemodialysis
- Leukemia
- Acute miliary tuberculosis
- Pancreatitis
- Thrombotic thrombocytopenic purpura
- Uremia
- Venous air embolism.

Pathophysiology

Injury in ARDS involves both the alveolar epithelium and the pulmonary capillary epithelium. Damage can occur directly — by aspiration of gastric contents or inhalation of noxious gases — or indirectly — from chemical mediators released in response to systemic disease. The causative agent triggers a cascade of cellular and biochemical changes. Once initiated, this agent triggers neutrophils, macrophages, monocytes, and lymphocytes to produce various cytokines — which promote cellular activation, chemotaxis, and adhesion — and inflammatory mediators, including oxidants, proteases, kinins, growth factors, and neuropeptides, which initiate the complement cascade, intravascular coagulation, and fibrinolysis.

These cellular events increase vascular permeability to proteins, increasing the hydrostatic pressure gradient of the capillary. Elevated capillary pressure, as results from fluid overload or cardiac dysfunction, greatly increases interstitial and alveolar edema, which is evident on chest X-rays as whitened areas in the lower lung. Alveolar closing pressure then exceeds pulmonary pressures, and the alveoli begin to collapse.

Phase 1. Fluid accumulation in the lung interstitium, the alveolar spaces, and the small airways causes the lungs to stiffen, thus impairing ventilation and reducing oxygenation of the pulmonary capillary blood, resulting in reduced blood flow to the lungs. Platelets begin to aggregate and release substances, such as serotonin, bradykinin, and histamine, which attract and activate neutrophils.

Phase 2. These substances inflame and damage the alveolar membrane and later increase capillary permeability. Additional chemotactic factors released include endotoxins, tumor necrosis factor, and interleukin-1 (IL-1). The activated neutrophils release several inflammatory mediators and platelet aggravating factors that damage the alveolar capillary membrane and increase capillary permeability, allowing fluids to move into the interstitial space.

Phase 3. As capillary permeability increases, proteins, blood cells, and more fluid leak out, increasing interstitial osmotic pressure and causing pulmonary edema.

(Text continues on page 80.)

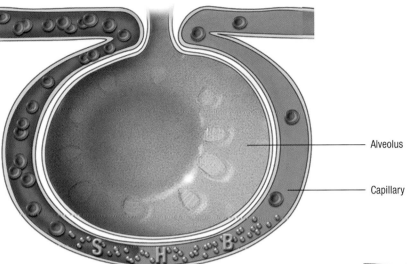

Phase 1. Injury reduces normal blood flow to the lungs. Platelets aggregate and release histamine (H), serotonin (S), and bradykinin (B).

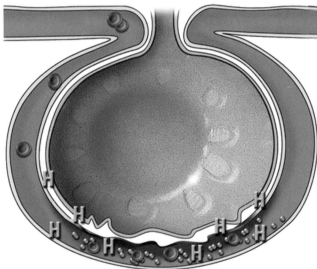

Phase 2. Those substances, especially histamine, inflame and damage the alveolocapillary membrane, increasing capillary permeability. Fluids then shift into the interstitial space.

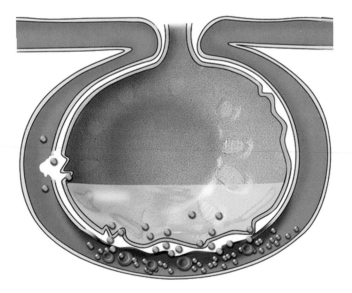

Phase 3. As capillary permeability increases, proteins and fluids leak out, increasing interstitial osmotic pressure and causing pulmonary edema.

Adult respiratory distress syndrome   **79**

Phase 4. The resulting pulmonary edema and hemorrhage significantly reduce lung compliance and impair alveolar ventilation.

Phase 5. Mediators released by neutrophils and macrophages also cause varying degrees of pulmonary vasoconstriction, resulting in pulmonary hypertension. The result of these changes is a mismatch in the ventilation-perfusion (V/Q) ratio. Although the patient responds with an increased respiratory rate, sufficient oxygen cannot cross the alveolar capillary membrane. Carbon dioxide continues to cross easily and is lost with every exhalation.

Phase 6. Pulmonary edema worsens and hyaline membranes form. Inflammation leads to fibrosis, which further impedes gas exchange. Fibrosis progressively obliterates alveoli, respiratory bronchioles, and the interstitium. Functional residual capacity decreases and shunting becomes more serious. Hypoxemia leads to metabolic acidosis. At this stage, the patient develops increasing $PaCO_2$, decreasing pH and PaO_2, decreasing bicarbonate levels, and mental confusion. The end result is respiratory failure.

Signs and symptoms
- Rapid, shallow breathing and dyspnea
- Increased rate of ventilation
- Intercostal and suprasternal retractions
- Crackles and rhonchi
- Restlessness, apprehension, and mental sluggishness
- Motor dysfunction
- Tachycardia
- Respiratory acidosis
- Metabolic acidosis.

Diagnostic tests
- Arterial blood gas analysis
- Pulmonary artery catheterization
- Pulmonary artery mixed venous blood sampling
- Serial chest X-rays
- Sputum analysis
- Blood cultures
- Toxicology testing
- Serum amylase.

Treatment
Therapy is focused on correcting the causes of ARDS and preventing progression of hypoxemia and respiratory acidosis. Treatment includes:
- mechanical ventilation and intubation
- positive end-expiratory pressure
- pressure-controlled inverse ratio ventilation
- permissive hypercapnia
- sedatives, narcotics, and neuromuscular blockers
- high-dose corticosteroids
- sodium bicarbonate
- I.V. fluid administration
- vasopressors
- antimicrobial drugs
- diuretics
- correction of electrolyte and acid–base imbalances
- fluid restrictions.

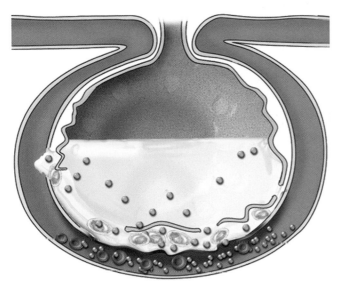

Phase 4. Decreased blood flow and fluids in the alveoli damage surfactant and impair the cell's ability to produce more. As a result, alveoli collapse, impeding gas exchange and decreasing lung compliance.

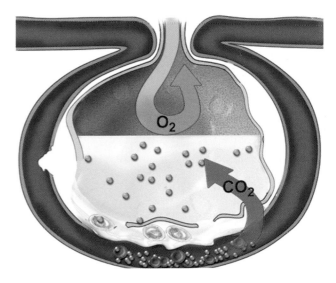

Phase 5. Sufficient oxygen can't cross the alveolocapillary membrane, but carbon dioxide (CO_2) can and is lost with every exhalation. Oxygen (O_2) and CO_2 levels decrease in the blood.

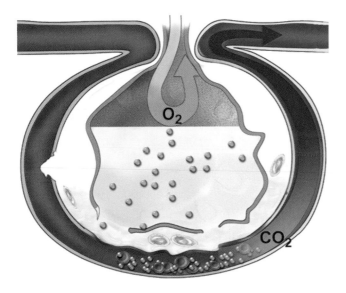

Phase 6. Pulmonary edema worsens, inflammation leads to fibrosis, and gas exchange is further impeded.

Adult respiratory distress syndrome **81**

ASTHMA

Asthma is a chronic reactive airway disorder that causes episodic airway obstruction. Such obstruction results from bronchospasms, increased mucus secretion, and mucosal edema. It is a type of chronic obstructive pulmonary disease, a group of lung diseases characterized by increased airflow resistance.

AGE ALERT
Although this common condition can strike at any age, half of all cases first occur in children under age 10; in this age-group asthma affects twice as many boys as girls.

Causes

Asthma may result from sensitivity to extrinsic or intrinsic allergens. Extrinsic, or atopic, asthma begins in childhood; typically, patients are sensitive to specific external allergens.

Extrinsic allergens include:
- pollen
- animal dander
- house dust or mold
- kapok or feather pillows
- food additives, including sulfites and some dyes
- noxious fumes.

Patients with intrinsic, or nonatopic, asthma react to internal, nonallergenic factors; external substances cannot be implicated in patients with intrinsic asthma. Most episodes occur after a severe respiratory tract infection, especially in adults.

Intrinsic allergens include:
- irritants
- emotional stress, anxiety
- fatigue
- endocrine changes
- temperature or humidity variations
- coughing or laughing
- genetic factors.

Many asthmatics, especially children, have both intrinsic and extrinsic asthma.

Pathophysiology

Two genetic influences are identified with asthma, namely the ability of an individual to develop asthma (atopy) and the tendency to develop hyperresponsiveness of the airways independent of atopy. A locus on chromosome 11 associated with atopy contains an abnormal gene that encodes a part of the immunoglobulin E (IgE) receptor. Environmental factors interact with inherited factors to cause asthmatic reactions and associated bronchospasms.

In asthma, bronchial linings overreact to various stimuli, causing smooth muscle spasms that severely constrict the airways. When the hypersensitive patient inhales a triggering substance, abnormal antibodies stimulate mast cells in the lung interstitium to release both histamine and the slow-reacting substance of anaphylaxis (SRS-A). Histamine attaches to receptor sites in the larger bronchi, where it causes swelling in smooth muscles. SRS-A attaches to receptor sites in the smaller bronchi and causes swelling of smooth muscle there. SRS-A also causes fatty acids called prostaglandins to travel by way of

the bloodstream to the lungs, where they enhance histamine's effects. Histamine stimulates the mucous membranes to secrete excessive mucus, further narrowing the bronchial lumen. On inhalation, the narrowed bronchial lumen can still expand slightly, allowing air to reach the alveoli. On exhalation, increased intrathoracic pressure closes the bronchial lumen completely. Mucus fills the lung bases, inhibiting alveolar ventilation. Blood, shunted to alveoli in other lung parts, still can't compensate for diminished ventilation.

CLINICAL TIP
When status asthmaticus occurs, hypoxia worsens, expiratory flow slows, and expiratory volumes decrease. If treatment is not initiated, the patient begins to tire. Acidosis develops as arterial carbon dioxide increases. The situation becomes life-threatening when no air movement is audible on auscultation (a silent chest) and $Paco_2$ rises to over 70 mm Hg.

Signs and symptoms

Mild asthma:
- Asymptomatic between attacks
- Wheezing
- Coughing; thick, clear or yellow mucus
- Dyspnea on exertion.
  Moderate asthma:
- Respiratory distress at rest
- Hyperpnea
- Barrel chest
- Diminished breath sounds.
  Severe asthma:
- Marked respiratory distress, wheezing
- Absent breath sounds
- Pulsus paradoxus greater than 10 mm Hg
- Chest wall contractions.

Diagnostic tests

- Pulmonary function studies
- Serum IgE
- Sputum analysis
- Complete blood count with differential
- Chest X-ray
- Arterial blood gas analysis
- Skin testing
- Bronchial challenge testing
- Electrocardiography.

Treatment

- Identification and avoidance of precipitating factors
- Desensitization to specific antigens
- Bronchodilators
- Corticosteroids
- Subcutaneous epinephrine
- Mast cell stabilizers
- Low-flow humidified oxygen
- Mechanical ventilation
- Relaxation exercises.

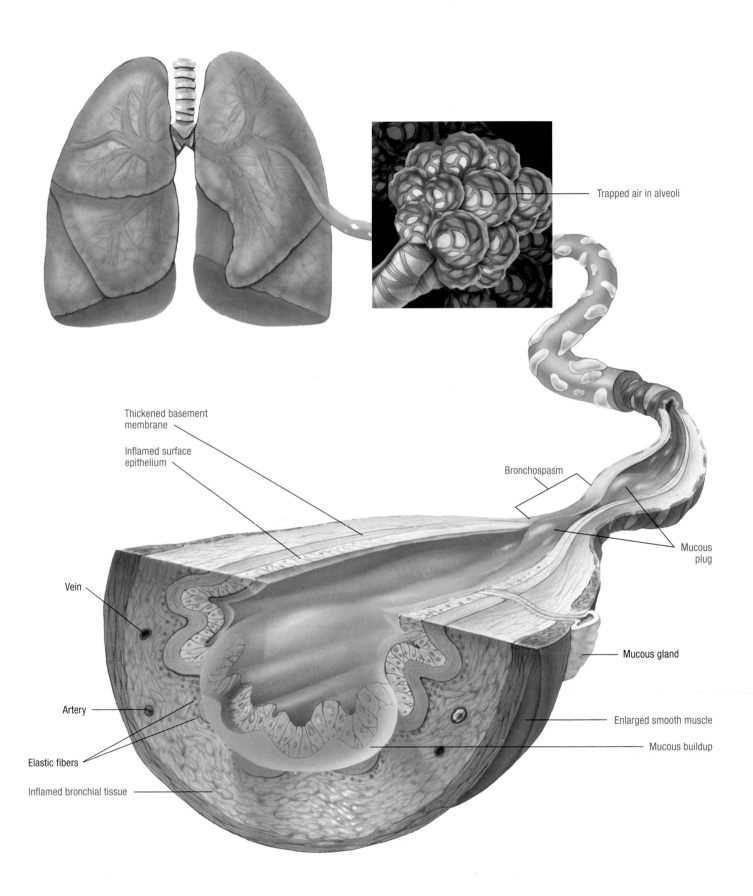

Trapped air in alveoli

Thickened basement membrane

Inflamed surface epithelium

Bronchospasm

Mucous plug

Vein

Mucous gland

Artery

Enlarged smooth muscle

Mucous buildup

Elastic fibers

Inflamed bronchial tissue

CHRONIC BRONCHITIS

Bronchitis is acute or chronic inflammation of the bronchi caused by irritants or infection. The distinguishing characteristic of bronchitis is obstruction of airflow. In chronic bronchitis, a form of chronic obstructive pulmonary disease (COPD), hypersecretion of mucus and chronic productive cough are present during three months of the year for at least two consecutive years.

 AGE ALERT
Children of parents who smoke are at higher risk for respiratory tract infection that can lead to chronic bronchitis.

Causes
- Cigarette smoking
- Exposure to irritants
- Genetic predisposition
- Exposure to organic or inorganic dusts
- Exposure to noxious gases
- Respiratory tract infection.

Pathophysiology

Chronic bronchitis develops when irritants are inhaled for a prolonged time. The irritants inflame the tracheobronchial tree, leading to increased mucus production and a narrowed or blocked airway. As the inflammation continues, changes in the cells lining the respiratory tract increase resistance in the small airways, and severe imbalance in the ventilation-perfusion $(\dot{V}/\dot{Q})$ ratio decreases arterial oxygenation.

Chronic bronchitis causes hypertrophy of airway smooth muscle and hyperplasia of the mucous glands, increased numbers of goblet cells, ciliary damage, squamous metaplasia of the columnar epithelium, and chronic leukocytic and lymphocytic infiltration of bronchial walls. Hypersecretion of the goblet cells blocks the free movement of the cilia, which normally sweep dust, irritants, and mucus away from the airways. Accumulating mucus and debris impair the defenses and increase the likelihood of respiratory tract infections.

Additional effects include narrowing and widespread inflammation within the airways. Bronchial walls become inflamed and thickened from edema and accumulation of inflammatory cells, and smooth muscle bronchospasm further

narrows the lumen. Initially, only large bronchi are involved, but eventually all airways are affected. Airways become obstructed and close, especially on expiration, trapping the gas in the distal portion of the lung. Consequent hypoventilation leads to a $\dot{V}/\dot{Q}$ mismatch and resultant hypoxemia.

Signs and symptoms
- Copious gray, white, or yellow sputum
- Dyspnea, tachypnea
- Cyanosis
- Use of accessory muscles
- Pedal edema
- Neck vein distention
- Weight gain due to edema or weight loss due to difficulty eating and increased metabolic rate
- Wheezing, prolonged expiratory time, rhonchi
- Pulmonary hypertension.

Diagnostic tests
- Sputum analysis
- Chest X-ray
- Pulmonary function studies
- Arterial blood gas analysis
- Electrocardiography (may show changes consistent with right heart enlargement).

Treatment
- Smoking cessation
- Avoidance of air pollutants
- Antibiotics
- Bronchodilators
- Adequate hydration
- Chest physiotherapy
- Ultrasonic or mechanical nebulizers
- Corticosteroids
- Diuretics
- Oxygen therapy.

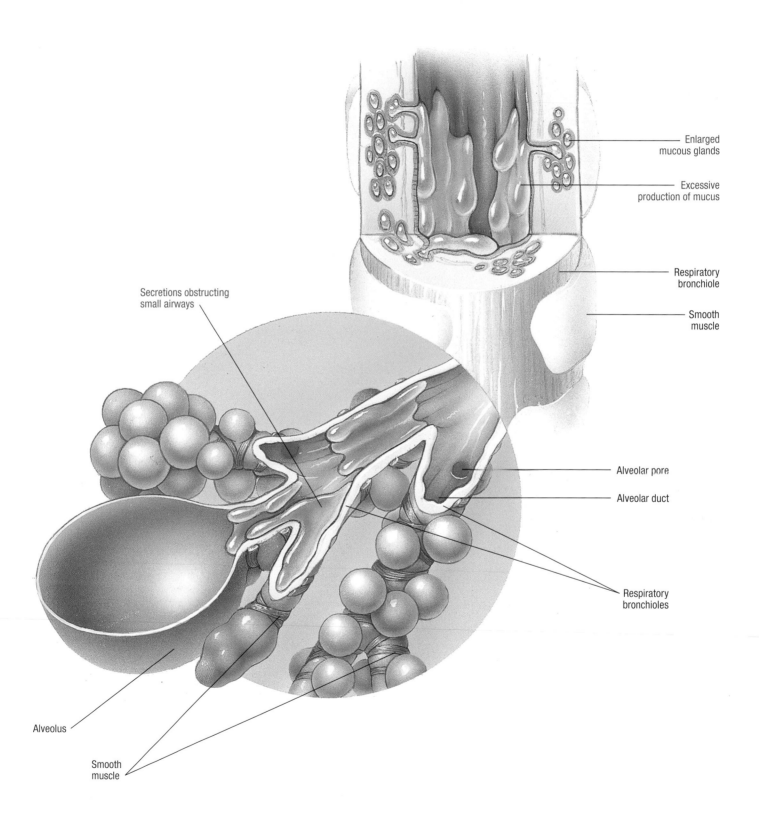

Enlarged
mucous glands

Excessive
production of mucus

Respiratory
bronchiole

Smooth
muscle

Secretions obstructing
small airways

Alveolar pore

Alveolar duct

Respiratory
bronchioles

Alveolus

Smooth
muscle

CYSTIC FIBROSIS

In cystic fibrosis (CF) , dysfunction of the exocrine glands affects multiple organ systems. The disorder is characterized by chronic airway infection leading to bronchiectasis, bronchiolectasis, exocrine pancreatic insufficiency, intestinal dysfunction, abnormal sweat gland function, and reproductive dysfunction. CF is accompanied by many complications and now carries an average life expectancy of 28 years. The disease affects males and females and is the most common fatal genetic disease in children of European ancestry.

Causes

Inherited as an autosomal recessive trait, the responsible gene, on chromosome 7q, encodes a membrane-associated protein called the cystic fibrosis transmembrane regulator (CFTR). The exact function of CFTR remains unknown, but it appears to help regulate chloride and sodium transport across epithelial membranes.

Pathophysiology

Most cases arise from the mutation that affects the genetic coding for a single amino acid, resulting in a protein (CFTR) that doesn't function properly. CFTR resembles other transmembrane transport proteins, but it lacks the phenylalanine in the protein produced by normal genes. This regulator interferes with cAMP-regulated chloride channels and other ions by preventing adenosine triphosphate from binding to the protein or by interfering with activation by protein kinase.

The mutation affects volume-absorbing epithelia (in the airways and intestines), salt-absorbing epithelia (in sweat ducts), and volume-secretory epithelia (in the pancreas). Lack of phenylalanine leads to dehydration, increasing the viscosity of mucus-gland secretions, leading to obstruction of glandular ducts. CF has a variable effect on electrolyte and water transport.

Signs and symptoms

- Failure to thrive: poor weight gain, poor growth, distended abdomen, thin extremities, and sallow skin with poor turgor
- Thick secretions and dehydration
- Chronic airway infections
- Dyspnea, paroxysmal cough
- Crackles, wheezes
- Retention of bicarbonate and water
- Obstruction of small and large intestines; biliary cirrhosis
- Fatal shock and arrhythmias
- Clotting problems, retarded bone growth, and delayed sexual development.

Diagnostic tests

- Sodium chloride levels in sweat
- Sputum culture
- Electrolyte status
- Stool analysis
- DNA testing.

AGE ALERT
The sweat test may be inaccurate in very young infants because they may not produce enough sweat for a valid test. The test may need to be repeated.

Treatment

- Increased fat, increased sodium diet
- Salt supplements
- Pancreatic enzyme replacement
- Breathing exercises and chest percussion
- Inhaled beta-adrenergic agonists
- Recombinant human DNase
- Antibiotics
- Sodium-channel blocker
- Uridine triphosphate
- Transplantation of heart or lungs.

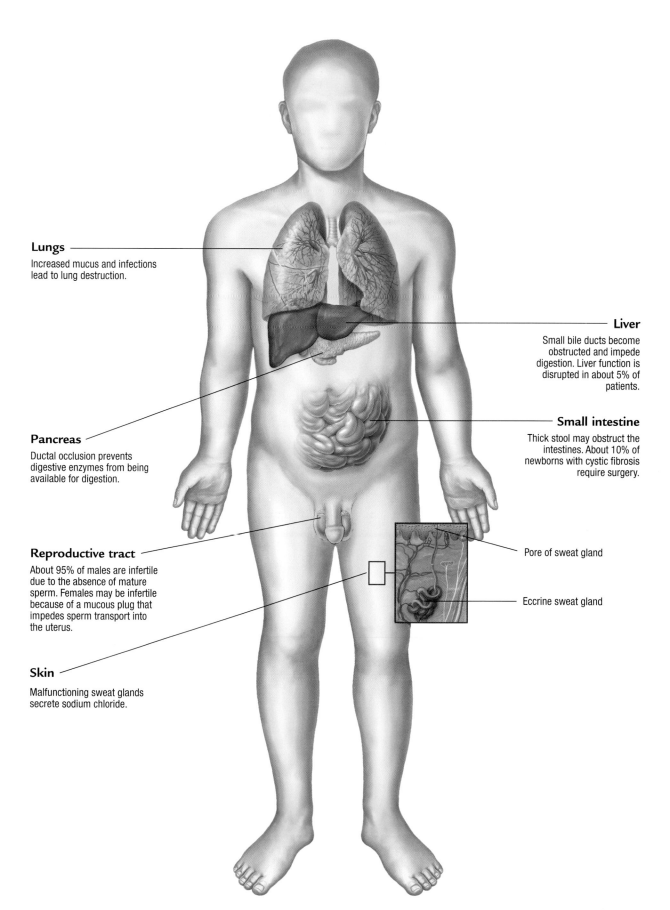

Lungs

Increased mucus and infections lead to lung destruction.

Liver

Small bile ducts become obstructed and impede digestion. Liver function is disrupted in about 5% of patients.

Small intestine

Thick stool may obstruct the intestines. About 10% of newborns with cystic fibrosis require surgery.

Pancreas

Ductal occlusion prevents digestive enzymes from being available for digestion.

Pore of sweat gland

Reproductive tract

About 95% of males are infertile due to the absence of mature sperm. Females may be infertile because of a mucous plug that impedes sperm transport into the uterus.

Eccrine sweat gland

Skin

Malfunctioning sweat glands secrete sodium chloride.

EMPHYSEMA

Emphysema, a form of chronic obstructive pulmonary disease, is the abnormal, permanent enlargement of the acini accompanied by destruction of alveolar walls. Obstruction results from tissue changes rather than mucus production, which occurs in asthma and chronic bronchitis. The distinguishing characteristic of emphysema is airflow limitation caused by lack of elastic recoil in the lungs.

 AGE ALERT
Aging is a risk factor for emphysema. Senile emphysema results from degenerative changes that cause stretching without destruction of the smooth muscle. Connective tissue is not usually affected.

Causes
- Cigarette smoking
- Deficiency of alpha$_1$-antitrypsin.

Pathophysiology
Primary emphysema has been linked to an inherited deficiency of the enzyme alpha$_1$-antitrypsin, a major component of alpha$_1$-globulin. Alpha$_1$-antitrypsin inhibits the activation of several proteolytic enzymes; its deficiency is an autosomal recessive trait that predisposes a person to emphysema.

In emphysema, recurrent inflammation is associated with the release of proteolytic enzymes from lung cells. This causes irreversible enlargement of the air spaces distal to the terminal bronchioles. Enlargement of air spaces destroys the alveolar walls, which results in a breakdown of elasticity and loss of fibrous and muscle tissue, making the lungs less compliant.

The alveolar septa are initially destroyed, eliminating a portion of the capillary bed and increasing air volume in the acinus. This breakdown leaves the alveoli unable to recoil normally after expanding and results in bronchiolar collapse on expiration. The damaged or destroyed alveolar walls cannot support the airways to keep them open. The amount of air that can be exhaled passively is diminished, trapping air in the lungs and leading to overdistention. Hyperinflation of the alveoli produces bullae and air spaces adjacent to the pleura.

Signs and symptoms
- Tachypnea
- Dyspnea on exertion
- Barrel chest
- Prolonged expiration and grunting
- Crackles and wheezing on inspiration
- Decreased breath sounds
- Hyperresonance
- Clubbed fingers and toes
- Decreased tactile fremitus
- Decreased chest expansion.

Diagnostic tests
- Chest X-ray
- Pulmonary function studies
- Arterial blood gas analysis
- Electrocardiography (may show signs of right ventricular hypertrophy)
- Complete blood count.

Treatment
- Avoiding tobacco smoke and air pollution
- Bronchodilators
- Antibiotics
- Flu vaccine to prevent influenza
- Pneumovax to prevent pneumococcal pneumonia
- Adequate hydration
- Chest physiotherapy
- Oxygen therapy
- Mucolytics
- Aerosolized or systemic corticosteroids.

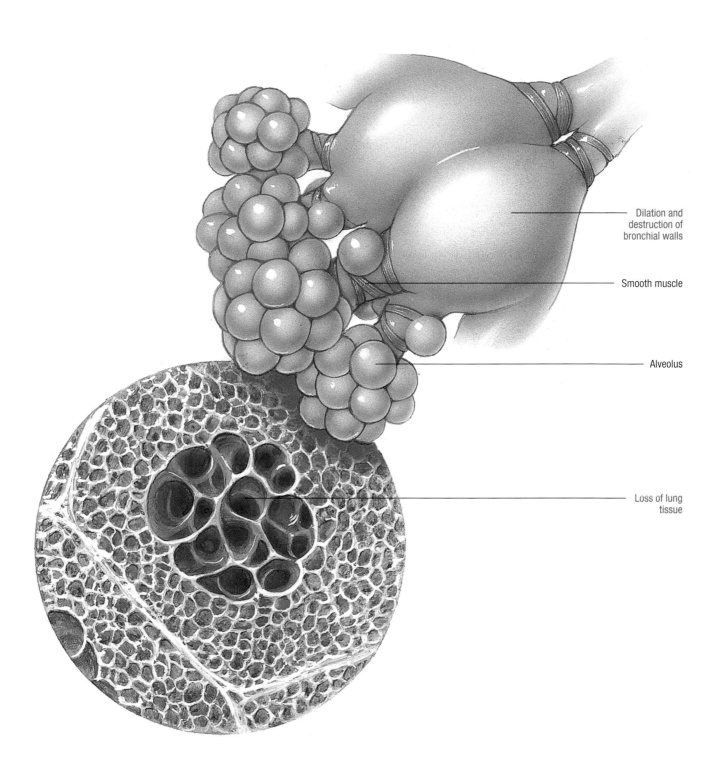

Dilation and destruction of bronchial walls

Smooth muscle

Alveolus

Loss of lung tissue

IDIOPATHIC PULMONARY FIBROSIS

Idiopathic pulmonary fibrosis (IPF) is a chronic and usually fatal interstitial pulmonary disease. Once thought to be a rare condition, it's now diagnosed with much greater frequency. IPF has been known by several other names over the years, including cryptogenic fibrosing alveolitis, diffuse interstitial fibrosis, idiopathic interstitial pneumonitis, and Hamman-Rich syndrome.

Causes

Unknown.

Pathophysiology

IPF reflects the accumulation of excessive fibrous or connective tissue in the lung parenchyma. IPF is the result of a cascade of inflammatory, immune, and fibrotic processes in the lung. Despite many studies, the stimulus that begins the progression remains unknown. Speculation has revolved around viral and genetic causes, but no good evidence has been found to support either theory. However, it's clear that chronic inflammation plays an important role. Inflammation develops the injury and the fibrosis that ultimately distorts and impairs the structure and function of the alveolocapillary gas exchange surface. The lungs become stiff and difficult to ventilate, and the diffusion capacity of the alveolocapillary membrane decreases, leading to hypoxemia.

Signs and symptoms

- Dyspnea; rapid, shallow breathing
- Dry, hacking cough
- End-expiratory crackles, bronchial breath sounds
- Clubbed fingers and toes
- Cyanosis
- Pulmonary hypertension
- Profound hypoxemia and severe, debilitating dyspnea in advanced disease.

Diagnostic tests

Diagnosis begins with a thorough patient history to exclude any of the more common causes of interstitial lung disease, such as:

- environmental or occupational exposure: coal dust, asbestos, silica, beryllium
- connective tissue diseases: scleroderma, rheumatoid arthritis
- drug use: amiodarone, tocainide, crack cocaine.
  The following confirm the diagnosis:
- lung biopsy
- chest X-ray
- high-resolution computed tomography
- pulmonary function tests
- bronchoalveolar lavage.

Treatment

- Oxygen therapy
- Corticosteroids
- Immunosuppressive-cytotoxic agents
- Colchicine
- Lung transplantation.

Because IPF generally responds poorly to treatment, and drug therapies cause so many adverse reactions, research studies are currently aimed at learning which factors may improve the patient's response to treatment. The chances of a positive response to therapy and extended survival seem to be best for young female patients with less-than-average dyspnea and hypoxemia, more normal lung function, and no history of smoking. Evidence of inflammation (lymphocytes in bronchoalveolar lavage fluid, circulating immune complexes, and positive response to corticosteroids) also seems to predict a better outcome. Indicators of a poor prognosis are irreversible lung destruction and fibrosis (severe hypoxemia, decreased diffusing capacity for carbon monoxide [DLCO], and neutrophils and eosinophils in bronchoalveolar lavage fluid).

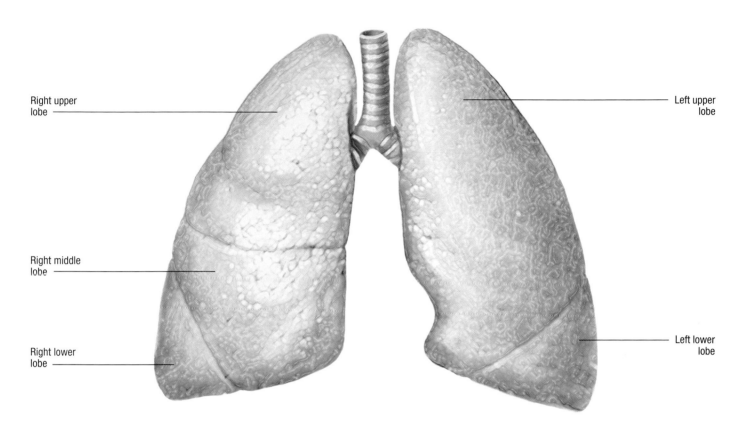

Right upper
lobe

Left upper
lobe

Right middle
lobe

Right lower
lobe

Left lower
lobe

Normal lungs

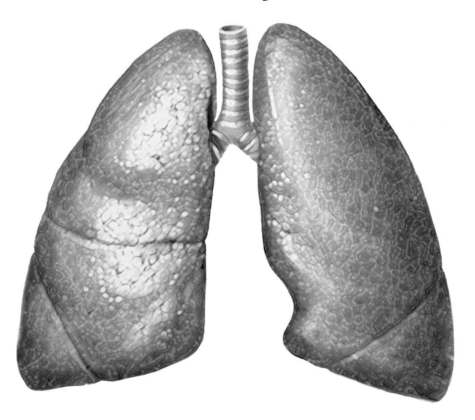

LUNG CANCER

Lung cancer has long been the most common cause of cancer death in men, and since 1987, it's been the most common cause of cancer death in women. Lung cancer usually develops in the wall or epithelium of the bronchial tree. Its most common types are epidermoid (squamous cell), adenocarcinoma, small cell (oat cell), and large cell (anaplastic).

Causes
- Tobacco smoke
- Carcinogenic industrial and air pollutants (asbestos, uranium, arsenic, nickel, iron oxides, chromium, radioactive dust, coal dust)
- Familial susceptibility.

Pathophysiology
Lung cancer begins with the transformation of one epithelial cell of the airway. Some lung cancers originating in the bronchi, and certain portions of the bronchi, such as the segmental bifurcations and sites of mucus production, are thought to be more vulnerable to injury from carcinogens.

As a lung tumor grows, it can partially or completely obstruct the airway, resulting in lobar collapse distal to the tumor. A lung tumor can also hemorrhage, causing hemoptysis. Early metastasis may occur to other thoracic structures, such as hilar lymph nodes or the mediastinum. Distant metastasis can occur to the brain, liver, bone, and adrenal glands.

Signs and symptoms
Because early-stage lung cancer usually produces no symptoms, this disease is often in an advanced state at diagnosis. The following late-stage signs and symptoms often lead to diagnosis:
- *Epidermoid and small cell carcinomas:* smoker's cough, hoarseness, wheezing, dyspnea, hemoptysis, and chest pain
- *Adenocarcinoma and large cell carcinoma:* fever, weakness, weight loss, anorexia, and shoulder pain.

In addition to their obvious interference with respiratory function, lung tumors may also alter the production of hormones that regulate body function or homeostasis, such as:
- *Gynecomastia* in large cell carcinoma
- *Hypertrophic pulmonary osteoarthropathy* (bone and joint pain from cartilage erosion due to abnormal production of growth hormone) in large cell carcinoma or adenocarcinoma
- *Cushing's* and *carcinoid syndromes* in small cell carcinoma
- *Hypercalcemia* in epidermoid tumors.

Metastatic signs and symptoms vary greatly, depending on the effect of tumors on intrathoracic and distant structures:
- *Bronchial obstruction*: hemoptysis, atelectasis, pneumonitis, dyspnea
- *Recurrent nerve invasion*: hoarseness, vocal cord paralysis
- *Chest wall invasion*: piercing chest pain, increasing dyspnea, severe shoulder pain, radiating down arm
- *Local lymphatic spread*: cough, hemoptysis, stridor, pleural effusion
- *Phrenic nerve involvement*: dyspnea, shoulder pain, unilateral paralyzed diaphragm, with paradoxical motion
- *Esophageal compression*: dysphagia
- *Vena caval obstruction*: venous distention and edema of face, neck, chest, and back
- *Pericardial involvement*: pericardial effusion, tamponade, arrhythmias
- *Cervical thoracic sympathetic nerve involvement*: miosis, ptosis, exophthalmos, reduced sweating.

Distant metastases may involve any part of the body, most commonly the central nervous system, liver, and bone.

Diagnostic tests
Typical clinical findings may strongly suggest lung cancer, but firm diagnosis requires further evidence. The following diagnostic tests may be used:
- chest X-ray
- sputum cytology
- computed tomography (CT) scan of the chest
- bronchoscopy
- needle or tissue biopsy
- thoracentesis
- preoperative mediastinoscopy or mediastinotomy to rule out involvement of mediastinal lymph nodes (which would preclude curative pulmonary resection)
- bone scan, bone marrow biopsy (recommended in small cell carcinoma), CT scan of the brain or abdomen to detect metastases.

Treatment
- Surgery
- Radiation
- Chemotherapy
- Laser therapy.

Right lung — Anterior view

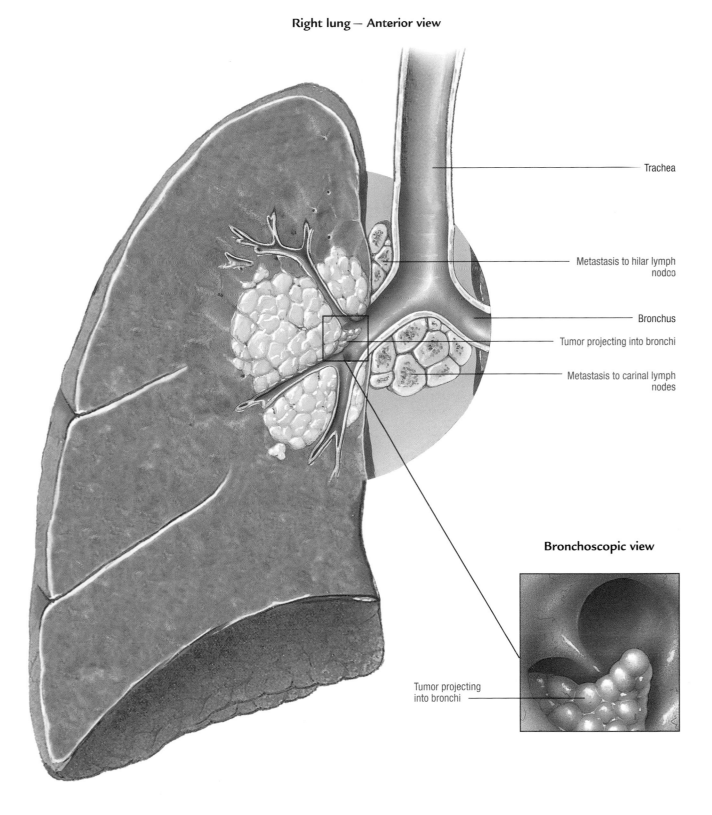

Trachea

Metastasis to hilar lymph nodes

Bronchus

Tumor projecting into bronchi

Metastasis to carinal lymph nodes

Bronchoscopic view

Tumor projecting into bronchi

PLEURAL EFFUSION

Pleural effusion is an excess of fluid in the pleural space. Normally, this space contains a small amount of extracellular fluid that lubricates the pleural surfaces. Increased production or inadequate removal of this fluid results in transudative or exudative pleural effusion. Empyema is the accumulation of pus and necrotic tissue in the pleural space.

Causes
Transudative pleural effusions:
- Heart failure
- Hepatic disease with ascites
- Peritoneal dialysis
- Hypoalbuminemia
- Disorders causing expanded intravascular volume.
  Exudative pleural effusions:
- Tuberculosis
- Subphrenic abscess
- Pancreatitis
- Bacterial or fungal pneumonitis or empyema
- Malignancy
- Pulmonary embolism with or without infarction
- Collagen disease
- Myxedema
- Chest trauma.
  Empyema:
- Idiopathic
- Pneumonitis
- Carcinoma
- Perforation
- Esophageal rupture.

Pathophysiology
The balance of osmotic and hydrostatic pressures in parietal pleural capillaries normally results in fluid movement into the pleural space. Balanced pressures in visceral pleural capillaries promote reabsorption of this fluid. Excessive hydrostatic pressure or decreased osmotic pressure can cause excessive amounts of fluid to pass across intact capillaries. The result is a *transudative pleural effusion*, an ultrafiltrate of plasma containing low concentrations of protein.

Exudative pleural effusions result when capillary permeability increases with or without changes in hydrostatic and colloid osmotic pressures, allowing protein-rich fluid to leak into the pleural space.

Empyema is usually associated with infection in the pleural space.

Signs and symptoms
- Characteristically related to underlying pathologic condition
- Dyspnea
- Pleuritic chest pain
- Fever
- Malaise
- Displaced point of maximum impulse, based on size of effusion.

Diagnostic tests
- Chest X-ray
- Thoracentesis.

Treatment
- Thoracentesis
- Chest tube insertion
- Injection of a sclerosing agent, such as talc
- Decortication
- Rib resection
- Parenteral antibiotics
- Oxygen therapy.

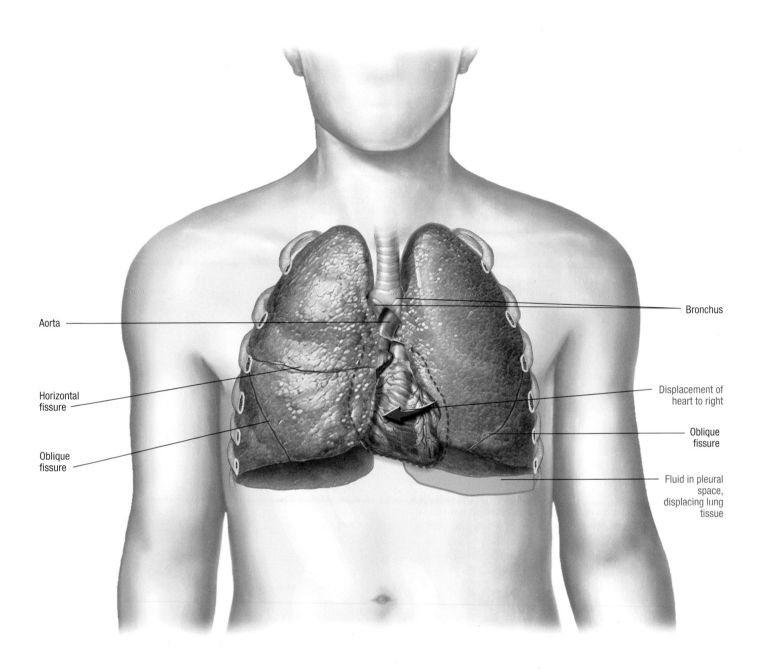

Aorta

Horizontal
fissure

Oblique
fissure

Bronchus

Displacement of
heart to right

Oblique
fissure

Fluid in pleural
space,
displacing lung
tissue

PNEUMONIA

Pneumonia is an acute infection of the lung parenchyma that commonly impairs gas exchange. The prognosis is generally good for people who have normal lungs and adequate host defenses before the onset of pneumonia. Pneumonia is often classified according to location: *bronchopneumonia* involves distal airways and alveoli; *lobular pneumonia*, part of a lobe; *lobar pneumonia*, an entire lobe.

Causes

Primary:
- Inhalation or aspiration of a pathogen, including pneumococcal, viral, and mycoplasmal pneumonia.

   Secondary:
- After initial damage from a noxious chemical or other insult (superinfection)
- Hematogenous spread of bacteria from a distant focus.

Pathophysiology

In bacterial pneumonia, an infection initially triggers alveolar inflammation and edema. This produces an area of low ventilation with normal perfusion. Capillaries become engorged with blood, causing stasis. As the alveolocapillary membrane breaks down, alveoli fill with blood and exudate, resulting in atelectasis.

In viral pneumonia, the virus first attacks bronchiolar epithelial cells. This causes interstitial inflammation and desquamation. The virus also invades bronchial mucous glands and goblet cells. It then spreads to the alveoli, which fill with blood and fluid. In advanced infection, a hyaline membrane may form.

In aspiration pneumonia, inhalation of gastric juices or hydrocarbons triggers inflammatory changes and also inactivates surfactant over a large area. Decreased surfactant leads to alveolar collapse. Acidic gastric juices may damage the airways and alveoli. Particles containing aspirated gastric juices may obstruct the airways and reduce airflow, leading to secondary bacterial pneumonia.

Signs and symptoms
- Coughing
- Sputum production
- Pleuritic chest pain
- Shaking chills
- Fever
- Wide range of physical signs, from diffuse, fine crackles to signs of localized or extensive consolidation and pleural effusion.

Diagnostic tests
- Chest X-ray
- Sputum analysis
- Pleurocentesis
- Transtracheal aspirate
- Bronchoscopy
- White blood cell count.

Treatment
- Antimicrobial therapy, varies with causative agent
- Humidified oxygen therapy
- Mechanical ventilation
- High-calorie diet and adequate fluid intake
- Bed rest
- Analgesics
- Positive end-expiratory pressure to facilitate adequate oxygenation in patients on mechanical ventilation for severe pneumonia.

TYPES OF PNEUMONIA

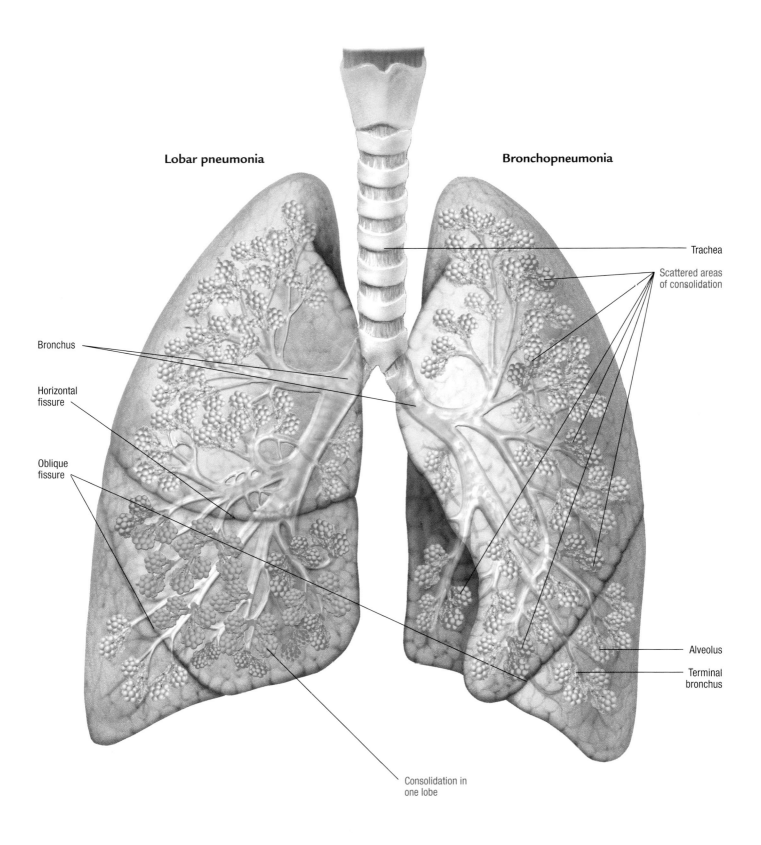

Lobar pneumonia

Bronchopneumonia

Trachea

Scattered areas of consolidation

Bronchus

Horizontal fissure

Oblique fissure

Alveolus

Terminal bronchus

Consolidation in one lobe

PNEUMOTHORAX

Pneumothorax is an accumulation of air in the pleural cavity that leads to partial or complete lung collapse. When the air between the visceral and parietal pleurae collects and accumulates, increasing tension in the pleural cavity can cause the lung to progressively collapse. The amount of air trapped in the intrapleural space determines the degree of lung collapse. Venous return to the heart may be impeded to cause a life-threatening condition called tension pneumothorax. The most common types of pneumothorax are *open*, *closed*, and *tension*.

Causes

Open pneumothorax:
- Penetrating chest injury (gunshot or stab wound)
- Insertion of a central venous catheter
- Chest surgery
- Transbronchial biopsy
- Thoracentesis or closed pleural biopsy.
  Closed pneumothorax:
- Blunt chest trauma
- Air leakage from ruptured blebs
- Rupture resulting from barotrauma
- Tubercular or cancerous lesions
- Interstitial lung disease.
  Tension pneumothorax:
- Penetrating chest wound treated with an air-tight dressing
- Fractured ribs
- Mechanical ventilation
- High-level positive end-expiratory pressure
- Chest tube occlusion or malfunction.

Pathophysiology

A rupture in the visceral or parietal pleura and chest wall causes air to accumulate and separate the visceral and parietal pleurae. Negative pressure is destroyed and the elastic recoil forces are affected. The lung recoils by collapsing toward the hilus.

Open pneumothorax (also called sucking chest wound or communicating pneumothorax) results when atmospheric air (positive pressure) flows directly into the pleural cavity (negative pressure). As the air pressure in the pleural cavity becomes positive, the lung collapses on the affected side, resulting in decreased total lung capacity, vital capacity, and lung compliance. Imbalances in the ventilation-perfusion ($\dot{V}/\dot{Q}$) ratio lead to hypoxia.

Closed pneumothorax occurs when air enters the pleural space from within the lung, causing increased pleural pressure, which prevents lung expansion during normal inspiration. Spontaneous pneumothorax is another type of closed pneumothorax.

 AGE ALERT
Spontaneous pneumothorax is common in older patients with chronic pulmonary disease, but it may also occur in healthy, young adults.

Tension pneumothorax results when air in the pleural space is under higher pressure than air in the adjacent lung. The air enters the pleural space from the site of pleural rupture, which acts as a one-way valve. Air is allowed to enter into the pleural space on inspiration but cannot escape as the rupture site closes on expiration. More air enters on inspiration and air pressure begins to exceed barometric pressure. Increasing air pressure pushes against the recoiled lung, causing compression atelectasis. Air also presses against the mediastinum, compressing and displacing the heart and great vessels. The air cannot escape, and the accumulating pressure causes the lung to collapse. As air continues to accumulate and intrapleural pressures rise, the mediastinum shifts away from the affected side and decreases venous return.

Signs and symptoms

- Sudden, sharp pleuritic pain exacerbated by chest movement, breathing, or coughing
- Asymmetrical chest wall movement
- Shortness of breath; respiratory distress
- Cyanosis
- Decreased vocal fremitus
- Absent breath sounds and chest rigidity on the affected side
- Tachycardia
- Subcutaneous emphysema.
  Tension pneumothorax (produces the most severe respiratory symptoms):
- Decreased cardiac output; hypotension; compensatory tachycardia
- Tachypnea
- Lung collapse
- Mediastinal shift; tracheal deviation to the opposite side
- Distended neck veins.

Diagnostic tests

- Chest X-ray
- Arterial blood gas analysis.

Treatment

Spontaneous pneumothorax with less than 30% lung collapse, no signs of increased pleural pressure, and no dyspnea or indications of physiologic compromise:
- Bed rest
- Monitoring of blood pressure and pulse
- Monitoring of respiratory rate
- Oxygen therapy
- Aspiration of air with a large-bore needle attached to a syringe.
  Pneumothorax with more than 30% lung collapse:
- Thoracostomy tube connected to underwater seal or to low-pressure suction
- Thoracotomy and pleurectomy.
  Open (traumatic) pneumothorax:
- Chest tube drainage
- Surgical repair of the lung.
  Tension pneumothorax:
- Immediate treatment with large-bore needle insertion
- Insertion of a thoracostomy tube, connected to underwater seal or to low-pressure suction
- Analgesics.

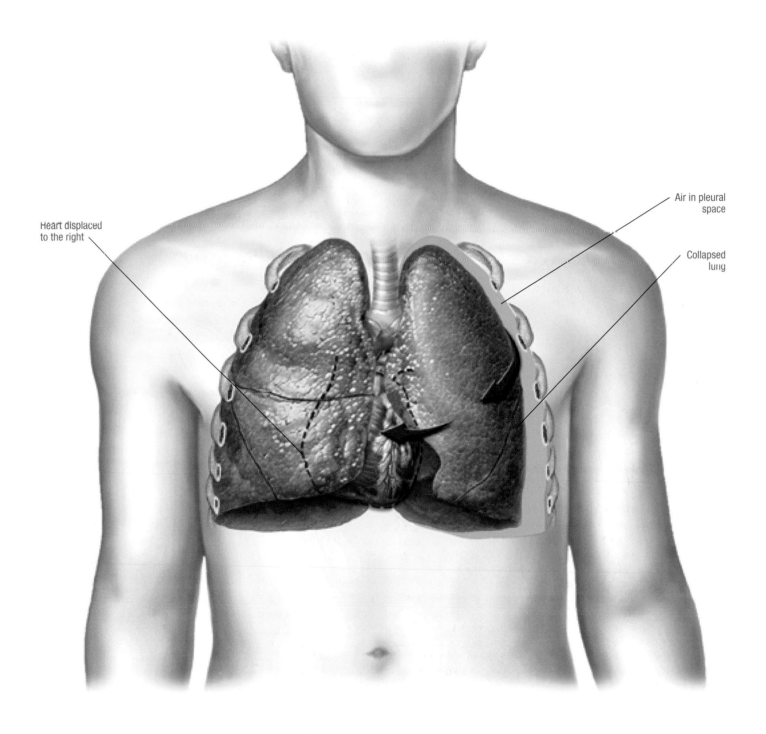

Air in pleural space

Collapsed lung

Heart displaced to the right

PULMONARY EDEMA

Pulmonary edema is an accumulation of fluid in the extravascular spaces of the lungs. It is a common complication of cardiac disorders and may occur as a chronic condition or may develop quickly and rapidly become fatal.

Causes
Left-sided heart failure:
- Arteriosclerosis
- Cardiomyopathy
- Hypertension
- Valvular heart disease.
  Predisposing factors:
- Barbiturate or opiate poisoning
- Cardiac failure
- Excessive volume or too-rapid infusion of I.V. fluids
- Impaired pulmonary lymphatic drainage
- Inhalation of irritating gases
- Mitral stenosis and left atrial myxoma
- Pneumonia
- Pulmonary veno-occlusive disease.

Pathophysiology
Normally, pulmonary capillary hydrostatic pressure, capillary oncotic pressure, capillary permeability, and lymphatic drainage are in balance. When this balance changes, or the lymphatic drainage system is obstructed, fluid infiltrates into the lung and pulmonary edema results. If pulmonary capillary hydrostatic pressure increases, the compromised left ventricle requires increased filling pressures to maintain adequate cardiac output. These pressures are transmitted to the left atrium, pulmonary veins, and pulmonary capillary bed, forcing fluids and solutes from the intravascular compartment into the interstitium of the lungs. As the interstitium overloads with fluid, the fluid floods the peripheral alveoli and impairs gas exchange.

If colloid osmotic pressure decreases, the hydrostatic force that regulates intravascular fluids (the natural pulling force) is lost because there is no opposition. Fluid flows freely into the interstitium and alveoli, impairing gas exchange and leading to pulmonary edema.

Lymphatic vessels may be blocked by edema or tumor fibrotic tissue or by increased systemic venous pressure. Hydrostatic pressure in the large pulmonary veins rises, the pulmonary lymphatic system cannot drain into the pulmonary veins, and excess fluid moves into the interstitial space. Pulmonary edema then results from the accumulation of fluid.

Capillary injury and consequent increased permeability may occur in adult respiratory distress syndrome or after inhalation of toxic gases. Plasma proteins and water leak out of the injured capillary and into the interstitium, increasing the interstitial oncotic pressure, which is normally low. As interstitial oncotic pressure begins to equal capillary oncotic pressure, the water begins to move out of the capillary and into the lungs, resulting in pulmonary edema.

Signs and symptoms
Early stage:
- Dyspnea on exertion, paroxysmal nocturnal dyspnea, orthopnea
- Cough
- Mild tachypnea
- Increased blood pressure
- Dependent crackles
- Neck vein distention
- Tachycardia.
  Later stages:
- Labored, rapid respiration
- More diffuse crackles
- Cough, producing frothy, bloody sputum
- Increased tachycardia, arrhythmias, thready pulse
- Cold, clammy skin, diaphoresis
- Cyanosis
- Hypotension.

Diagnostic tests
- Arterial blood gas analysis
- Chest X-ray
- Pulse oximetry
- Pulmonary artery catheterization
- Electrocardiography.

Treatment
- High concentrations of oxygen, assisted ventilation
- Diuretics
- Positive inotropic agents
- Vasopressors
- Arterial vasodilators
- Antiarrhythmics
- Morphine.

NORMAL ALVEOLI

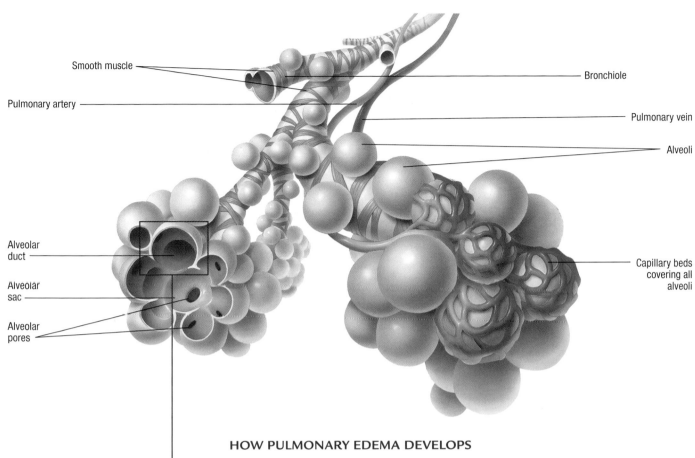

Smooth muscle

Pulmonary artery

Bronchiole

Pulmonary vein

Alveoli

Alveolar duct

Alveolar sac

Alveolar pores

Capillary beds covering all alveoli

HOW PULMONARY EDEMA DEVELOPS

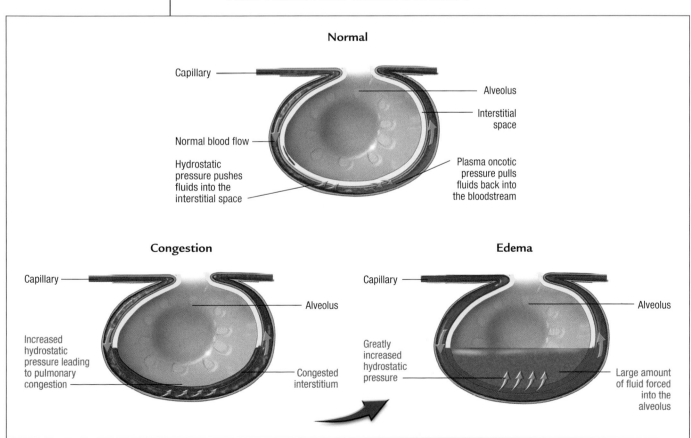

Normal

Capillary

Alveolus

Interstitial space

Normal blood flow

Hydrostatic pressure pushes fluids into the interstitial space

Plasma oncotic pressure pulls fluids back into the bloodstream

Congestion

Capillary

Alveolus

Increased hydrostatic pressure leading to pulmonary congestion

Congested interstitium

Edema

Capillary

Alveolus

Greatly increased hydrostatic pressure

Large amount of fluid forced into the alveolus

PULMONARY EMBOLISM

A complication in hospitalized patients, pulmonary embolism is an obstruction of the pulmonary arterial bed by a dislodged thrombus, heart valve vegetation, or foreign substance.

Causes
- Dislodged thrombi, originating in the leg veins (most common)
- Other sites where thrombi may originate:
- pelvic veins
- renal veins
- hepatic vein
- right side of heart
- upper extremities.
  Predisposing factors:
- Long-term immobility
- Chronic pulmonary disease
- Heart failure or atrial fibrillation
- Deep vein thrombosis
- Polycythemia vera, thrombocytosis
- Autoimmune hemolytic anemia, sickle cell disease
- Varicose veins
- Recent surgery, lower extremity fractures
- Advanced age
- Pregnancy
- Burns
- Obesity
- Vascular injury
- Cancer
- I.V. drug abuse
- Oral contraceptives.

Pathophysiology
Thrombus formation results directly from vascular wall damage, venostasis, or hypercoagulability of the blood. Trauma, clot dissolution, sudden muscle spasm, intravascular pressure changes, or a change in peripheral blood flow can cause the thrombus to loosen or fragmentize. Then the thrombus — now called an embolus — floats to the heart's right side and enters the lung through the pulmonary artery. There, the embolus may dissolve, continue to fragmentize, or grow.

If the embolus occludes the pulmonary artery, it prevents alveoli from producing enough surfactant to maintain alveolar integrity. As a result, alveoli collapse and atelectasis develops. If the embolus enlarges, it may clog most or all of the pulmonary vessels and cause death.

Rarely, the emboli contain air, fat, bacteria, amniotic fluid, talc (from drugs intended for oral administration, injected intravenously by addicts), or tumor cells.

Signs and symptoms
Total occlusion of the main pulmonary artery is rapidly fatal; smaller or fragmented emboli produce symptoms that vary with the size, number, and location, as follows:
- dyspnea
- pleuritic chest pain
- tachycardia
- productive cough (sputum may be blood-tinged)
- low-grade fever
- pleural effusion.
  Less common signs include:
- massive hemoptysis
- splinting of the chest
- leg edema
- cyanosis, syncope, distended neck veins
- pleural friction rub
- signs of circulatory collapse (weak, rapid pulse and hypotension)
- signs of hypoxia (restlessness and anxiety).

Diagnostic tests
- Chest X-ray
- Lung scan
- Pulmonary angiography
- Electrocardiography
- Arterial blood gas analysis.

 CLINICAL TIP
A triad of deep vein thrombosis (DVT) formation is stasis, endothelial injury, and hypercoaguability. Risk factors include long car or plane trips, cancer, pregnancy, hypercoaguability, and prior DVT or pulmonary emboli.

Treatment
Treatment is designed to maintain adequate cardiovascular and pulmonary function during resolution of the obstruction and to prevent recurrence of embolic episodes. Because most emboli resolve within 10 to 14 days, treatment may consist of:
- oxygen therapy
- fibrinolytic therapy, anticoagulation
- vasopressors
- antibiotics
- vena caval ligation, plication, or insertion of a device to filter blood returning to the heart and lungs, against future pulmonary emboli.

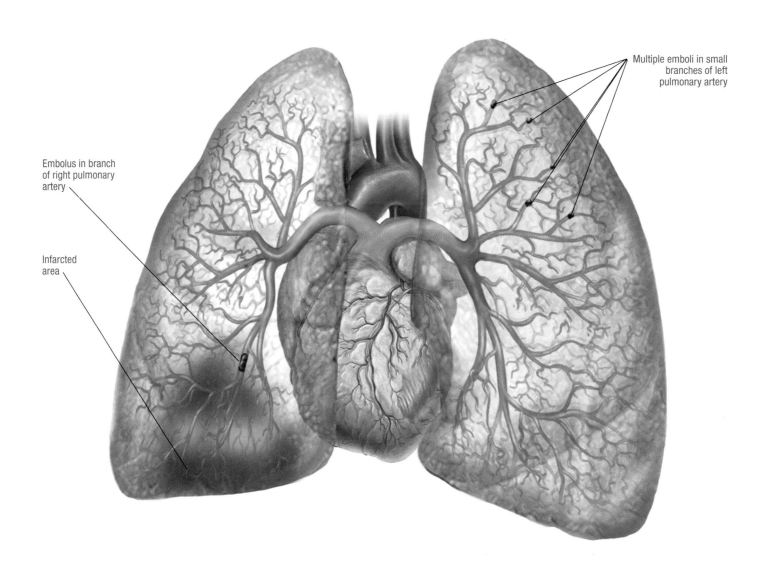

Multiple emboli in small branches of left pulmonary artery

Embolus in branch of right pulmonary artery

Infarcted area

PULMONARY HYPERTENSION

Pulmonary hypertension is a resting systolic pulmonary artery pressure (PAP) above 30 mm Hg and a mean PAP above 18 mm Hg. Primary or idiopathic pulmonary hypertension is characterized by increased PAP and increased pulmonary vascular resistance.

 AGE ALERT
Primary pulmonary hypertension is most common in women ages 20 to 40 and is usually fatal within 3 to 4 years. Mortality is highest in pregnant women.

Secondary pulmonary hypertension results from existing cardiac or pulmonary disease, or both. The prognosis in secondary pulmonary hypertension depends on the severity of the underlying disorder.

Causes
Primary pulmonary hypertension:
- Unknown, but may include:
- hereditary factors
- altered immune mechanisms.
  Secondary pulmonary hypertension:
- Conditions causing alveolar hypoventilation:
- chronic obstructive pulmonary disease
- sarcoidosis
- diffuse interstitial pneumonia
- malignant metastases
- scleroderma
- obesity
- kyphoscoliosis
- Conditions causing vascular obstruction:
- pulmonary embolism
- vasculitis
- left atrial myxoma
- idiopathic veno-occlusive disease
- fibrosing mediastinitis
- mediastinal neoplasm
- Conditions causing primary cardiac disease:
- patent ductus arteriosus
- atrial septal defect
- ventricular septal defect
- Conditions causing acquired cardiac disease:
- rheumatic valvular disease
- mitral stenosis.

Pathophysiology
In primary pulmonary hypertension, the smooth muscle in the pulmonary artery wall hypertrophies for no known reason, narrowing or obliterating the artery or arteriole. Fibrous lesions form around the vessels, impairing distensibility and increasing vascular resistance. Pressures in the left ventricle, which receives blood from the lungs, remain normal. However, the increased pressures generated in the lungs are transmitted to the right ventricle, which supplies the pulmonary artery. Eventually, the right ventricle fails (cor pulmonale).

Alveolar hypoventilation can result from diseases caused by alveolar destruction or from disorders that prevent the chest wall from expanding sufficiently to allow air into the alveoli. The resulting decreased ventilation increases pulmonary vascular resistance. Hypoxemia resulting from this ventilation-perfusion ($\dot{V}/\dot{Q}$) mismatch also causes vasoconstriction, further increasing vascular resistance and resulting in pulmonary hypertension.

Signs and symptoms
- Increasing dyspnea on exertion
- Fatigue and weakness
- Syncope
- Shortness of breath
- Ascites
- Neck vein distention
- Restlessness and agitation, decreased level of consciousness, confusion, and memory loss
- Decreased diaphragmatic excursion and respiration
- Possible displacement of point of maximal impulse
- Peripheral edema
- Easily palpable right ventricular lift
- Reduced carotid pulse
- Palpable and tender liver
- Tachycardia
- Systolic ejection murmur
- Split S_2; S_3 and S_4 sounds
- Decreased breath sounds
- Loud, tubular breath sounds.

Diagnostic tests
- Arterial blood gas analysis
- Electrocardiography
- Cardiac catheterization
- Pulmonary angiography
- Pulmonary function studies
- Radionuclide imaging
- Open lung biopsy
- Echocardiography
- Perfusion lung scanning.

Treatment
- Treatment of the underlying cause
- Oxygen therapy
- Fluid restriction
- Digoxin
- Diuretics
- Vasodilators
- Pulmonary vasodilators
- Calcium channel blockers
- Bronchodilators
- Beta-adrenergic blockers
- Lung transplant or heart-lung transplant.

NORMAL PULMONARY ARTERY

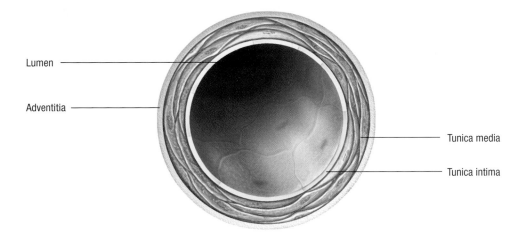

Lumen

Adventitia

Tunica media

Tunica intima

EARLY PULMONARY HYPERTENSION

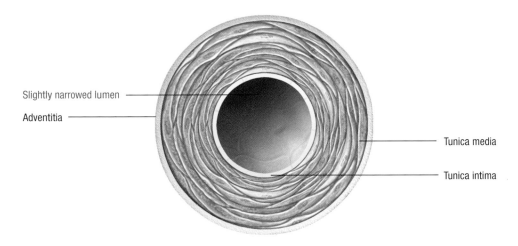

Slightly narrowed lumen

Adventitia

Tunica media

Tunica intima

LATE PULMONARY HYPERTENSION

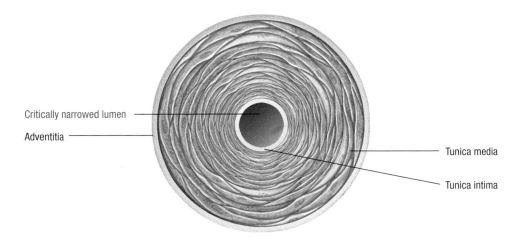

Critically narrowed lumen

Adventitia

Tunica media

Tunica intima

SARCOIDOSIS

Sarcoidosis is a multisystem, granulomatous disorder that characteristically produces lymphadenopathy, pulmonary infiltration, and skeletal, liver, eye, or skin lesions.

Causes

Unknown.

Possible factors:

● *Hypersensitivity response* (possibly from T-cell imbalance) to such agents as atypical mycobacteria, fungi, and pine pollen
● *Genetic predisposition* (suggested by a slightly higher incidence of sarcoidosis within the same family)
● *Chemicals,* such as zirconium and beryllium, that can lead to illnesses resembling sarcoidosis, suggesting an extrinsic cause for this disease.

Pathophysiology

Organ dysfunction results from an accumulation of T lymphocytes, mononuclear phagocytes, and nonsecreting epithelial granulomas, which distort normal tissue architecture (causing alveolitis). Patients with sarcoidosis exhibit a combination of decreased cell-mediated immunity and increased humoral system activity. The absolute number of circulating T cells is decreased; B lymphocytes may be normal or increased.

Signs and symptoms

Initial symptoms of sarcoidosis include arthralgia (in the wrists, ankles, and elbows), fatigue, malaise, and weight loss. Sarcoidosis is characterized by formation of granulomatous tissue leading to pulmonary fibrosis. Other clinical features vary according to the extent and location of the fibrosis:

● *Respiratory:* breathlessness, cough (usually nonproductive), substernal pain; complications in advanced pulmonary disease include pulmonary hypertension and cor pulmonale
● *Cutaneous:* erythema nodosum, subcutaneous skin nodules with maculopapular eruptions, and extensive nasal mucosal lesions

● *Ophthalmic:* anterior uveitis (common); glaucoma
● *Lymphatic:* bilateral hilar and right paratracheal lymphadenopathy and splenomegaly
● *Musculoskeletal:* muscle weakness, polyarthralgia, pain, and punched-out lesions on phalanges
● *Hepatic:* granulomatous hepatitis, usually asymptomatic
● *Genitourinary:* hypercalciuria
● *Cardiovascular:* arrhythmias and, rarely, cardiomyopathy
● *Central nervous system (CNS):* cranial or peripheral nerve palsies, basilar meningitis, seizures, and pituitary and hypothalamic lesions producing diabetes insipidus.

Diagnostic tests

● Chest X-ray
● Lymph node, skin, or lung biopsy
● Pulmonary function tests
● Arterial blood gas analysis.

CLINICAL TIP
A positive Kveim-Stilzbach skin test supports the diagnosis. In this test, the patient receives an intradermal injection of an antigen prepared from human sarcoidal spleen or lymph nodes from patients with sarcoidosis. If the patient has active sarcoidosis, granuloma develops at the injection site in 2 to 6 weeks.

Treatment

● No treatment for asymptomatic sarcoidosis
● With ophthalmic, respiratory, CNS, cardiovascular, or systemic symptoms or destructive skin lesions: systemic or topical steroids, usually for 1 to 2 years, but possibly lifelong
● With hypercalcemia: low-calcium diet and avoidance of direct exposure to sunlight.

Normal lungs and alveoli

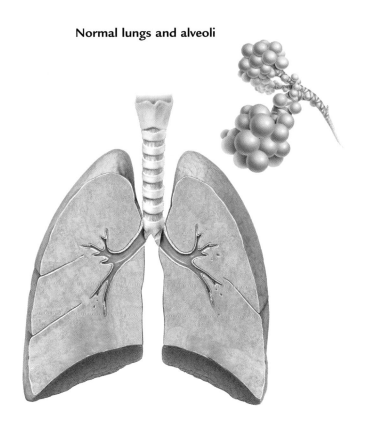

Granulomatous tissue formation

Alveolitis

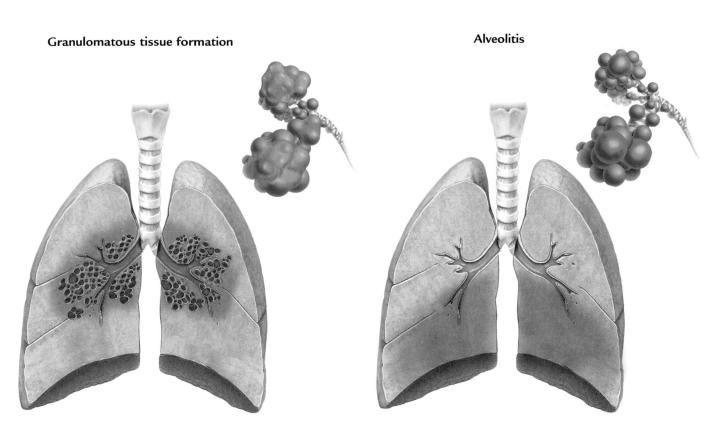

TUBERCULOSIS

An acute or chronic infection caused by *Mycobacterium tuberculosis,* tuberculosis (TB) is characterized by pulmonary infiltrates, formation of granulomas with caseation, fibrosis, and cavitation. People who live in crowded, poorly ventilated conditions and those who are immunocompromised are most likely to become infected. In patients with strains that are sensitive to the usual antitubercular agents, the prognosis is excellent with correct treatment. However, in those with strains that are resistant to two or more of the major antitubercular agents, mortality is 50%. The incidence of TB has been increasing in the United States secondary to homelessness, drug abuse, and human immunodeficiency virus (HIV) infection. Globally, TB is the leading infectious cause of morbidity and mortality, generating 8 to 10 million new cases each year.

Causes

Although the primary infection site is the lungs, mycobacteria commonly exist in other parts of the body. A number of factors increase the risk of infection, including:

- gastrectomy
- uncontrolled diabetes mellitus
- Hodgkin's disease
- leukemia
- silicosis
- HIV infection
- treatment with corticosteroids or immunosuppressants.

Pathophysiology

After exposure to *M. tuberculosis,* roughly 5% of infected people develop active tuberculosis within 1 year; in the remainder, microorganisms cause a latent infection. Transmission of active disease is by droplet nuclei produced when infected persons cough or sneeze. The host's immune system usually controls the tubercle bacillus by killing it or walling it up in a tiny nodule (tubercle). However, the bacillus may lie dormant within the tubercle for years and later reactivate and spread. Persons with a cavitary lesion (large, granulomatous lesion) are particularly infectious because their sputum usually contains 1 million to 100 million bacilli per milliliter. If an inhaled tubercle bacillus settles in an alveolus, infection occurs, with alveolocapillary dilation and endothelial cell swelling. Alveolitis results, with replication of tubercle bacilli and influx of polymorphonuclear leukocytes. These organisms spread through the lymph system to the circulatory system and then throughout the body.

Cell-mediated immunity to the mycobacteria, which develops 3 to 6 weeks later, usually contains the infection and arrests the disease. If the infection reactivates, the body's response characteristically leads to caseation — the conversion of necrotic tissue to a cheeselike material. The caseum may localize, undergo fibrosis, or excavate and form cavities, the walls of which are studded with multiplying tubercle bacilli. If this happens, infected caseous debris may spread throughout the lungs by the tracheobronchial tree. Sites of extrapulmonary TB include the pleurae, meninges, joints, lymph nodes, peritoneum, genitourinary tract, and bowel.

Signs and symptoms

After an incubation period of 4 to 8 weeks, TB is usually asymptomatic in primary infection but may produce nonspecific symptoms, such as:

- fatigue
- weakness
- anorexia
- weight loss
- night sweats
- low-grade fever.

In reactivation, symptoms may include a cough that produces mucopurulent sputum, occasional hemoptysis, and chest pains.

AGE ALERT
Fever and night sweats, the typical hallmarks of TB, may not be present in elderly patients, who instead may exhibit a change in activity or weight.

Diagnostic tests

- Auscultation
- Chest percussion
- Chest X-ray
- Tuberculin skin test
- Stains and cultures (of sputum, cerebrospinal fluid, urine, drainage from abscess, or pleural fluid).

Treatment

Antitubercular therapy is the main treatment. After 2 to 3 weeks of continuous medication, the disease generally is no longer infectious, and the patient can resume his normal lifestyle while taking medication.

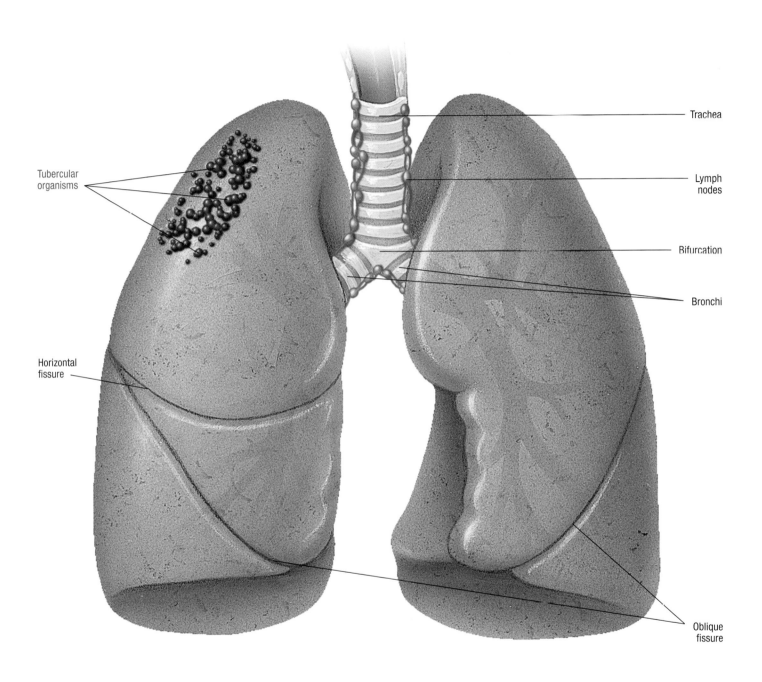

Trachea

Tubercular
organisms

Lymph
nodes

Bifurcation

Bronchi

Horizontal
fissure

Oblique
fissure

UPPER RESPIRATORY TRACT INFECTION

Upper respiratory tract infection (also known as the common cold or acute coryza) is an acute, usually afebrile viral infection that causes inflammation of the upper respiratory tract. It is the most common infectious disease. Although a cold is benign and self-limiting, it can lead to secondary bacterial infections.

Causes

About 90% of colds stem from a viral infection of the upper respiratory passages and consequent mucous membrane inflammation; occasionally, colds result from a mycoplasmal infection. Over a hundred viruses can cause the common cold. Major offenders include:

- rhinoviruses
- coronaviruses
- myxoviruses
- adenoviruses
- coxsackieviruses
- echoviruses.

Pathophysiology

Infection occurs when the offending organism gains entry into the upper respiratory tract, proliferates, and begins an inflammatory reaction. Acute inflammation of the upper airway structures, including the sinuses, nasopharynx, pharynx, larynx, and trachea are seen. The presence of the pathogen triggers infiltration of the mucus membranes by inflammatory and infection fighting cells. Mucosal swelling and secretion of a serous or mucupurulent exudate result.

Signs and symptoms

After a 1- to 4-day incubation period, the common cold produces:

- pharyngitis
- nasal congestion
- coryza
- headache
- burning, watery eyes.
  Additional effects may include:
- fever
- chills
- myalgia
- arthralgia
- malaise
- lethargy
- hacking, nonproductive, or nocturnal cough.
  As the cold progresses, clinical features develop more fully. After a day, symptoms include a feeling of fullness with a copious nasal discharge that commonly irritates the nose, adding to discomfort.

Diagnostic tests

No explicit diagnostic test exists to isolate the specific organism responsible for the common cold. Consequently, diagnosis rests on the typically mild, localized, and afebrile upper respiratory symptoms. Diagnosis must rule out allergic rhinitis, measles, rubella, and other disorders that produce similar early symptoms.

Treatment

The primary treatments — aspirin or acetaminophen, fluids, and rest — are purely symptomatic because the common cold has no cure.

Other treatments may include:

- decongestants
- throat lozenges
- steam.

COMPLICATIONS OF THE COMMON COLD

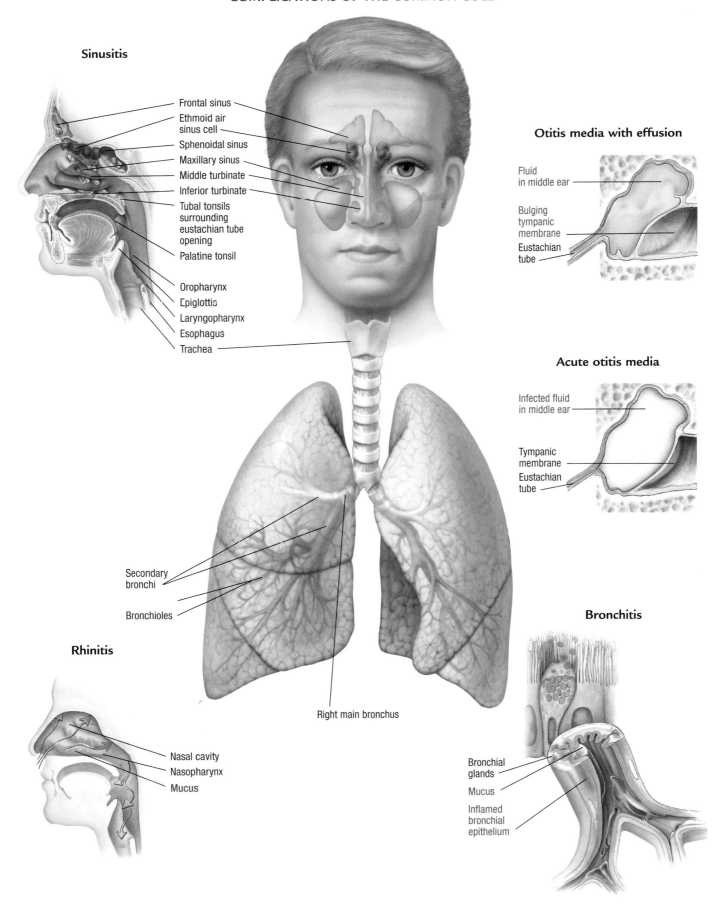

Sinusitis

Frontal sinus
Ethmoid air sinus cell
Sphenoidal sinus
Maxillary sinus
Middle turbinate
Inferior turbinate
Tubal tonsils surrounding eustachian tube opening
Palatine tonsil
Oropharynx
Epiglottis
Laryngopharynx
Esophagus
Trachea

Otitis media with effusion

Fluid in middle ear
Bulging tympanic membrane
Eustachian tube

Acute otitis media

Infected fluid in middle ear
Tympanic membrane
Eustachian tube

Secondary bronchi
Bronchioles

Right main bronchus

Rhinitis

Nasal cavity
Nasopharynx
Mucus

Bronchitis

Bronchial glands
Mucus
Inflamed bronchial epithelium

Upper respiratory tract infection   **111**

ACCELERATION-DECELERATION INJURIES

Acceleration–deceleration cervical injuries (commonly known as whiplash) result from sharp hyperextension and flexion of the neck that damages muscles, ligaments, disks, and nerve tissue. The prognosis for this type of injury is usually excellent; symptoms usually subside with treatment of symptoms.

Causes
- Motor vehicle and other transportation accidents
- Falls
- Sports-related accidents
- Crimes and assaults.

Pathophysiology
The brain is shielded by the cranial vault (hair, skin, bone, meninges, and cerebrospinal fluid), which intercepts the force of a physical blow. Below a certain level of force (the absorption capacity), the cranial vault prevents energy from affecting the brain. The degree of traumatic head injury usually is proportional to the amount of force reaching the cranial tissues. Furthermore, unless ruled out, neck injuries should be presumed present in patients with traumatic head injury.

In acceleration-deceleration cervical injuries, the head is propelled in a forward and downward motion in hyperflexion. A wedge-shaped deformity of the bone may be created if the anterior portions of the vertebrae are crushed. Intervertebral disks may be damaged; they may bulge or rupture, irritating spinal nerves. Then, the head is forced backward. A tear in the anterior ligament may pull pieces of bone from cervical vertebrae. Spinous processes of the vertebrae may be fractured. Intervertebral disks may be compressed posteriorly and torn anteriorly. Vertebral arteries may be stretched, pinched, or torn, causing reduced blood flow to the brain. Nerves of the cervical sympathetic chain may also be injured.

A complex arrangement of ligaments holds the vertebrae in place. Some of the ligaments are barely a centimeter long and all are only a few millimeters thick. In a whiplash injury, ligaments may be badly stretched, partially torn, or completely ruptured (arrows). Injuries of neck muscles may range from minor strains and microhemorrhages to severe tears. The anterior longitudinal ligament, running vertically along the anterior surface of the vertebrae, may be injured during hyperextension. The posterior longitudinal ligament, running on the posterior surface of the vertebral bodies, may be injured in hyperflexion. The broad ligamentum nuchae may also be stretched or torn.

Closed trauma is typically a sudden acceleration-deceleration or *coup/contrecoup* injury. In coup/contrecoup, the head hits a relatively stationary object, injuring cranial tissues near the point of impact (coup); then the remaining force pushes the brain against the opposite side of the skull, causing a second impact and injury (contrecoup). Contusions and lacerations may also occur during contrecoup as the brain's soft tissues slide over the rough bone of the cranial cavity. In addition, rotational shear forces on the cerebrum may damage the upper midbrain and areas of the frontal, temporal, and occipital lobes.

Signs and symptoms
Although symptoms may develop immediately, they're often delayed 12 to 24 hours if the injury is mild. Whiplash produces moderate to severe anterior and posterior neck pain. Within several days, the anterior pain diminishes, but the posterior pain persists or even intensifies, causing patients to seek medical attention if they did not do so before. Whiplash may also cause:
- dizziness, gait disturbances
- vomiting
- headache, nuchal rigidity, neck muscle asymmetry
- rigidity or numbness in the arms.

Diagnostic tests
- Full cervical spine X-rays
- Physical examination focusing on motor ability and sensation below the cervical spine to detect signs of nerve root compression
- Computed tomography scan
- Magnetic resonance imaging.

Treatment

CLINICAL TIP

In all suspected spinal injuries, assume that the spine is injured until proven otherwise. Any patient with suspected whiplash or other injuries requires careful transportation from the accident scene. To do this, place him in a supine position on a spine board and immobilize his neck with tape and a hard cervical collar or sandbags.

Until an X-ray rules out a cervical fracture, move the patient as little as possible. Before the X-ray is taken, carefully remove any ear and neck jewelry. Don't undress the patient; cut clothes away, if necessary. Warn him against movements that could injure his spine.

Symptomatic treatment includes:
- immobilization with a soft, padded cervical collar for several days or weeks
- ice or cool compresses to the neck
- a mild analgesic and possibly a muscle relaxant
- in severe muscle spasms, short-term cervical traction.

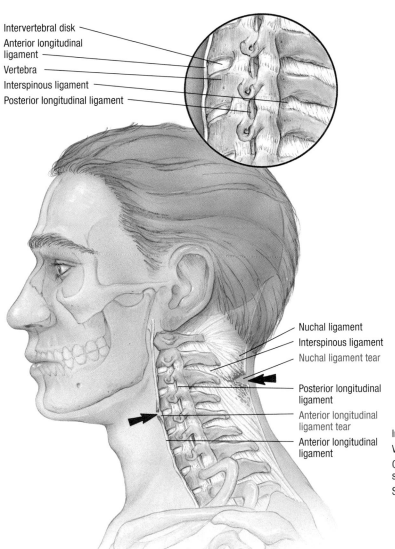

Intervertebral disk

Anterior longitudinal ligament

Vertebra

Interspinous ligament

Posterior longitudinal ligament

Nuchal ligament

Interspinous ligament

Nuchal ligament tear

Posterior longitudinal ligament

Anterior longitudinal ligament tear

Anterior longitudinal ligament

Hyperflexion

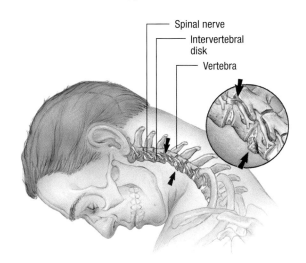

Spinal nerve

Intervertebral disk

Vertebra

Hyperextension

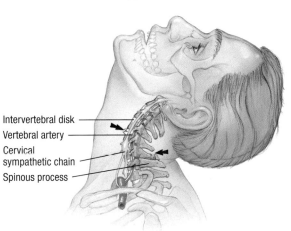

Intervertebral disk

Vertebral artery

Cervical sympathetic chain

Spinous process

Muscle injury

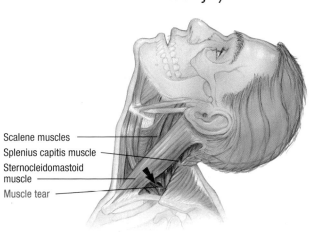

Scalene muscles

Splenius capitis muscle

Sternocleidomastoid muscle

Muscle tear

ALZHEIMER'S DISEASE

Alzheimer's disease is a degenerative disorder of the cerebral cortex, especially the frontal lobe. It affects approximately 4 million Americans; by 2040, that figure may exceed 6 million.

AGE ALERT
In the elderly, Alzheimer's disease accounts for over 50% of all cases of dementia. The highest prevalence is among those over age 85. About 5% of people over the age of 65 have a severe form of this disease, and 12% have a mild to moderate form. It is the fourth leading cause of death among the elderly, after heart disease, cancer, and stroke.

This primary progressive disease has a poor prognosis. Typically, the duration of illness is 8 years, and patients die 2 to 5 years after onset of debilitating brain symptoms.

Causes

The exact cause is unknown.
Associated factors:
- *Neurochemical:* deficiencies in the neurotransmitters acetylcholine, somatostatin, substance P, and norepinephrine
- *Environmental:* repeated head trauma
- *Genetic:* abnormalities on chromosomes 14 or 21; deposits of beta amyloid protein.

Pathophysiology

At autopsy, the brain tissue of patients with Alzheimer's disease exhibits three characteristic features:
- neurofibrillatory tangles (fibrous proteins)
- neuritic plaques (composed of degenerating axons and dendrites)
- granulovascular changes (degneration).

Neurofibrillar tangles (fibrous proteins) are bundles of filaments (in the neuron) that abnormally twist around one another. Tangles are numerous in areas of the brain associated with memory and learning (hippocamus), fear and aggression (amygdala), and thinking (cerebral cortex).

Amyloid plaques (senile plaques) are found outside neurons in the extracellular space of the cerebral cortex and hippocamus. Amyloid plaques contain a core of beta amyloid protein surrounded by abnormal nerve endings, or *neurites*. Amyloid also accumulates in the walls of cerebral blood vessels, causing the condition called amyloid angiopathy.

Granulovascular degeneration affects the neurons of the hippocampus. Fluid-filled spaces, called vacuoles, enlarge the cell body, causing malfunction or death.

Other structural changes include cortical atrophy, ventricular dilation, deposition of amyloid (a glycoprotein) around the cortical blood vessels, and selective loss of cholinergic neurons in the pathways to the frontal lobes and hippocampus, areas that are important for memory and cognitive functions. Autopsy commonly reveals an atrophic brain, which may weigh less than 1000 g (normal, 1380 g).

Signs and symptoms

The typical signs and symptoms reflect neurologic abnormalities associated with the disease, including:
- gradual loss of recent and remote memory, loss of sense of smell, and flattening of affect and personality
- difficulty with learning new information
- deterioration in personal hygiene
- inability to concentrate
- increasing difficulty with abstraction and judgment
- impaired communication
- loss of coordination
- personality changes, wanderings
- nocturnal awakenings
- loss of eye contact and fearful look
- acute confusion, agitation, compulsiveness or fearfulness when overwhelmed with anxiety
- disorientation and emotional lability
- progressive deterioration of physical and intellectual ability.

Diagnostic tests

- Confirmed by autopsy revealing definitive pathological changes in the brain.
  Suggestive tests:
- Positron emission tomography
- Computed tomography scan
- Magnetic resonance imaging
- Electroencephalography
- Cerebral blood flow studies.

Treatment

No cure or definitive treatment currently exists.
Useful therapy may include:
- cerebral vasodilators such as ergoloid mesylates, isoxsuprine, and cyclandelate
- pychostimulants, such as methylphenidate
- antidepressants
- tacrine, an anticholinesterase agent.

TISSUE CHANGES IN ALZHEIMER'S DISEASE

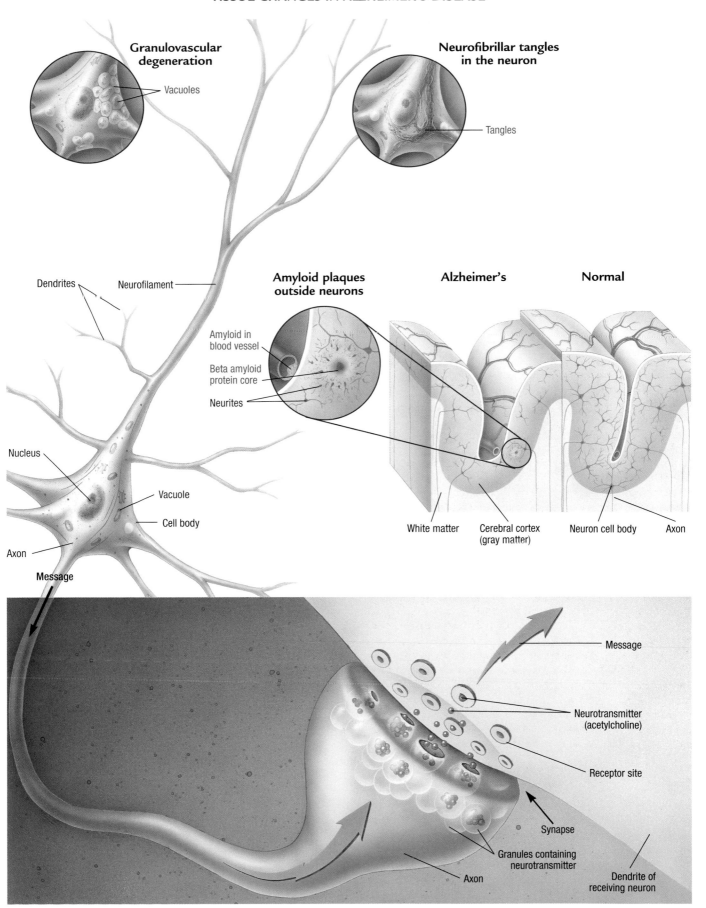

Granulovascular degeneration

Vacuoles

Neurofibrillar tangles in the neuron

Tangles

Dendrites

Neurofilament

Amyloid plaques outside neurons

Amyloid in blood vessel

Beta amyloid protein core

Neurites

Alzheimer's

Normal

Nucleus

Vacuole

Cell body

Axon

Message

White matter

Cerebral cortex (gray matter)

Neuron cell body

Axon

Message

Neurotransmitter (acetylcholine)

Receptor site

Synapse

Granules containing neurotransmitter

Axon

Dendrite of receiving neuron

AMYOTROPHIC LATERAL SCLEROSIS

Commonly called *Lou Gehrig's disease,* after the New York Yankees first baseman who died of this disorder, amyotrophic lateral sclerosis (ALS) is the most common of the motor neuron diseases causing muscular atrophy. A chronic, progressively debilitating disease, ALS may be fatal in less than 1 year or continue for 10 years or more, depending on the muscles affected. More than 30,000 Americans have ALS; about 5,000 new cases are diagnosed each year, and the disease affects three times as many men as women.

 AGE ALERT
Onset usually occurs between ages 40 and 70.

Causes
Exact cause unknown.
Possible associated factors:
- Genetic component in about 5% to 10% of cases — an autosomal dominant trait that affects men and women equally
- Slow-acting virus
- Nutritional deficiency related to disturbance in enzyme metabolism
- Metabolic interference in the production of nucleic acid by nerve fibers
- Autoimmune disorder
- Precipitating factors for acute deterioration include trauma, viral infections, and physical exhaustion.

Pathophysiology
ALS progressively destroys the upper and lower motor neurons. It does not affect cranial nerves III, IV, and VI, and therefore some facial movements, such as blinking, persist. Intellectual and sensory functions are not affected.

Some believe that glutamate — the primary excitatory neurotransmitter of the central nervous system (CNS) — accumulates to toxic levels at the synapses. The affected motor units are no longer innervated and progressive degeneration of axons causes loss of myelin. Some nearby motor nerves may sprout axons in an attempt to maintain function, but, ultimately, nonfunctional scar tissue replaces normal neuronal tissue.

Signs and symptoms
- Fasciculations, spasticity, atrophy, weakness, loss of functioning motor units (especially in forearms and hands)
- Impaired speech, chewing, and swallowing; choking; drooling
- Difficulty breathing, especially if the brain stem is affected
- Muscle atrophy
- Reactive depression.

Diagnostic tests
None specific to ALS.
May be suggestive:
- Electromyography
- Nerve conduction studies
- Muscle biopsy
- Computed tomography scan
- Electroencephalography.

Treatment
No cure.
Supportive treatment may include:
- diazepam, dantrolene, baclofen
- quinidine
- thyrotropin-releasing hormone (I.V. or intrathecally)
- riluzole (an antiglutamate agent that acts in the CNS)
- respiratory, speech, physical therapy
- psychological support.

Normal nerve cell and muscle

ALS-affected nerve cell and muscle

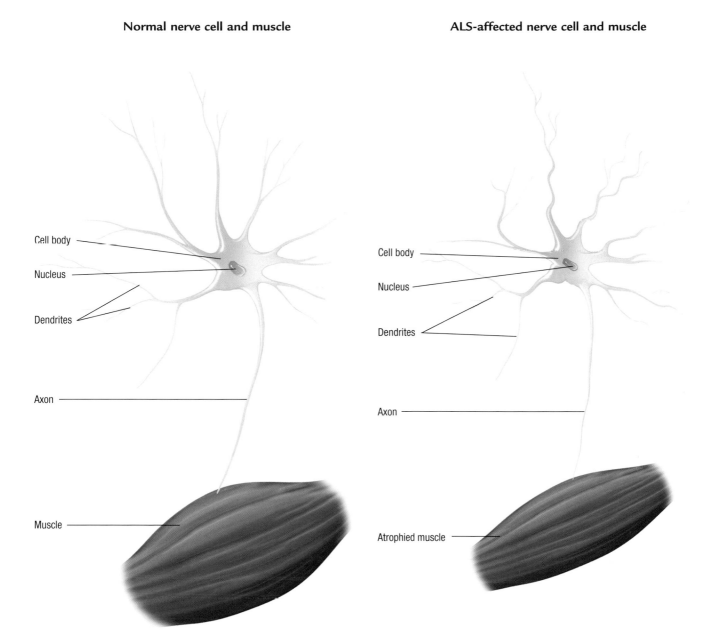

ARTERIOVENOUS MALFORMATION

Arteriovenous malformations (AVMs) are tangled masses of thin-walled, dilated blood vessels between arteries and veins that are not connected by capillaries. AVMs are common in the brain, primarily in the posterior portion of the cerebral hemispheres. Abnormal channels between the arterial and venous system mix oxygenated and unoxygenated blood, and thereby prevent adequate perfusion of brain tissue.

AVMs range in size from a few millimeters to large malformations extending from the cerebral cortex to the ventricles. Usually more than one AVM is present. Males and females are affected equally, and some evidence exists that AVMs occur in families.

 AGE ALERT
Most AVMs are present at birth; however, symptoms typically do not occur until the person is 10 to 20 years of age.

Causes
- Congenital: caused by a hereditary defect
- Acquired: caused by trauma, such as penetrating injuries.

Pathophysiology
AVMs lack the typical structural characteristics of the blood vessels. The vessel walls of an AVM are very thin; one or more arteries feed into the AVM, causing it to appear dilated and torturous. The typically high-pressured arterial flow moves into the venous system through the connecting channels to increase venous pressure, engorging and dilating the venous structures. An aneurysm may develop. If the AVM is large enough, the shunting can deprive the surrounding tissue of adequate blood flow. Additionally, the thin-walled vessels may ooze small amounts of blood or actually rupture, causing hemorrhage into the brain or subarachnoid space.

Signs and symptoms
Typically, few or none.
If AVM is large, leaks, or ruptures:
- Chronic headache and confusion
- Seizures
- Systolic bruit over carotid artery, mastoid process, or orbit
- Focal neurologic deficits (depending on location of AVM)
- Hydrocephalus.

 CLINICAL TIP
Symptoms of intracranial hemorrhage, indicating AVM rupture, include sudden severe headache, seizures, confusion, lethargy, and meningeal irritation.

Diagnostic tests
- Cerebral arteriography
- Doppler ultrasonography of cerebrovascular system
- Magnetic resonance imaging
- Magnetic resonance angiography.

Treatment
- Supportive measures, including aneurysm precautions
- Surgery, including block dissection, laser, or ligation
- Embolization or radiation therapy.

Cerebral cortex — Sagittal section

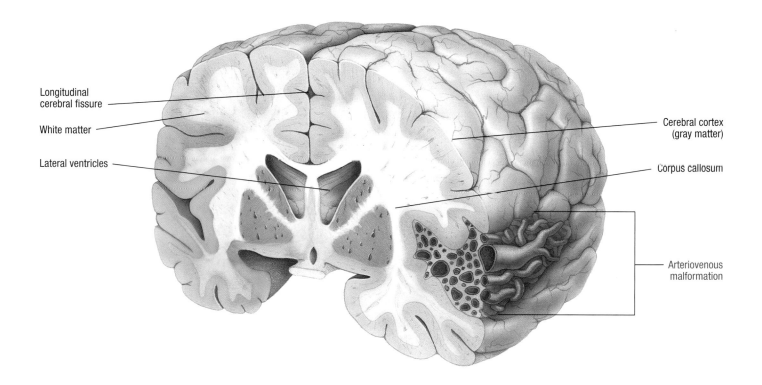

Longitudinal cerebral fissure

White matter

Lateral ventricles

Cerebral cortex (gray matter)

Corpus callosum

Arteriovenous malformation

BELL'S PALSY

Bell's palsy is a disease of the facial nerve (cranial nerve VII) that produces unilateral or bilateral facial weakness. Onset is rapid. In 80% to 90% of patients, it subsides spontaneously and recovery is complete in 1 to 8 weeks. If recovery is partial, contractures may develop on the paralyzed side of the face. Bell's palsy may recur on the same or opposite side of the face.

 AGE ALERT
Although Bell's palsy affects all age groups, it occurs most often in people under age 60. Recovery may be slower in the elderly.

Causes
- Infection
- Hemorrhage
- Tumor
- Meningitis
- Local trauma.

Pathophysiology
Bell's palsy reflects an inflammatory reaction around the seventh cranial nerve, usually at the internal auditory meatus where the nerve leaves bony tissue. The characteristic unilateral or bilateral facial weakness results from the lack of appropriate neural stimulation to the muscle by the motor fibers of the facial nerve.

Signs and symptoms
- Distorted facial appearance and inability to raise the eyebrow, close the eyelid, smile, show the teeth, or puff out the cheek
- Unilateral facial weakness, occasionally with aching pain around the angle of the jaw or behind the ear
- Drooping mouth on the affected side (causing the patient to drool saliva from the corner of his mouth)
- Distorted taste perception over the affected anterior portion of the tongue
- Ringing in the ear.

 CLINICAL TIP
When the patient tries to close the affected eye, it rolls upward (Bell's phenomenon) and shows excessive tearing.

Diagnostic tests
After 10 days, electromyography helps predict the level of expected recovery by distinguishing temporary conduction defects from a pathologic interruption of nerve fibers.

Treatment
- Prednisone to reduce facial nerve edema and to improve nerve conduction and blood flow
- Sometimes, antiviral agents.

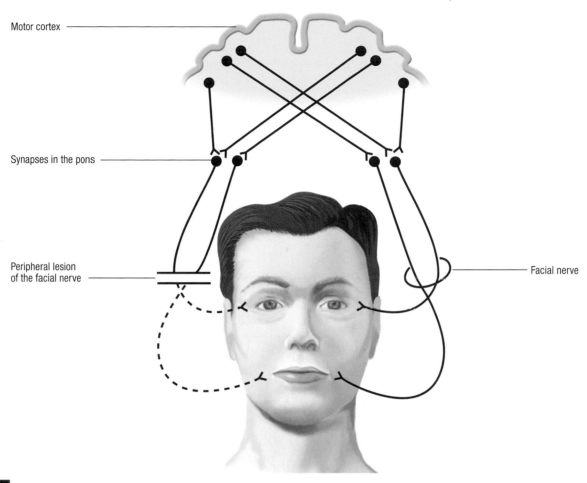

Motor cortex

Synapses in the pons

Peripheral lesion
of the facial nerve

Facial nerve

> CLINICAL TIP

DIAGNOSING BELL'S PALSY

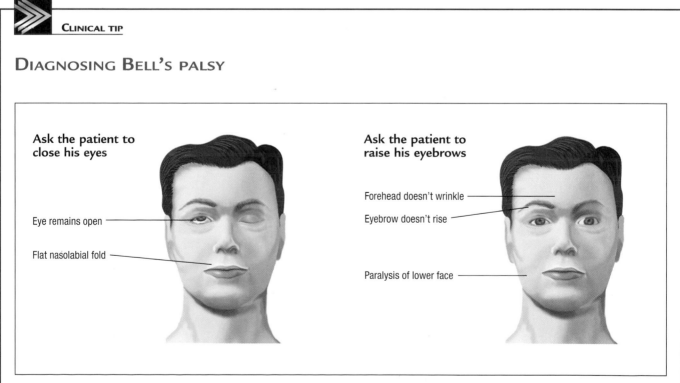

**Ask the patient to
close his eyes**

Eye remains open

Flat nasolabial fold

**Ask the patient to
raise his eyebrows**

Forehead doesn't wrinkle

Eyebrow doesn't rise

Paralysis of lower face

BRAIN TUMORS

Malignant brain tumors occur in about 4.5 persons per 100,000. The incidence is slightly higher in men than in women. These tumors may occur at any age.

 AGE ALERT
In adults, incidence is generally highest between ages 40 and 60. The most common tumor types in adults are gliomas and meningiomas, which usually occur supratentorially (above the covering of the cerebellum).

In children, incidence is generally highest before age 1 and again between ages 2 and 12. The most common types in children are astrocytomas, medulloblastomas, ependymomas, and brain stem gliomas. In children, brain tumors are one of the most common causes of death from cancer.

Causes
- Unknown in most cases
- Exposure to ionizing radiation, a known environmental risk
- Metastatic in 20% to 40% of patients with other cancers
- Some believed to be familial.

Pathophysiology
Brain tumors are growths within the intracranial space and include tumors of the brain tissue, meninges, pituitary gland, and blood vessels. Brain tumors are classified based on histology or grade of cell malignancy. Symptoms of brain tumors are caused by displacement of cerebral tissue and obstruction of cerebrospinal fluid (CSF). As the tumor grows, edema develops in surrounding tissues and intracranial pressure (ICP) increases. As the tumor continues to grow it may interfere with the normal flow and drainage of CSF causing an increase in ICF.

The brain compensates for increases by regulating the volume of the three substances in the following ways: limiting blood flow to the head, displacing CSF into the spinal canal, and increasing absorption or decreasing production of CSF.

Signs and symptoms
Generally those of increased ICP:
- Headache
- Decreased motor strength and coordination
- Seizures
- Altered vital signs
- Nausea and vomiting
- Papilledema
- Insidious onset.

Diagnostic tests
- Tissue biopsy performed by stereotactic surgery guided by computed tomography (CT) scan or magnetic resonance imaging (MRI)
- Neurologic assessment
- Skull X-ray, CT scan, MRI
- Cerebral angiography
- Lumbar puncture.

Treatment
- Surgical removal of resectable tumor
- Reducing size of nonresectable tumor by chemotherapy, radiation, or both
- Relieving cerebral edema, increased ICP, and other symptoms with:
- diuretics, corticosteroids
- possibly ventriculoatrial or ventriculoperitoneal shunting of CSF.

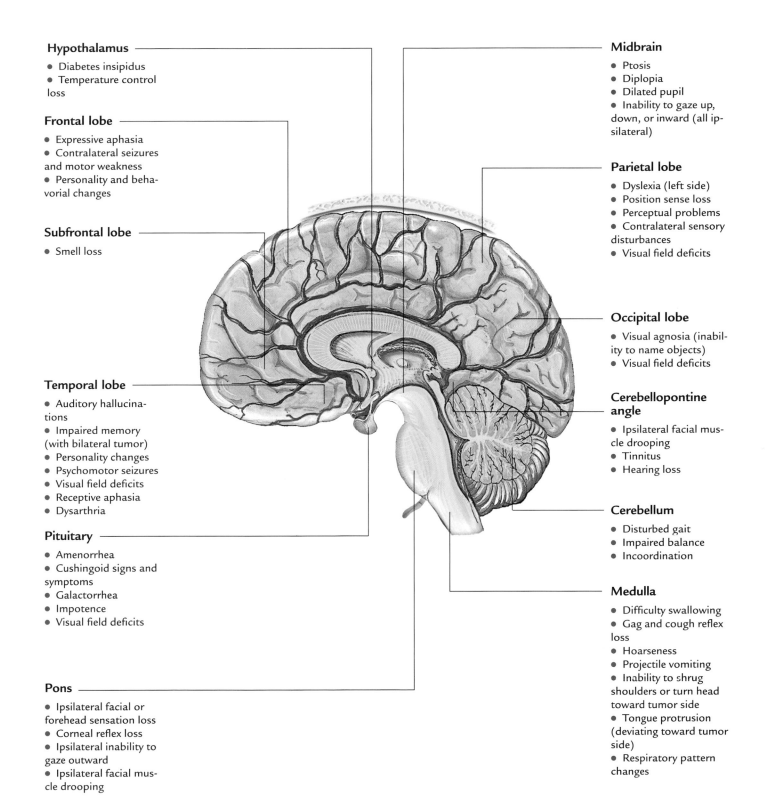

Hypothalamus
- Diabetes insipidus
- Temperature control loss

Frontal lobe
- Expressive aphasia
- Contralateral seizures and motor weakness
- Personality and behavorial changes

Subfrontal lobe
- Smell loss

Temporal lobe
- Auditory hallucinations
- Impaired memory (with bilateral tumor)
- Personality changes
- Psychomotor seizures
- Visual field deficits
- Receptive aphasia
- Dysarthria

Pituitary
- Amenorrhea
- Cushingoid signs and symptoms
- Galactorrhea
- Impotence
- Visual field deficits

Pons
- Ipsilateral facial or forehead sensation loss
- Corneal reflex loss
- Ipsilateral inability to gaze outward
- Ipsilateral facial muscle drooping

Midbrain
- Ptosis
- Diplopia
- Dilated pupil
- Inability to gaze up, down, or inward (all ipsilateral)

Parietal lobe
- Dyslexia (left side)
- Position sense loss
- Perceptual problems
- Contralateral sensory disturbances
- Visual field deficits

Occipital lobe
- Visual agnosia (inability to name objects)
- Visual field deficits

Cerebellopontine angle
- Ipsilateral facial muscle drooping
- Tinnitus
- Hearing loss

Cerebellum
- Disturbed gait
- Impaired balance
- Incoordination

Medulla
- Difficulty swallowing
- Gag and cough reflex loss
- Hoarseness
- Projectile vomiting
- Inability to shrug shoulders or turn head toward tumor side
- Tongue protrusion (deviating toward tumor side)
- Respiratory pattern changes

CEREBRAL ANEURYSM

In an intracranial, or cerebral, aneurysm, a weakness in the wall of a cerebral artery causes localized dilation. Cerebral aneurysms usually arise at an arterial junction in the circle of Willis, the circular anastomosis connecting the major cerebral arteries at the base of the brain. Many cerebral aneurysms rupture and cause subarachnoid hemorrhage.

AGE ALERT
Incidence is slightly higher in women than in men, especially those in their late 40s or early to mid-50s, but a cerebral aneurysm may occur at any age in either sex.

Causes
- Congenital defect
- Degenerative process, such as atherosclerosis
- Hypertension
- Trauma.

Pathophysiology
Blood flow exerts pressure against a congenitally weak arterial wall, stretching it like an overblown balloon and making it likely to rupture. Such a rupture is followed by a subarachnoid hemorrhage, in which blood spills into the space normally occupied by cerebrospinal fluid. Sometimes, blood also spills into brain tissue, where a clot can cause potentially fatal increased intracranial pressure and brain tissue damage.

Signs and symptoms
- Premonitory symptoms resulting from oozing of blood into the subarachnoid space:
- headache, intermittent nausea
- nuchal rigidity
- stiff back and legs.

- Rupture usually occurs abruptly and may cause:
- sudden severe headache
- nausea and projectile vomiting
- altered level of consciousness, including deep coma
- meningeal irritation, resulting in nuchal rigidity, back and leg pain, fever, restlessness, irritability, seizures, photophobia, blurred vision
- hemiparesis, hemisensory defects, dysphagia, visual defects
- diplopia, ptosis, dilated pupil, and inability to rotate the eye.

Diagnostic tests
- Cerebral angiography (the test of choice)
- Computed tomography scan
- Magnetic resonance imaging, magnetic resonance angiography
- Skull X-ray.

Treatment
- Bed rest in a quiet, darkened room with minimal stimulation
- Surgical repair by clipping, ligation, or wrapping
- Avoidance of caffeine or other stimulants, and aspirin
- Codeine or another analgesic as needed
- Hydralazine or other antihypertensive agent, if indicated.

TYPICAL SITES OF CEREBRAL ANEURYSM

Circle of Willis

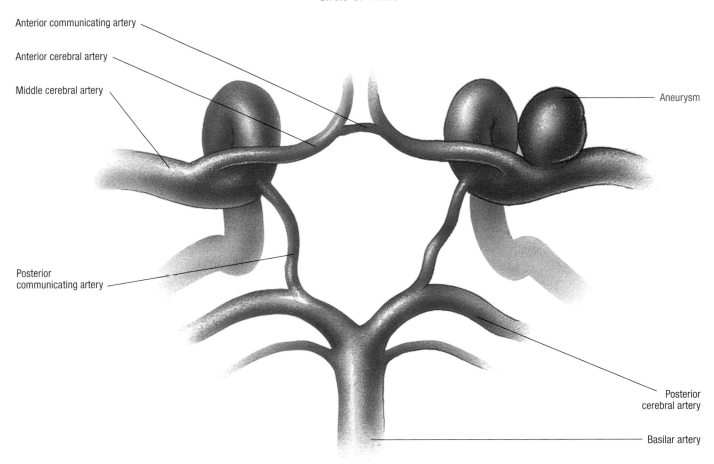

Anterior communicating artery

Anterior cerebral artery

Middle cerebral artery

Aneurysm

Posterior communicating artery

Posterior cerebral artery

Basilar artery

Vessels of the brain — Inferior view

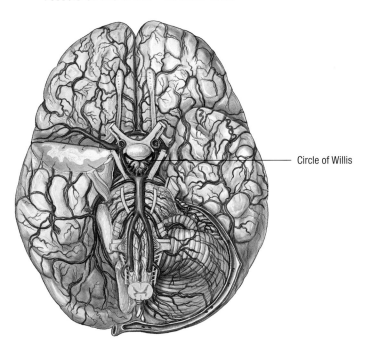

Circle of Willis

CEREBROVASCULAR ACCIDENT

A cerebrovascular accident (CVA), also known as a stroke, is a sudden impairment of cerebral circulation in one or more blood vessels. CVA interrupts or diminishes oxygen supply, and often causes serious damage or necrosis in the brain tissues.

Causes
- Thrombosis of the cerebral arteries supplying the brain, or of the intracranial vessels occluding blood flow
- Embolism from thrombus outside the brain, such as in the heart, aorta, or common carotid artery
- Hemorrhage from an intracranial artery or vein, such as from hypertension, ruptured aneurysm, arteriovenous malformation trauma, hemorrhagic disorder, or septic embolism.

Pathophysiology
Regardless of the cause, the underlying event is deprivation of oxygen and nutrients. Normally, if the arteries become blocked, autoregulatory mechanisms help maintain cerebral circulation until collateral circulation develops to deliver blood to the affected area. If the compensatory mechanisms become overworked, or if cerebral blood flow remains impaired for more than a few minutes, oxygen deprivation leads to infarction of brain tissue.

A thrombotic or embolic stroke causes ischemia. Some of the neurons served by the occluded vessel die from lack of oxygen and nutrients, resulting in cerebral infarction. Injury to surrounding cells disrupts metabolism and leads to changes in ionic transport, localized acidosis, and free radical formation. Calcium, sodium, and water accumulate in injured cells, and excitatory neurotransmitters are released. Consequent continued cellular injury and swelling may cause further damage.

When hemorrhage is the cause, impaired cerebral perfusion causes infarction, and the blood itself acts as a space-occupying mass. The brain's regulatory mechanisms attempt to maintain equilibrium by increasing blood pressure to maintain cerebral perfusion pressure. The increased intracranial pressure (ICP) forces cerebrospinal fluid out, thus restoring the balance. If the hemorrhage is small, this may be enough to keep the patient alive with only minimal neurologic deficits. However, if the bleeding is heavy, ICP increases rapidly and perfusion stops. Even if the pressure returns to normal, many brain cells die.

Signs and symptoms
The clinical features of CVA vary according to the affected artery and the region of the brain it supplies, the severity of the damage, and the extent of collateral circulation developed. A CVA in one hemisphere causes signs and symptoms on the opposite side of the body; one that damages cranial nerves affects structures on the same side.

General symptoms:
- Unilateral limb weakness, unilateral numbness
- Speech difficulties
- Headache, visual disturbances (diplopia, hemianopia, ptosis)
- Dizziness, anxiety
- Altered level of consciousness.

Anterior cerebral artery:
- Confusion, personality changes
- Weakness, numbness
- Incontinence, impaired motor and sensory functions
- Loss of coordination.

Middle cerebral artery:
- Aphasia, dysphasia
- Visual field deficits
- Hemiparesis of affected side (more severe in face and arm than leg).

Posterior cerebral artery:
- Visual field deficits, cortical blindness, sensory impairment
- Dyslexia, perseveration
- Coma.

Carotid artery:
- Weakness, paralysis, numbness, ptosis
- Sensory changes
- Visual disturbances on affected side
- Altered level of consciousness
- Bruits, headaches
- Aphasia.

Vertebrobasilar artery:
- Weakness, dizziness, ataxia, poor coordination
- Numbness around lips and mouth, slurred speech
- Visual field deficits, diplopia, nystagmus
- Dysphagia
- Amnesia.

Diagnostic tests
- Computed tomography scan, magnetic resonance imaging
- Cerebral angiography, digital subtraction angiography
- Single-photon emission computed tomography (SPECT) scan, positron emission tomography (PET) scan
- Electroencephalography
- Carotid duplex scan, transesophageal echocardiography
- Lumbar puncture
- Ophthalmoscopy.

Treatment
General:
- ICP management with monitoring, hyperventilation, osmotic diuretics, and corticosteroids
- Anticonvulsants
- Surgery for large cerebellar infarction
- Aneurysm repair
- Percutaneous transluminal angioplasty or stent insertion
- Stool softeners.

Ischemic CVA:
- Thrombolytic therapy within 3 hours after onset of symptoms
- Anticoagulant therapy.

Transient ischemic attacks:
- Antiplatelet agents
- Carotid endarterectomy.

Hemorrhagic CVA:
- Analgesics such as acetaminophen.

ISCHEMIC CVA

Common sites of plaque formation, embolism, and infarction

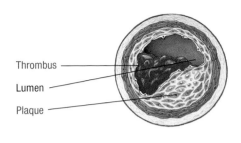

Thrombus
Lumen
Plaque

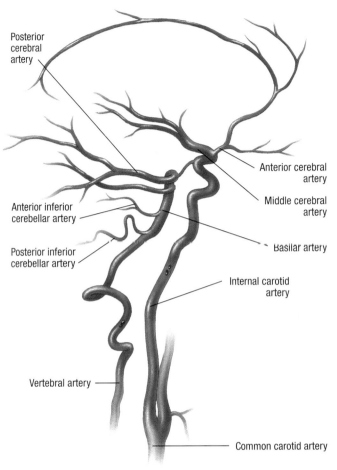

Posterior cerebral artery

Anterior cerebral artery

Middle cerebral artery

Anterior inferior cerebellar artery

Basilar artery

Posterior inferior cerebellar artery

Internal carotid artery

Vertebral artery

Common carotid artery

Common sites of cardiac thrombosis

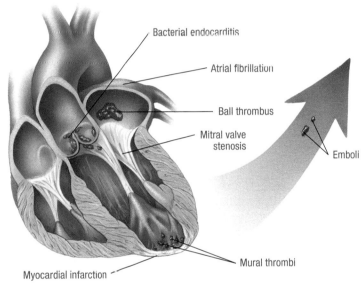

Bacterial endocarditis

Atrial fibrillation

Ball thrombus

Mitral valve stenosis

Emboli

Myocardial infarction

Mural thrombi

HEMORRHAGIC CVA
Common sites of cerebral hemorrhage

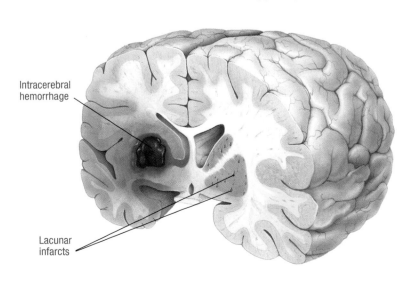

Intracerebral hemorrhage

Lacunar infarcts

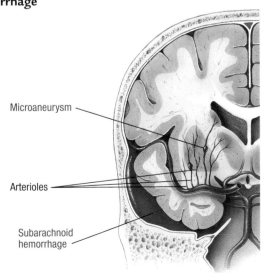

Microaneurysm

Arterioles

Subarachnoid hemorrhage

EPILEPSY

Epilepsy is a condition of the brain characterized by susceptibility to recurrent seizures — paroxysmal events associated with abnormal electrical discharges of neurons in the brain.

The brain is made up of billions of cells, including a network of cells called neurons. This neural network enables communication within the brain and between the brain and the rest of the body.

The brain's ability to turn electrical impulses "on" and "off" allows it to control messages and work effectively. In people with epilepsy, however, this fine balance is upset, making the brain unable to limit the spread of electrical activity.

Generalized seizures affect both hemispheres of the brain at the same time, and abnormal activity is not focused in one specific area. The two types of partial seizures, called simple and complex, are based on whether a person remains fully conscious during a seizure.

Causes
- Idiopathic in about half of all cases.
  Possible causes of other cases:
- Birth trauma (inadequate oxygen supply to the brain, blood incompatibility, or hemorrhage), perinatal infection
- Infectious diseases (meningitis, encephalitis, or brain abscess)
- Ingestion of toxins (mercury, lead, or carbon monoxide)
- Brain tumors, head injury or trauma
- Inherited disorders or degenerative disease, such as phenylketonuria or tuberous sclerosis
- Cerebrovascular accident (hemorrhage, thrombosis, or embolism).

Pathophysiology
Some neurons in the brain may depolarize easily or be hyperexcitable; this *epileptogenic focus* fires more readily than normal when stimulated. In these neurons, the membrane potential at rest is less negative or inhibitory connections are missing, possibly because of decreased gamma-amino butyric acid activity or localized shifts in electrolytes.

On stimulation, the epileptogenic focus fires and spreads electrical current toward the synapse and surrounding cells. These cells fire in turn and the impulse cascades to one side of the brain (a partial seizure), both sides of the brain (a generalized seizure), or cortical, subcortical, or brain stem areas.

The brain's metabolic demand for oxygen increases dramatically during a seizure. If this demand isn't met, hypoxia and brain damage ensue. Firing of inhibitory neurons causes the excitatory neurons to slow their firing and eventually stop.

If this inhibitory action doesn't occur, the result is status epilepticus: one prolonged seizure or one seizure occurring right after another and another. Without treatment, this may be fatal.

Signs and symptoms
The hallmark of epilepsy is recurring seizures. There are generally six types of seizures.
  Simple partial seizure:
- Sensory symptoms (lights flashing, smells, auditory hallucinations)
- Autonomic symptoms (sweating, flushing, pupil dilation)
- Psychic symptoms (dream states, anger, fear).
  Complex partial seizure:
- Altered level of consciousness
- Amnesia.
  Absence seizure:
- Brief change in level of consciousness indicated by blinking or rolling of the eyes, a blank stare, and slight mouth movements.
  Myoclonic seizure:
- Brief involuntary muscular jerks of the body or extremities.
  Generalized tonic-clonic seizure:
- Typically begin with a loud cry
- Change in level of consciousness
- Body stiffens and alternates between muscle spasm and relaxation
- Tongue biting, incontinence, labored breathing, apnea, and cyanosis
- After awakening, patient may be confused and have difficulty talking
- May complain of drowsiness, fatigue, headache, muscle soreness, and weakness.
  Atonic seizure:
- General loss of postural tone
- Temporary loss of consciousness.

Diagnostic tests
- Electroencephalography
- Computed tomography scan, magnetic resonance imaging
- Skull X-ray
- Serum electrolytes, liver enzymes, blood alcohol.

Treatment
- Tonic-clonic and complex partial seizures — phenytoin, fosphenytoin, carbamazepine, phenobarbital, primidone
- Demonstrated focal lesion or underlying cause, such as a tumor, abscess, or vascular problem — surgery
- Focal seizures — vagus nerve stimulator implant
- Status epilepticus — I.V. diazepam, lorazepam, phenytoin, or phenobarbital
- Hypoglycemic seizure — dextrose
- Chronic alcoholism or withdrawal — thiamine and benzodiazepines.

TYPES OF SEIZURES

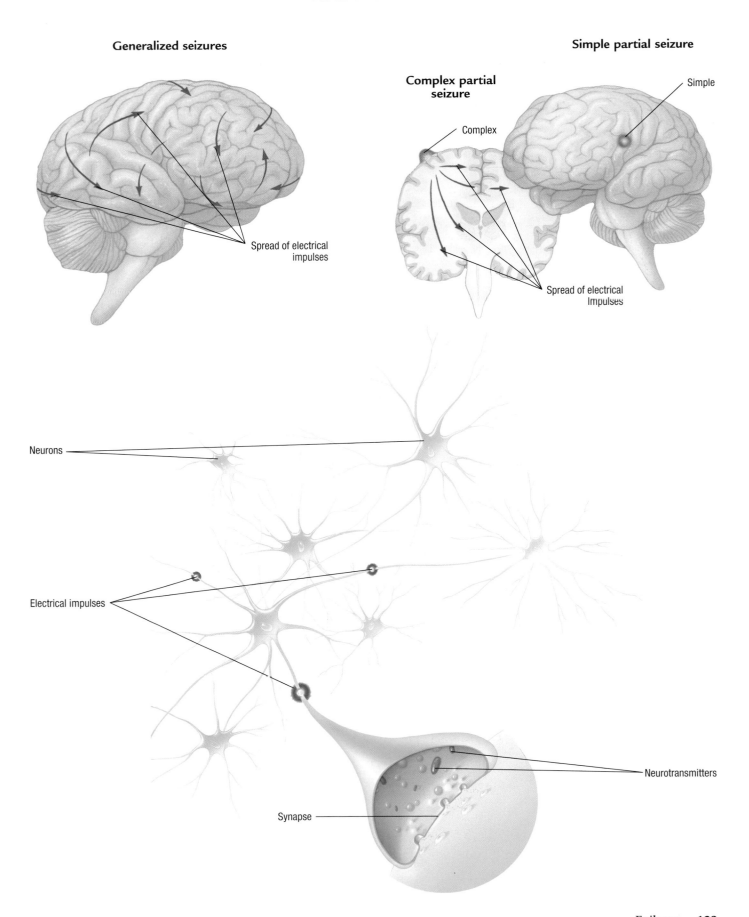

Generalized seizures

Spread of electrical impulses

Complex partial seizure

Simple partial seizure

Complex

Simple

Spread of electrical Impulses

Neurons

Electrical impulses

Neurotransmitters

Synapse

GUILLAIN-BARRÉ SYNDROME

Also known as infectious polyneuritis, Landry-Guillain-Barré syndrome, or acute idiopathic polyneuritis, Guillain-Barré syndrome is an acute, rapidly progressive, and potentially fatal form of polyneuritis that causes muscle weakness and mild distal sensory loss. About 50% of patients with Guillain-Barré syndrome have a recent history of minor febrile illness, usually an upper respiratory tract infection or, less often, gastroenteritis. When infection precedes the onset of Guillain-Barré syndrome, signs of infection subside before neurologic features appear.

This syndrome occurs in three phases:
- *Acute:* begins with onset of first definitive symptom and ends 1 to 3 weeks later; further deterioration does not occur after the acute phase
- *Plateau:* several days to 2 weeks
- *Recovery:* remyelinization and regrowth of axonal processes; generally lasts 4 to 6 months, but up to 3 years if disease was severe.

Causes

Unknown; may be a cell-mediated immune response to a virus.
Possible precipitating factors:
- Surgery
- Rabies or swine influenza vaccination
- Hodgkin's or other malignant disease
- Systemic lupus erythematosus.

Pathophysiology

The major pathologic manifestation is segmental demyelination of the peripheral nerves. This prevents normal transmission of electrical impulses. Because this syndrome causes inflammation and degenerative changes in both the posterior (sensory) and the anterior (motor) nerve roots, signs of sensory and motor losses occur simultaneously. Additionally, autonomic nerve transmission may be impaired.

Signs and symptoms
- Symmetrical muscle weakness (major neurologic sign) appearing in the legs first (ascending type) and then extending to the arms and facial nerves within 24 to 72 hours
- Muscle weakness developing in the arms first (descending type), or in the arms and legs simultaneously
- Paresthesia, sometimes preceding muscle weakness but vanishing quickly
- Diplegia, possibly with ophthalmoplegia
- Dysphagia, dysarthria
- Hypotonia and areflexia.

Diagnostic tests
- Cerebrospinal fluid analysis by lumbar puncture
- Complete blood count, serum immunoglobulin levels
- Electromyography
- Nerve conduction velocity studies.

Treatment
Primarily supportive, including:
- Endotracheal intubation or tracheotomy, as indicated to clear secretions
- Trial of prednisone to reduce inflammatory response
- Plasmapheresis
- Continuous electrocardiogram monitoring.

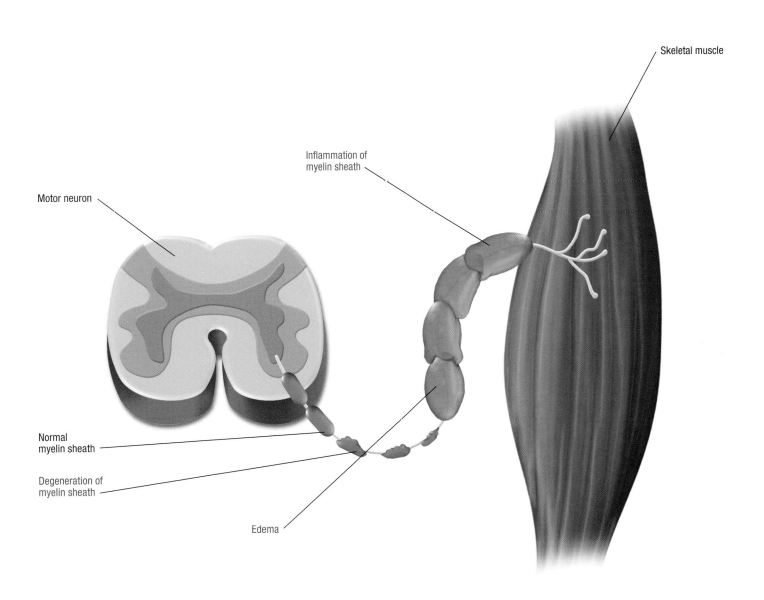

Skeletal muscle

Inflammation of
myelin sheath

Motor neuron

Normal
myelin sheath

Degeneration of
myelin sheath

Edema

HEADACHE

Headache is the most common patient complaint. Ninety percent of all headaches are vascular, muscle contraction, or a combination; 10% are due to an underlying intracranial, systemic, or psychological disorder.

Migraine headaches, probably the most intensively studied, are throbbing, vascular headaches that usually begin to appear in childhood or adolescence and recur throughout adulthood. Affecting up to 10% of Americans, they're more common in females and have a strong familial incidence.

Causes

Most chronic headaches result from tension (muscle contraction), which may be caused by:
- emotional stress or fatigue
- menstruation
- environmental stimuli (noise, crowds, or bright lights).
  Other possible causes include:
- glaucoma
- inflammation of the eyes or mucosa of the nasal or paranasal sinuses
- diseases of the scalp, teeth, extracranial arteries, or external or middle ear
- vasodilators (nitrates, alcohol, and histamine)
- systemic disease
- hypertension
- head trauma or tumor
- intracranial bleeding, abscess, or aneurysm.

Pathophysiology

Headaches are believed to be associated with constriction and dilation of intracranial and extracranial arteries. Certain biochemical abnormalities are thought to occur during a *migraine* attack. These include local leakage of a vasodilator polypeptide called neurokinin through the dilated arteries and a decrease in the plasma level of serotonin.

Headache pain may emanate from the pain-sensitive structures of the skin, scalp, muscles, arteries, and veins; cranial nerves V, VII, IX, and X; or cervical nerves 1, 2, and 3. *Intracranial* mechanisms of headaches include traction or displacement of arteries, venous sinuses, or venous tributaries and inflammation or direct pressure on the cranial nerves with afferent pain fibers.

The evolution of a *headache* has four distinct phases. In the *normal phase,* cerebral and temporal arteries are innervated extracranial; parenchymal arteries are noninnervated.

In the *vasoconstriction (aura) phase,* stress-related neurogenic local vasoconstriction of innervated cerebral arteries reduces cerebral blood flow (localized ischemia). Systemically, the prostaglandin thromboxane causes platelet aggregation and release of serotonin, a potent vasoconstrictor, and perhaps of other vasoactive substances.

In the *parenchymal artery dilation phase,* noninnervated parenchymal vessels dilate in response to local acidosis and anoxia (ischemia). Neurogenic or biologic factors may cause preformed arteriovenous (AV) shunts to open. Increased blood flow, increased internal pressure, and enhanced pulsations short-circuit the normal nutritive capillaries and cause pain.

In the *vasodilation (headache) phase,* compensatory mechanisms cause marked vasodilation of the innervated arteries resulting in headache. Systemic platelet aggregation decreases, and falling serotonin levels result in vasodilation. A painful sterile perivascular inflammation develops and persists into a postheadache phase.

Signs and symptoms

Muscle contraction and traction-inflammatory vascular headaches:
- Dull, persistent ache
- Tender spots on the head and neck
- Feeling of tightness around the head, with a characteristic "hatband" distribution
- Severe and unrelenting pain.
  Intracranial bleeding:
- Neurologic deficits such as paresthesia and muscle weakness
- Pain, possibly unresponsive to narcotics.
  Tumor:
- Pain is most severe when patient awakens.
  Migraine headaches:
- Unilateral, pulsating pain, which later becomes more generalized
- Premonitory aura of scintillating scotoma, hemianopsia, unilateral paresthesia, speech disorders
- Irritability, anorexia, nausea, vomiting, photophobia.

Diagnostic tests
- Cervical spine and sinus X-rays
- Electroencephalography
- Computed tomography scan (performed before lumbar puncture to rule out increased intracranial pressure)
- Magnetic resonance imaging
- Lumbar puncture.

Treatment

Symptomatic relief:
- Analgesics ranging from aspirin to codeine or meperidine
- Identification and elimination of causative factors.
  Chronic tension headaches:
- Muscle relaxants
- Stress management therapy.
  Migraine:
- Ergotamine alone or with caffeine (contraindicated in pregnant women because they stimulate uterine contractions)
- These drugs and others, such as metoclopramide or naproxen, work best when taken early in the course of an attack. If nausea and vomiting make oral administration impossible, drugs may be given as rectal suppositories.
  Acute migraine or cluster headaches:
- Sumatriptan or another in the same class.
  Migraine prevention:
- Propranolol, atenolol, clonidine, amitriptyline.

VASCULAR CHANGES IN HEADACHE

Normal

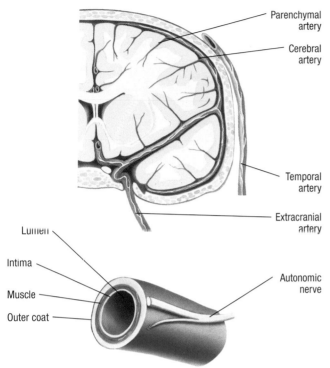

Parenchymal artery

Cerebral artery

Temporal artery

Extracranial artery

Lumen

Intima

Muscle

Outer coat

Autonomic nerve

Vasoconstriction (aura) phase

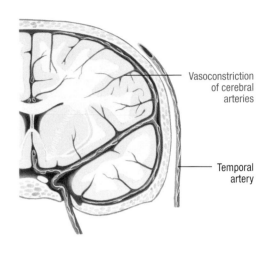

Vasoconstriction of cerebral arteries

Temporal artery

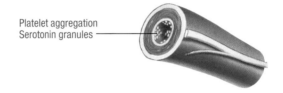

Platelet aggregation
Serotonin granules

Parenchymal artery dilation

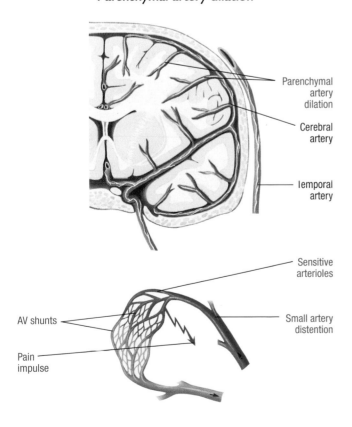

Parenchymal artery dilation

Cerebral artery

Temporal artery

Sensitive arterioles

AV shunts

Pain impulse

Small artery distention

Vasodilation (headache) phase

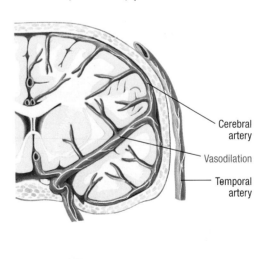

Cerebral artery

Vasodilation

Temporal artery

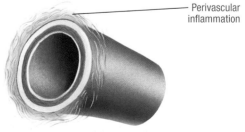

Perivascular inflammation

HYDROCEPHALUS

Hydrocephalus is an excessive accumulation of cerebrospinal fluid (CSF) within the ventricular spaces of the brain.

 AGE ALERT
Hydrocephalus occurs most often in neonates. It can also occur in adults because of injury or disease. In infants, hydrocephalus enlarges the head, and in both infants and adults, the resulting compression can damage brain tissue.

Causes
- Obstruction of CSF flow (*noncommunicating* hydrocephalus)
- Faulty absorption of CSF (*communicating* hydrocephalus).
  Risk factors in infants:
- Intrauterine infection
- Intracranial hemorrhage from birth trauma or prematurity.
  Risk factors in older children and adults:
- Meningitis
- Mastoiditis, chronic otitis media
- Brain tumors, intracranial hemorrhage.

Pathophysiology
In *noncommunicating* hydrocephalus, the obstruction occurs most commonly at the aqueduct of Sylvius, between the third and fourth ventricles, but it can also occur at the outlets of the fourth ventricle (foramina of Luschka and Magendie) or, rarely, at the foramen of Monro. This obstruction may result from fetal developmental error, infection (syphilis, granulomatous diseases, meningitis), a tumor, a cerebral aneurysm, or a blood clot (after intracranial hemorrhage).

In *communicating* hydrocephalus, faulty absorption of CSF may result from surgery to repair a myelomeningocele, adhesions between meninges at the base of the brain, or meningeal hemorrhage. Rarely, a tumor in the choroid plexus causes overproduction of CSF and consequent hydrocephalus.

In either type, both CSF pressure and volume increase. Obstruction in the ventricles causes dilation, stretching, and disruption of the lining. Underlying white matter atrophies. Compression of brain tissue and cerebral blood vessels may lead to ischemia and, eventually, cell death.

Signs and symptoms
In infants:
- Enlargement of the head clearly disproportionate to the infant's growth (most characteristic sign)
- Distended scalp veins
- Thin, shiny, fragile-looking scalp skin
- Depressed orbital roof with downward displacement of the eyes and prominent sclerae; widened skull
- High-pitched, shrill cry, irritability, abnormal muscle tone in legs
- Projectile vomiting.
  In adults and older children:
- Decreased level of consciousness
- Ataxia
- Incontinence
- Impaired intellect.

Diagnostic tests
- Skull X-rays
- Angiography, ventriculography
- Computed tomography, magnetic resonance imaging
- Lumbar puncture.

Treatment
The only treatment for hydrocephalus is surgical correction by insertion of a ventriculoperitoneal or ventriculoatrial shunt.

VENTRICLES OF THE BRAIN

Normal brain — Lateral view

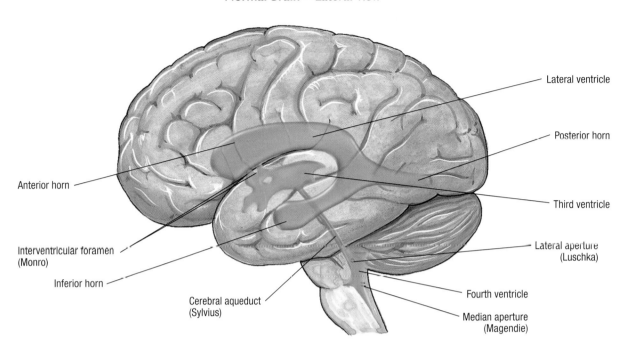

Lateral ventricle

Posterior horn

Third ventricle

Anterior horn

Interventricular foramen
(Monro)

Inferior horn

Cerebral aqueduct
(Sylvius)

Lateral aperture
(Luschka)

Fourth ventricle

Median aperture
(Magendie)

VENTRICULAR ENLARGEMENT IN HYDROCEPHALUS

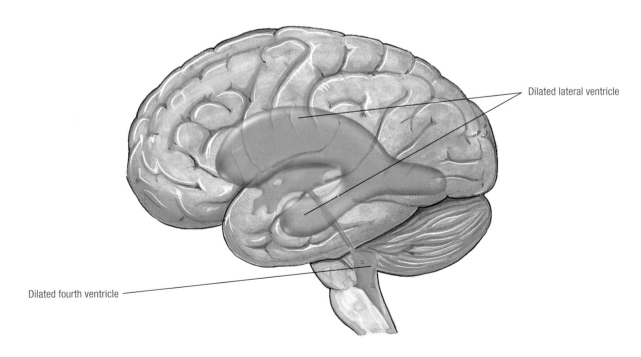

Dilated lateral ventricle

Dilated fourth ventricle

MENINGITIS

In meningitis, the brain and the spinal cord meninges become inflamed, usually because of bacterial infection. Such inflammation may involve all three meningeal membranes — the dura mater, arachnoid, and pia mater.

Causes
- Bacteremia from pneumonia, empyema, osteomyelitis, endocarditis
- Other infections, such as sinusitis, otitis media, encephalitis
- Brain abscess, usually caused by *Neisseria meningitidis*, *Haemophilus influenzae*, *Streptococcus pneumoniae*, *Escherichia coli*
- Viral or other infection
- May be idiopathic
- Trauma or invasive procedures, including, skull fracture, penetrating head wound, lumbar puncture, ventricular shunting.

Pathophysiology
Meningitis often begins as an inflammation of the pia and arachnoid, which may progress to congestion of adjacent tissues and destroy some nerve cells. The microorganism typically enters the central nervous system (CNS) by way of blood (most common); direct communication between cerebrospinal fluid (CSF) and the environment (trauma); along cranial or peripheral nerves; through the mouth or nose. Microorganisms can reach a fetus via the intrauterine environment.

The invading organism triggers an inflammatory response in the meninges. In an attempt to ward off the invasion, neutrophils gather in the area and produce an exudate in the subarachnoid space, causing the CSF to thicken. The thickened CSF flows less readily around the brain and spinal cord, and it can block the arachnoid villi, causing hydrocephalus.

The exudate can also:
- exacerbate the inflammatory response, increasing the pressure in the brain
- extend to the cranial and peripheral nerves, triggering additional inflammation
- irritate the meninges, disrupting their cell membranes and causing edema.

The consequences are elevated intracranial pressure (ICP), engorged blood vessels, disrupted cerebral blood supply, possible thrombosis or rupture, and, if ICP is not reduced, cerebral infarction. Encephalitis also may ensue as a secondary infection of the brain tissue.

In aseptic meningitis, lymphocytes infiltrate the pia and arachnoid, but usually not as severely as in bacterial meningitis, and no exudate is formed. Thus, this type of meningitis is self-limiting.

Signs and symptoms
- Fever, chills, malaise
- Headache, vomiting and, rarely, papilledema
- Signs of meningeal irritation:
- nuchal rigidity
- positive Brudzinski's and Kernig's signs
- exaggerated and symmetrical deep tendon reflexes
- opisthotonos
- Sinus arrhythmias; irritability; photophobia, diplopia, or other visual problems; delirium, deep stupor, coma.

CLINICAL TIP
An infant may show signs of infection, but most are simply fretful and refuse to eat. In an infant, vomiting can lead to dehydration, which prevents formation of a bulging fontanelle, an important sign of increased ICP.

Diagnostic tests
- Lumbar puncture
- Cultures of blood, urine, and nose and throat secretions
- Chest X-ray ; sinus and skull X-rays
- White blood cell count
- Computed tomography scan, magnetic resonance imaging.

Treatment
- I.V. antibiotics for at least 2 weeks, followed by oral antibiotics selected by culture and sensitivity testing
- Agents to control arrhythmias
- Mannitol
- Anticonvulsant (usually given I.V.) or a sedative
- Aspirin or acetaminophen.

CLINICAL TIP
Staff should take droplet precautions (in addition to standard precautions) for meningitis caused by *H. influenzae* or *N. meningitidis,* until 24 hours after the start of effective therapy.

MENINGES AND CEREBROSPINAL FLUID FLOW

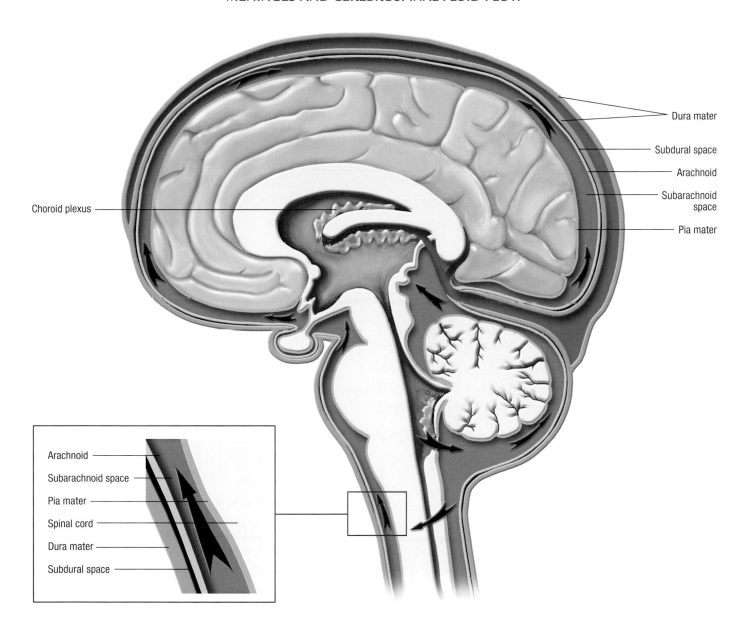

Dura mater

Subdural space

Arachnoid

Subarachnoid space

Pia mater

Choroid plexus

Arachnoid

Subarachnoid space

Pia mater

Spinal cord

Dura mater

Subdural space

INFLAMMATION IN MENINGITIS

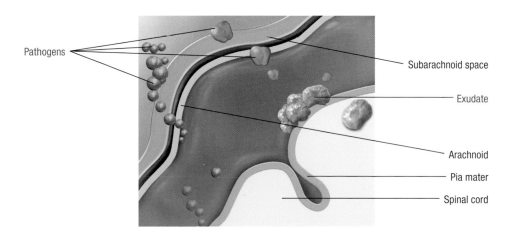

Pathogens

Subarachnoid space

Exudate

Arachnoid

Pia mater

Spinal cord

MULTIPLE SCLEROSIS

Multiple sclerosis (MS) causes demyelination of the white matter of the brain and spinal cord. The damage slows, blocks, or distorts transmission of nerve impulses.

Manifestations depend on the extent and site of myelin destruction, extent of remyelination, and adequacy of subsequent restored synaptic transmission. The prognosis varies. MS may progress rapidly, disabling the patient by early adulthood or causing death within months of onset. Alternatively, early symptoms may be mild, and years may elapse between onset and diagnosis. Flares may be bizarre and difficult for the patient to describe; transient or lasting hours or weeks, possibly waxing and waning with no predictable pattern, varying from day to day. Diagnosis of this disorder requires evidence of two or more neurologic attacks. About 70% of patients lead active, productive lives with prolonged remissions.

 AGE ALERT
Characterized by exacerbations and remissions, MS is a major cause of chronic disability in young adults. It usually becomes symptomatic between the ages of 20 and 40 (the average age of onset is 27).

Causes
- Exact cause unknown
- Autoimmune response to a slow-acting or latent viral infection
- Environmental or genetic factors.

Pathophysiology
In MS, axon demyelination and nerve fiber loss occur in patches throughout the central nervous system, inducing widely disseminated and varied neurologic dysfunction.

New evidence of nerve fiber loss may provide an explanation for the invisible neurologic deficits experienced by many patients with MS. The axons determine the presence or absence of function; loss of myelin does not correlate with loss of function.

Signs and symptoms
- Optic neuritis, diplopia, ophthalmoplegia, blurred vision, nystagmus
- Sensory impairment, such as burning, pins and needles, electrical sensations
- Fatigue (often the most debilitating symptom)
- Weakness, paralysis ranging from monoplegia to quadriplegia, spasticity, hyperreflexia, intention tremor, ataxia
- Incontinence, frequency, urgency, frequent urinary tract infections
- Involuntary evacuation or constipation
- Poorly articulated or scanning speech (syllables separated by pauses)
- Dysphagia.

Diagnostic tests
- Magnetic resonance imaging
- Electroencephalography
- Lumbar puncture
- Cerebrospinal fluid electrophoresis
- Evoked potential studies (visual, brain stem, auditory, and somatosensory).

Treatment
The aim of treatment is threefold: treat the acute exacerbation, treat the disease process, and treat the related signs and symptoms.
- I.V. methylprednisolone followed by oral therapy
- Interferon and glatiramen (a combination of 4 amino acids)
- Stretching and range-of-motion exercises, coupled with correct positioning, adaptive devices, physical therapy
- Baclofen and tizanidine
- Frequent rest periods, aerobic exercise, and cooling techniques (air conditioning, breezes, water sprays)
- Amantidine, pemoline, methylphenidate
- Low-dose tricyclic antidepressants, phenytoin, or carbamazepine
- Beta blockers, sedatives, diuretics
- Speech therapy, vision therapy, adaptive lenses
- Bladder problems (failure to store urine, failure to empty the bladder or, more commonly, both) are managed by such strategies as drinking cranberry juice, or insertion of an indwelling catheter and suprapubic tubes. Intermittent self-catheterization and postvoid catheterization programs are helpful, as are anticholinergic medications in some patients.
- Bowel problems (constipation and involuntary evacuation) are managed by such measures as increasing dietary fiber, using bulking agents, and bowel-training strategies, such as daily suppositories and rectal stimulation.

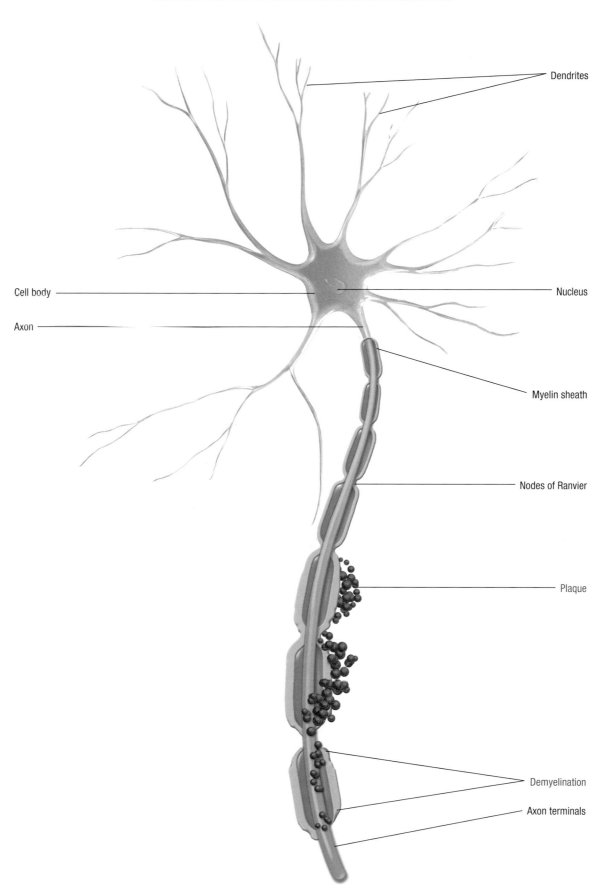

Dendrites

Nucleus

Cell body

Axon

Myelin sheath

Nodes of Ranvier

Plaque

Demyelination

Axon terminals

Myasthenia gravis

Myasthenia gravis causes sporadic but progressive weakness and abnormal fatigability of striated (skeletal) muscles; symptoms are exacerbated by exercise and repeated movement and relieved by anticholinesterase drugs. Usually, this disorder affects muscles innervated by the cranial nerves (face, lips, tongue, neck, and throat), but it can affect any muscle group.

Myasthenia gravis follows an unpredictable course of periodic exacerbations and remissions. There is no known cure. Drug treatment has improved the prognosis and allows patients to lead relatively normal lives, except during exacerbations. When the disease involves the respiratory system, it may be life-threatening.

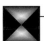
AGE ALERT
Myasthenia gravis affects 1 in 25,000 people at any age, but incidence peaks between the ages of 20 and 40. It's three times more common in women than in men in this age-group, but after age 40, the rate of incidence is similar.

Causes
- Exact cause unknown
- Possible mechanisms include autoimmune response, ineffective acetylcholine release from nerve terminals, inadequate muscle fiber response to acetylcholine.

Pathophysiology
Myasthenia gravis causes a failure in transmission of nerve impulses at the neuromuscular junction. The site of action is the postsynaptic membrane. Theoretically, antireceptor antibodies block, weaken, or reduce the number of acetylcholine receptors available at each neuromuscular junction and thereby impair muscle depolarization necessary for movement.

Signs and symptoms
- Weak eye closure, ptosis, and diplopia
- Skeletal muscle weakness and fatigue, increasing through the day but decreasing with rest; in the early stages, easy fatigability of certain muscles may appear with no other findings; later, it may be severe enough to cause paralysis
- Progressive muscle weakness and accompanying loss of function depending on muscle group affected; becoming more intense during menses and after emotional stress, prolonged exposure to sunlight or cold, or infections
- Blank, expressionless facial appearance and nasal vocal tones
- Frequent nasal regurgitation of fluids; difficulty chewing and swallowing
- Weak neck muscles (may become too weak to support the head without bobbing); patient tilts head back to see
- Weak respiratory muscles, low tidal volume and vital capacity.

CLINICAL TIP
Respiratory muscle weakness seen in myasthenic crisis may be severe enough to require emergency intubation and mechanical ventilation.

Diagnostic tests
- Tensilon test confirms diagnosis — temporarily improved muscle function within 30 to 60 seconds after I.V. injection of edrophonium or neostigmine and lasting up to 30 minutes
- Electromyography
- Serum antiacetylcholine antibody titer
- Chest X-ray reveals thymoma (in approximately 15% of patients).

Treatment
- Anticholinesterase drugs, such as neostigmine and pyridostigmine
- Immunosuppressant therapy with corticosteroids, azathioprine, cyclosporine, and cyclophosphamide used in a progressive fashion
- Immunoglobulin G during acute relapses or plasmapheresis in severe exacerbations
- Thymectomy
- Tracheotomy, positive-pressure ventilation, and vigorous suctioning
- Discontinue anticholinesterase drugs in myasthenic crisis until respiratory function improves.

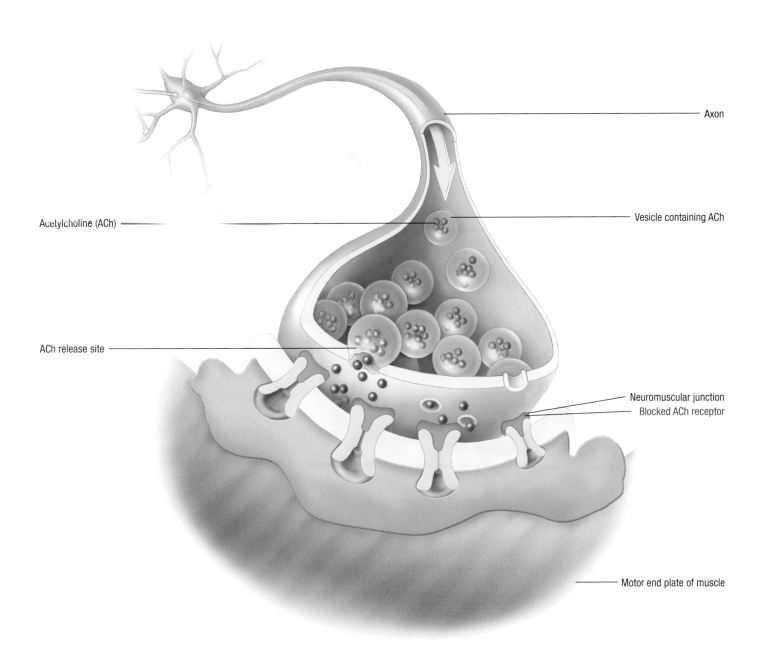

Axon

Vesicle containing ACh

Acetylcholine (ACh)

ACh release site

Neuromuscular junction
Blocked ACh receptor

Motor end plate of muscle

PARKINSON'S DISEASE

Parkinson's disease characteristically produces progressive muscle rigidity, akinesia, and involuntary tremor. Death may result from complications, such as aspiration pneumonia or other infection.

 AGE ALERT
Parkinson's disease is one of the most common crippling diseases in the United States. It strikes 1 in every 100 people over age 60 and affects men more often than women.

Causes
- Exact cause unknown
- In some cases, exposure to toxins, such as manganese dust or carbon monoxide.

Pathophysiology
Parkinson's disease is a degenerative process involving the dopaminergic neurons in the substantia nigra (the area of the basal ganglia that produces and stores the neurotransmitter dopamine). This area plays an important role in the extrapyramidal system, which controls posture and coordination of voluntary motor movements.

Dopamine allows for the transmission of electrical impulses from one nerve cell to another across a tiny gap called a synapse. Dendrites on one side of the synapse receive incoming messages and pass them to the the end of the axon, where granules containing dopamine are stimulated to release into the synapse. Dopamine crosses the synapse and binds to dopamine receptors on the other side. It stimulates the receptors to open, transmitting the message to the next nerve cell. After the message is sent, the receptors release the dopamine back into the synapse where it is reabsorbed into the axon. Dopamine can be broken down by a chemical called monoamine oxidase B. This "cleans" the synapse so it is ready for the next message.

Motor effects
The action of dopamine is opposed by another neurotransmitter called acetylcholine. The balance of dopamine and acetylcholine ensures smooth coordinated movement. In Parkinson's disease, the nerve cells that produce dopamine are dying. There is too little dopamine and too much acetylcholine; there are also high levels of glutamate, another neurotransmitter. With insufficient dopamine available to bind and open the dopamine receptors on the receiving nerve, the message is not correctly transmitted.

Normally, stimulation of the basal ganglia results in fine motor movement because acetylcholine (excitatory) and dopamine (inhibitory) release are balanced. Degeneration of the dopaminergic neurons and loss of available dopamine leads to an excess of excitatory acetylcholine at the synapse.

Other nondopaminergic neurons may be affected, possibly contributing to depression and the other nonmotor symptoms associated with this disease. In addition, the basal ganglia are interconnected to the hypothalamus, potentially affecting autonomic and endocrine function as well.

Current research on the pathogenesis of Parkinson's disease focuses on damage to the substantia nigra from oxidative stress, believed to diminish brain iron content, impair mitochondrial function, inhibit antioxidant and protective systems, reduce glutathione secretion, and damage lipids, proteins, and deoxyribonucleic acid. Brain cells are less capable of repairing oxidative damage than are other tissues.

Signs and symptoms
- Muscle rigidity, akinesia, and an insidious tremor beginning in the fingers (unilateral pill-roll tremor) that increases during stress or anxiety and decreases with purposeful movement and sleep
- Resistance to passive muscle stretching, which may be uniform (lead-pipe rigidity) or jerky (cogwheel rigidity)
- Akinesia causing difficulty walking (gait lacks normal parallel motion and may be retropulsive or propulsive)
- Drooling, excessive sweating
- Masklike facial expression
- Dysarthria, dysphagia, or both
- Oculogyric crises or blepharospasm
- Decreased motility of GI and genitourinary smooth muscle
- Orthostatic hypotension
- Oily skin.

Diagnostic tests
Generally, diagnostic tests are of little value in identifying Parkinson's disease. Diagnosis is based on the patient's age and history, and on the characteristic clinical picture. However, urinalysis may support the diagnosis by revealing decreased dopamine levels.

A conclusive diagnosis is possible only after ruling out other causes of tremor, involutional depression, cerebral arteriosclerosis, intracranial tumors, Wilson's disease, or phenothiazine or other drug toxicity.

Treatment
- Levodopa, a dopamine replacement most effective during early stages and given in increasing doses until symptoms are relieved or adverse effects appear
- Drugs that enhance the therapeutic effect of levodopa — anticholinergics, such as trihexyphenidyl; antihistamines such as diphenhydramine; amantidine, an antiviral agent; selegiline, an enzyme-inhibiting agent
- Stereotactic neurosurgery
- Physical therapy, including active and passive range-of-motion exercises, routine daily activities, walking, baths, and massage.

NEUROTRANSMITTER ACTION IN PARKINSON'S DISEASE

Brain — Coronal section

Motor cortex
(gray matter)

Thalamus

Striatum

Subthalamic
nucleus

Globus pallidus
interna

Optic nerve

Substantia
nigra

Cerebellum

Spinal cord

Brain — Lateral view

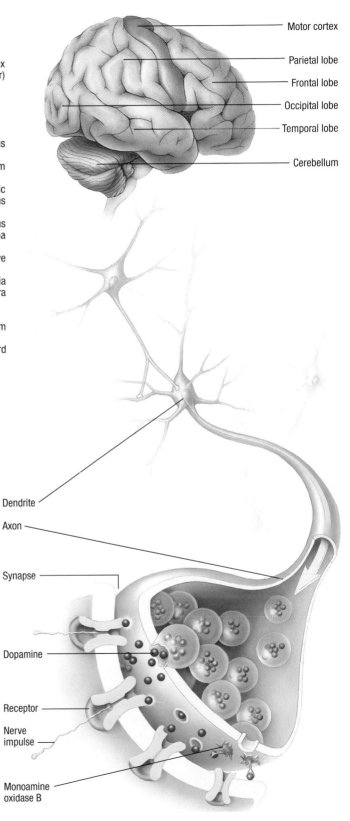

Motor cortex

Parietal lobe

Frontal lobe

Occipital lobe

Temporal lobe

Cerebellum

Dendrite

Axon

Synapse

Dopamine

Receptor

Nerve
impulse

Monoamine
oxidase B

Dopamine levels

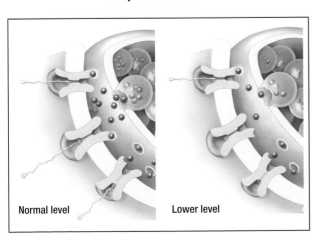

Normal level   Lower level

SPINA BIFIDA

Spina bifida and other neural tube defects (NTDs) are serious birth defects that involve the spine and spinal cord. In spina bifida, the neural tube fails to close at approximately 28 days after conception.

Causes
- Exact cause and most of the specific environmental triggers unknown
- Maternal folic acid deficiency
- Fetal exposure to a teratogen, such as valproic acid
- Multiple malformation syndrome (for example, chromosomal abnormalities such as trisomy 18 or 13 syndrome)
- Isolated NTDs (not due to a specific teratogen or associated with other malformations) believed to be caused by a combination of genetic and environmental factors.

Pathophysiology
Spina bifida occulta is the most common and least severe spinal cord defect. It's characterized by incomplete closure of one or more vertebrae without protrusion of the spinal cord or meninges.

However, in more severe forms of spina bifida, the spinal contents protrude in an external sac or cystic lesion (spina bifida cystica). *Spina bifida cystica* has two forms: *myelomeningocele (meningomyelocele)* and *meningocele*. In myelomeningocele, the external sac contains meninges, cerebrospinal fluid (CSF), and a portion of the spinal cord or nerve roots distal to the conus medullaris. When the spinal nerve roots end at the sac, motor and sensory function below the sac is abolished. Arnold-Chiari syndrome is a form of meningomyelocele in which part of the brain protrudes into the spinal canal. Meningocele, in which the sac contains only meninges and CSF, is less severe and may be asymptomatic.

Signs and symptoms
Spina bifida occulta:
- Depression or dimple, tuft of hair, soft fatty deposits, port-wine nevi, or a combination of these abnormalities on the skin over the spinal defect
- Occasionally associated with foot weakness or bowel and bladder disturbances.

Meningocele:
- Saclike structure protrudes over the spine
- Seldom causes neurologic deficit.

Myelomeningocele (meningomyelocele):
- Saclike protrusion containing nerve tissue
- Depending on the level of the defect, causes permanent neurologic dysfunction.

Associated disorders:
- Trophic skin disturbances (ulcerations, cyanosis), clubfoot, knee contractures, curvature of the spine, hydrocephalus (in about 90% of patients), and possibly mental retardation.

Diagnostic tests
- Amniocentesis
- Maternal screening for serum alpha-fetoprotein and other serum markers
- Ultrasonography.

Spina bifida occulta:
- May be palpable
- Spinal X-ray
- Myelography.

Myelomeningocele and meningocele:
- Transillumination — meningocele typically transilluminates; myelomeningocele doesn't
- Skull X-rays, cephalic measurements, and computed tomography scan to demonstrate associated hydrocephalus
- In patients with myelomeningocele — urinalysis, urine cultures, and tests for renal function starting in the neonatal period and continuing at regular intervals.

Treatment
- *Spina bifida occulta:* usually no treatment
- *Meningocele:* surgical closure of protruding sac
- *Myelomeningocele:* repair of the sac (does not reverse neurologic defects); shunt to relieve hydrocephalus if needed; supportive measures to promote independence and prevent further complications.

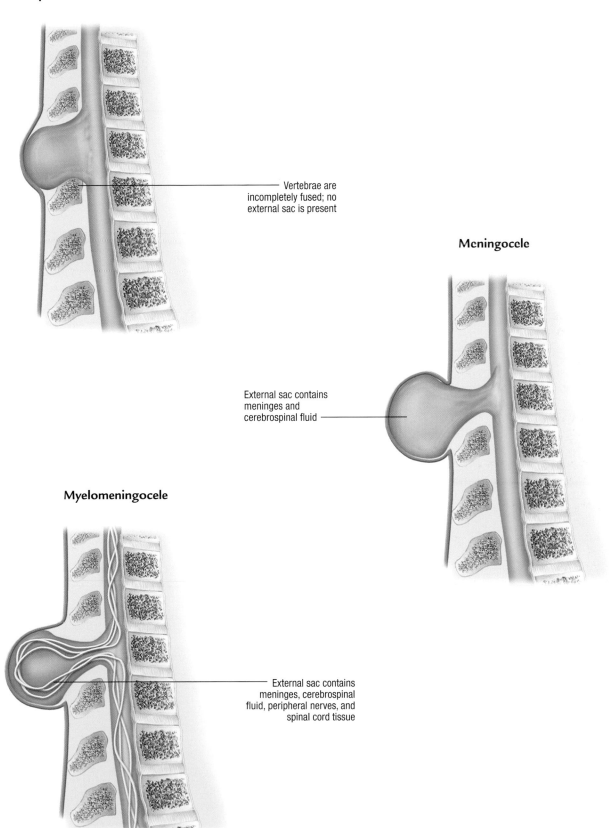

Spina bifida occulta

Vertebrae are incompletely fused; no external sac is present

Meningocele

External sac contains meninges and cerebrospinal fluid

Myelomeningocele

External sac contains meninges, cerebrospinal fluid, peripheral nerves, and spinal cord tissue

SPINAL CORD INJURY

Spinal injuries include fractures, contusions, and compressions of the vertebral column, usually as the result of trauma to the head or neck. The real danger lies in spinal cord damage — cutting, pulling, twisting, or compression. Damage may involve the entire cord or be restricted to one half, and it can occur at any level. Fractures of the C5, C6, C7, T12, and L1 vertebrae are most common.

Causes
Traumatic:
- Motor vehicle accidents
- Falls
- Sports injuries, diving into shallow water
- Gunshot or stab wounds
- Lifting heavy objects.
  Nontraumatic:
- Hyperparathyroidism
- Neoplastic lesions.

Pathophysiology
Like head trauma, spinal cord trauma results from acceleration, deceleration or other deforming forces usually applied from a distance.

Mechanisms triggered by spinal cord trauma include:
- *hyperextension*: acceleration-deceleration forces and sudden reduction in the anteroposterior diameter of the spinal cord
- *hyperflexion*: sudden and excessive force, propelling the neck forward or causing an exaggerated movement to one side
- *vertical compression*: upward or downward force along the vertical axis
- *rotation and shearing*: twisting.

Injury causes microscopic hemorrhages in the gray matter and pia-arachnoid. The hemorrhages gradually increase in size until all of the gray matter is filled with blood, which causes necrosis. From the gray matter, the blood enters the white matter, where it impedes the circulation within the spinal cord. Ensuing edema causes compression and decreases the blood supply. The edema and hemorrhage are greatest at the injury site and approximately two segments above and below it. The edema temporarily adds to the patient's dysfunction by increasing pressure and compressing the nerves. Edema near the C3 to C5 vertebrae may interfere with phrenic nerve-impulse transmission to the diaphragm and inhibit respiratory function.

In the white matter, circulation usually returns to normal in approximately 24 hours. However, in the gray matter, an inflammatory reaction prevents restoration of circulation. Phagocytes appear at the site within 36 to 48 hours after the injury, macrophages engulf degenerating axons, and collagen replaces the normal tissue. Scarring and meningeal thickening leave the nerves in the area blocked or tangled.

Signs and symptoms
- Muscle spasm and back pain that worsens with movement:
- in cervical fractures, pain may cause point tenderness
- in dorsal and lumbar fractures, pain may radiate to other body areas such as the legs
- Mild paresthesia to quadriplegia and shock, if the injury damages the spinal cord; in milder injury, such symptoms may be delayed several days or weeks.
  Specific to injury type or degree:
- Loss of motor function, muscle flaccidity
- Loss of reflexes and sensory function below the level of injury
- Bladder and bowel atony
- Loss of perspiration below the level of injury
- Respiratory impairment.

Diagnostic tests
- Spinal X-rays
- Lumbar puncture
- Computed tomography scan or magnetic resonance imaging.

Treatment
- Immediate immobilization to stabilize the spine and prevent cord damage (primary treatment), including use of sandbags on both sides of the patient's head, a hard cervical collar, or skeletal traction with skull tongs or a halo device for cervical spine injuries
- High doses of methylprednisolone
- Bed rest on firm support (such as a bed board), analgesics, and muscle relaxants
- Plaster cast or a turning frame
- Laminectomy and spinal fusion
- Neurosurgery
- Rehabilitation.

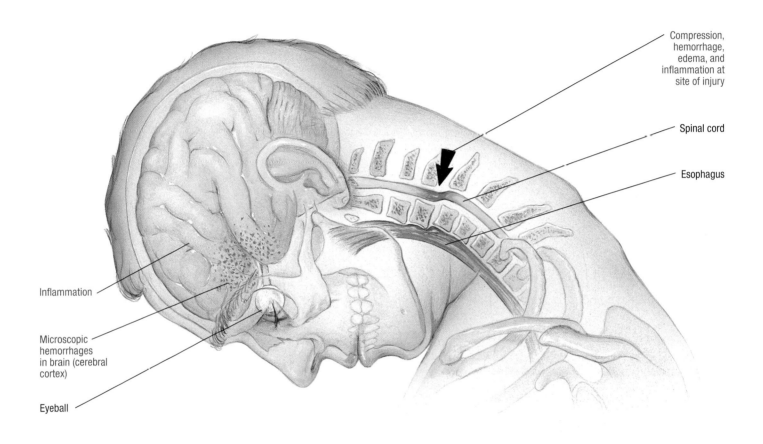

Compression,
hemorrhage,
edema, and
inflammation at
site of injury

Spinal cord

Esophagus

Inflammation

Microscopic
hemorrhages
in brain (cerebral
cortex)

Eyeball

VERTEBRAL DISK INJURY

A herniated disk, also called a ruptured or slipped disk or a herniated nucleus pulposus, occurs when all or part of the *nucleus pulposus* — the soft, gelatinous, central portion of an intervertebral disk — protrudes through the disk's weakened or torn outer ring (*anulus fibrosus*).

Herniated disks usually occur in adults (mostly men) under age 45. About 90% of herniated disks are lumbar or lumbosacral; 8%, cervical; and 1% to 2%, thoracic. Patients with a congenitally small lumbar spinal canal or with osteophyte formation along the vertebrae may be more susceptible to nerve root compression and more likely to have neurologic symptoms.

Causes
- Severe trauma or strain
- Intervertebral joint degeneration.

 AGE ALERT
In older patients whose disks have begun to degenerate, even minor trauma may cause herniation.

Pathophysiology
An intervertebral disk has two parts: the soft center called the *nucleus pulposus* and the tough, fibrous surrounding ring called the *anulus fibrosus*. The nucleus pulposus acts as a shock absorber, distributing the mechanical stress applied to the spine when the body moves.

Physical stress, usually a twisting motion, can tear or rupture the anulus fibrosus so that the nucleus pulposus herniates into the spinal canal. The vertebrae move closer together and in turn exert pressure on the nerve roots as they exit between the vertebrae. Pain and possibly sensory and motor loss follow. A herniated disk also can follow intervertebral joint degeneration; minor trauma may cause herniation.

Herniation occurs in three steps:
- *protrusion:* nucleus pulposus presses against the anulus fibrosus
- *extrusion:* nucleus pulposus bulges forcibly though the anulus fibrosus, pushing against the nerve root
- *sequestration:* anulus gives way as the disk's core bursts and presses against the nerve root.

Signs and symptoms
- Severe low back pain to the buttocks, legs, and feet, usually unilaterally
- Sudden pain after trauma, subsiding in a few days, and then recurring at shorter intervals and with progressive intensity
- Sciatic pain following trauma, beginning as a dull pain in the buttocks; Valsalva's maneuver, coughing, sneezing, and bending intensify the pain, which is often accompanied by muscle spasms
- Sensory and motor loss in the area innervated by the compressed spinal nerve root and, in later stages, weakness and atrophy of leg muscles.

Diagnostic tests
- Straight-leg-raising test
- Lasègue's test
- Spinal X-rays
- Myelography, computed tomography scan, and magnetic resonance imaging.

Treatment
- Heat applications
- Exercise program
- Nonsteroidal anti-inflammatory drugs, such as aspirin; rarely, corticosteroids such as dexamethasone; muscle relaxants, such as diazepam, methocarbamol, or cyclobenzaprine
- Surgery, including laminectomy to remove the protruding disk, spinal fusion to overcome segmental instability, or both to stabilize the spine
- Chemonucleolysis.

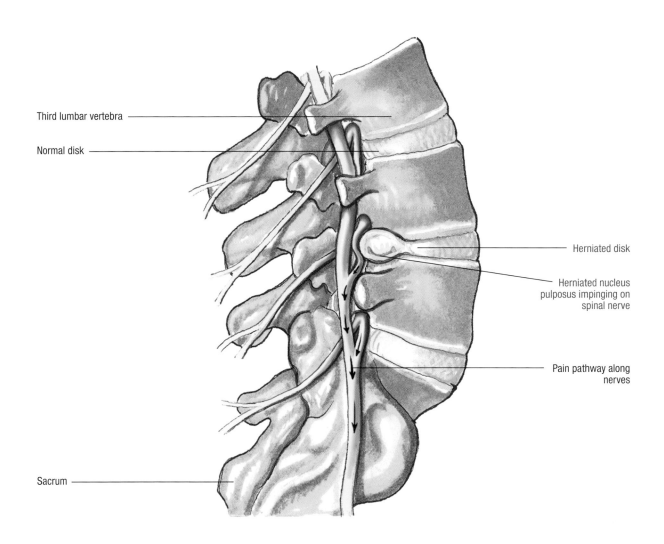

Third lumbar vertebra

Normal disk

Herniated disk

Herniated nucleus pulposus impinging on spinal nerve

Pain pathway along nerves

Sacrum

APPENDICITIS

The most common major surgical disease, appendicitis is inflammation and obstruction of the vermiform appendix. Since the advent of antibiotics, the incidence and the death rate of appendicitis have declined; if untreated, this disease is invariably fatal.

AGE ALERT
Appendicitis may occur at any age, and it affects both sexes equally; however, between puberty and age 25, it's more prevalent in men.

Causes
- Mucosal ulceration
- Fecal mass (fecalith)
- Stricture
- Barium ingestion
- Viral infection.

Pathophysiology
Mucosal ulceration triggers inflammation, which temporarily obstructs the appendix. The obstruction blocks mucus outflow. Pressure in the now distended appendix increases, and the appendix contracts. Bacteria multiply, and inflammation and pressure continue to increase, restricting blood flow to the organ and causing severe abdominal pain.

Inflammation can lead to infection, clotting, tissue decay, and perforation of the appendix. If the appendix ruptures or perforates, the infected contents spill into the abdominal cavity, causing peritonitis, the most common and dangerous complication.

Signs and symptoms
Appendicitis:
- Abdominal pain, which may become localized to the right lower right quadrant
- Rebound tenderness
- Anorexia after the onset of pain
- Nausea or vomiting
- Low-grade fever.
  Rupture:
- Pain
- Tenderness
- Spasm, followed by a brief cessation of abdominal pain.

Diagnostic tests
- White blood cell count
- X-ray with radiographic contrast agent.

Differential diagnosis rules out illnesses with similar symptoms, such as bladder infection, diverticulitis, gastritis, ovarian cyst, pancreatitis, renal colic, and uterine disease.

Treatment
- Nothing by mouth; parenteral fluids and electrolytes
- High Fowler's position
- Nasogastric intubation
- Appendectomy
- Antibiotics.

Small and large intestines

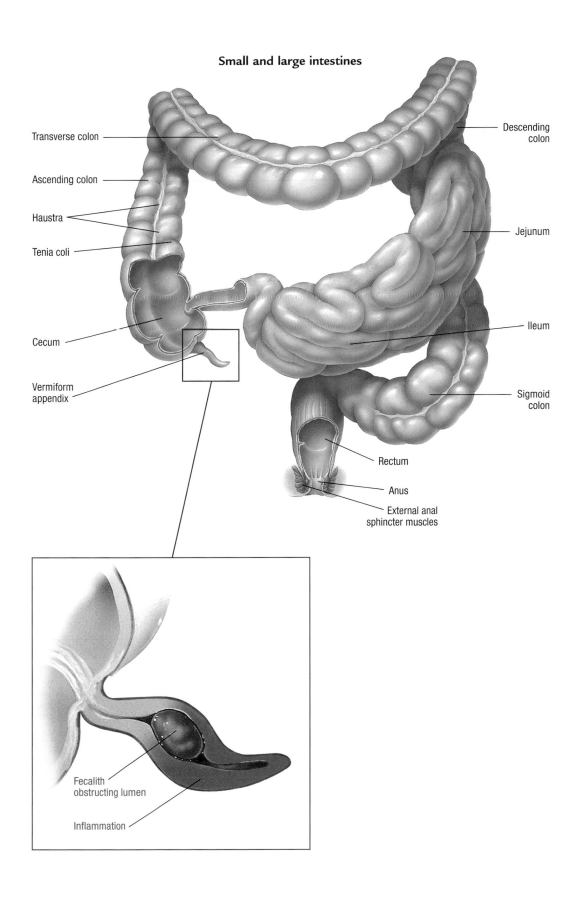

Transverse colon

Ascending colon

Haustra

Tenia coli

Cecum

Vermiform
appendix

Descending
colon

Jejunum

Ileum

Sigmoid
colon

Rectum

Anus

External anal
sphincter muscles

Fecalith
obstructing lumen

Inflammation

CHOLECYSTITIS

Cholecystitis — acute or chronic inflammation causing painful distention of the gallbladder — is usually associated with a gallstone impacted in the cystic duct. Cholecystitis accounts for 10% to 25% of all gallbladder surgery. The acute form is most common among middle-aged women; the chronic form, among the elderly. The prognosis is good with treatment.

Causes
- Gallstones (the most common cause)
- Poor or absent blood flow to the gallbladder
- Abnormal metabolism of cholesterol and bile salts.

Pathophysiology
In acute cholecystitis, inflammation of the gallbladder wall usually develops after a gallstone lodges in the cystic duct. Gallstones typically develop when metabolism of cholesterol and bile salts is abnormal. The liver usually makes bile continuously, and the gallbladder stores it until it's needed to help digest fat. Changes in the composition of bile may cause gallstones to form.

When gallstones block bile flow, the gallbladder becomes inflamed and distended. Growth of bacteria, usually *Escherichia coli*, may contribute to the inflammation and abscess formation or empyema.

Edema of the gallbladder (and sometimes the cystic duct) obstructs flow of bile, which chemically irritates the gallbladder. Cells in the gallbladder wall may become oxygen starved and die as the distended organ presses on vessels and impairs blood flow. The dead cells slough off, and an exudate covers ulcerated areas, causing the gallbladder to adhere to surrounding structures. Complications of cholecystitis include gangrene, hepatitis, pancreatitis, and cholangitis.

Signs and symptoms
- Acute abdominal pain in the right upper quadrant that may radiate to the back, between the shoulders, or to the front of the chest
- Colic
- Nausea and vomiting
- Chills, low-grade fever
- Jaundice.

Diagnostic tests
- X-ray
- White blood cell count
- Ultrasonography
- Technetium-labeled scan
- Percutaneous transhepatic cholangiography or cholesystoscopy
- Serum alkaline phosphate, lactate dehydrogenase, aspartate aminotransferase, amylase, total bilirubin, icteric index.

Treatment
- Cholecystectomy
- Choledochostomy
- Percutaneous transhepatic cholecytostomy
- Endoscopic retrograde cholangiopancreatography
- Lithotripsy
- Oral chenodeoxycholic acid or ursodeoxycholic acid
- Low-fat diet
- Vitamin K
- Antibiotics
- Nasogastric intubation.

Liver and gallbladder

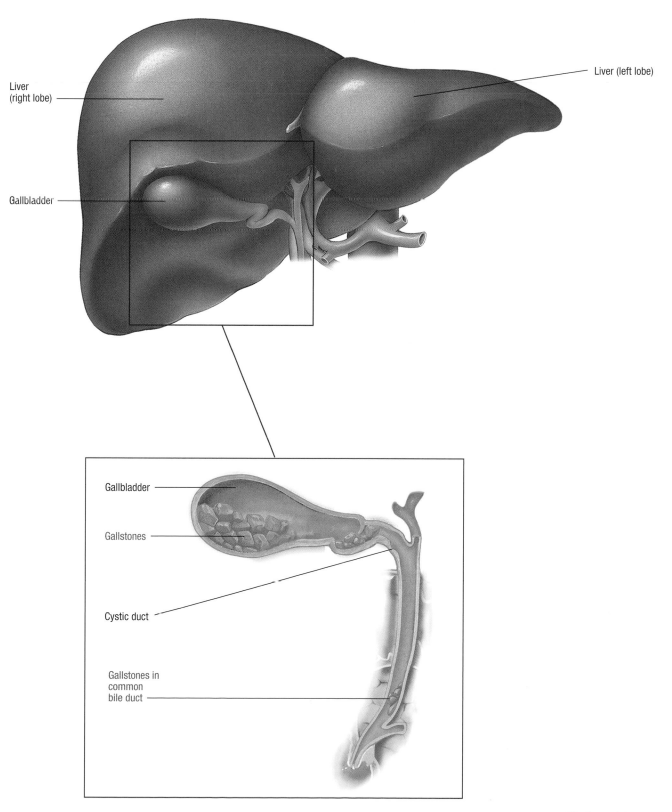

Liver (left lobe)

Liver (right lobe)

Gallbladder

Gallbladder

Gallstones

Cystic duct

Gallstones in common bile duct

CIRRHOSIS

Cirrhosis is a chronic disease characterized by diffuse destruction and fibrotic regeneration of hepatic cells. It's twice as common in men as in women, and is especially prevalent among malnourished persons over the age of 50 with chronic alcoholism. Mortality is high; many patients die within 5 years of onset. As cirrhosis progresses, complications can occur; these may include ascites, portal hypertension, jaundice, coagulopathy, hepatic encephalopathy, bleeding, esophageal varices, acute GI bleeding, liver failure, and renal failure.

Causes

Hepatocellular diseases:
- Postnecrotic cirrhosis: viral hepatitis, toxic exposure
- Laënnec's cirrhosis (portal, nutritional, or alcoholic cirrhosis; most common type of cirrhosis)
- Autoimmune disease, such as sarcoidosis or chronic inflammatory bowel disease.

Cholestatic diseases:
- Biliary cirrhosis: prolonged bile dict obstruction, inflammation.

Metabolic diseases:
- Wilson's disease (autosomal recessive disorder)
- Alpha₁antitrypsin deficiency
- Hemochromatosis (pigment cirrhosis; autosomal recessive disorder).

Other:
- Budd-Chiari syndrome: hepatic vein obstruction
- Cardiac cirrhosis (rare): right-sided heart failure
- Cryptogenic cirrhosis: unknown etiology.

Pathophysiology

The initial event in cirrhosis is hepatic scarring or fibrosis. The scar begins as an increase in extracellular matrix components — fibrin-forming collagens, proteoglycans, fibronectin, and hyaluronic acid. Hepatocyte function is eventually impaired as the matrix changes. Fat-storing cells are believed to be the source of the extracellular changes. Contraction of these cells may also contribute to disruption of the lobular architecture and obstruction of the flow of blood or bile. Cellular changes producing bands of scar tissue also disrupt the lobular structure.

Signs and symptoms

Early stage:
- Anorexia; nausea and vomiting; diarrhea
- Dull abdominal ache.

Late stage:
- Respiratory: pleural effusion, limited thoracic expansion, impaired gas exchange
- Central nervous system: progressive signs or symptoms of hepatic encephalopathy, including lethargy, extreme obtundation, coma
- Hematologic: bleeding tendency, anemia, splenomegaly, portal hypertension
- Endocrine: testicular atrophy, menstrual irregularities, gynecomastia, loss of chest and axillary hair
- Skin: severe pruritus, extreme dryness and poor tissue turgor, spider angiomas, palmar erythema
- Hepatic: jaundice, hepatomegaly, ascites and edema of the legs, hepatorenal syndrome
- Miscellaneous: musty breath, enlarged superficial abdominal veins, pain in the right upper abdominal quadrant that worsens when patient sits up or leans forward, temperature of 101° to 103° F (38° to 39° C)
- Hemorrhage from esophageal varices.

Diagnostic tests

- Liver biopsy
- Abdominal X-ray
- Computed tomography and liver scans
- Esophagogastroduodenoscopy
- Blood studies: liver enzymes, bilirubin, protein, complete blood count, electrolytes, coagulation factors, ammonia levels
- Urine bilirubin, urobilinogen
- Fecal urobilinogen.

Treatment

- Vitamins and nutritional supplements
- Antacids
- Potassium-sparing diuretics
- Vasopressin
- Esophagogastric intubation with multilumen tubes to control bleeding from esophageal varices or other hemorrhage sites
- Gastric lavage
- Esophageal balloon tamponade
- Paracentesis
- Surgical shunt placement
- Sclerosing agents
- Insertion of portosystemic shunts
- Liver transplantation .

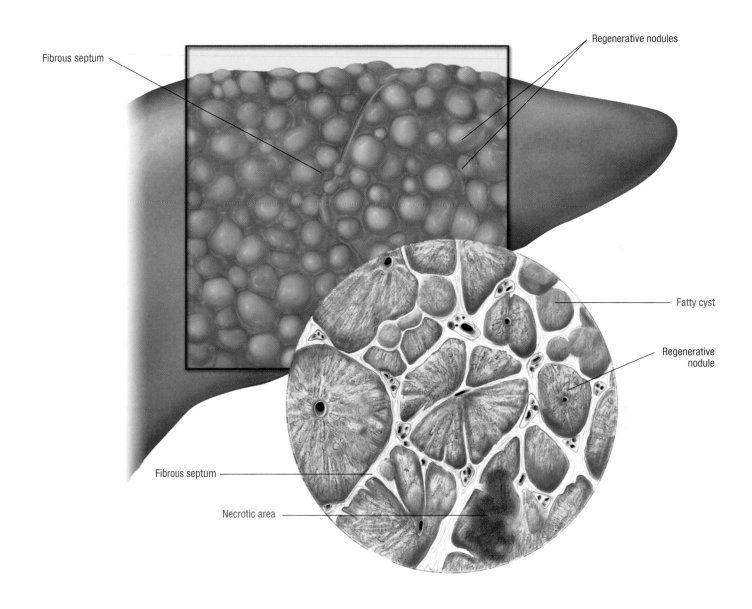

Fibrous septum

Regenerative nodules

Fatty cyst

Regenerative nodule

Fibrous septum

Necrotic area

COLONIC POLYPS

A polyp is a small tumorlike growth that projects from a mucous membrane surface. Types of polyps include common polypoid adenomas, villous adenomas, hereditary polyposis, focal polypoid hyperplasia, and juvenile polyps (hamartomas). Most rectal polyps are benign; however, villous and hereditary polyps tend to become malignant. Indeed, a striking feature of familial polyposis is its strong association with rectosigmoid adenocarcinoma.

 AGE ALERT
Juvenile polyps, usually occurring among children under age 10, are characterized by rectal bleeding. Villous adenomas are most prevalent in men over age 55; common polypoid adenomas, in white women between ages 45 and 60. Incidence of nonjuvenile polyps rises after age 70 in both sexes.

Causes
Unknown.
Predisposing factors:
- Heredity
- Age
- Infection
- Diet.

Pathophysiology
Colonic polyps are masses of tissue resulting from unrestrained cell growth in the upper epithelium that rise above the mucosal membrane and protrude into the GI tract.

Signs and symptoms
- Usually asymptomatic; discovered incidentally during a digital examination or rectosigmoidoscopy
- Rectal bleeding (high rectal polyps leave a streak of blood on the stool, whereas low rectal polyps bleed freely)
- Secondary fluid and electrolyte imbalances
- Secondary anemia.

 CLINICAL TIP
Although most are asymptomatic, polyps may cause symptoms by virtue of their protrusion into the bowel lumen. They may bleed, cause abdominal pain, or actually obstruct the intestine.

Diagnostic tests
- Barium enema
- Fecal occult blood
- Hemoglobin and hematocrit
- Serum electrolytes (to rule out villous adenomas)
- Proctosigmoidoscopy or colonoscopy and rectal biopsy.

Treatment
Common polypoid adenomas:
- Less than 1 cm in size: polypectomy, commonly by fulguration during endoscopy
- Over 4 cm: abdominoperineal resection or low anterior resection.
  Invasive villous adenomas:
- Abdominoperineal resection
- Low anterior resection.
  Focal polypoid hyperplasia:
- Obliterated by biopsy.
  Hereditary polyps:
- Total abdominoperineal resection with permanent ileostomy
- Subtotal colectomy with ileoproctostomy
- Ileoanal anastomosis.
  Juvenile polyps:
- Often autoamputate
- Snare removal during colonoscopy.

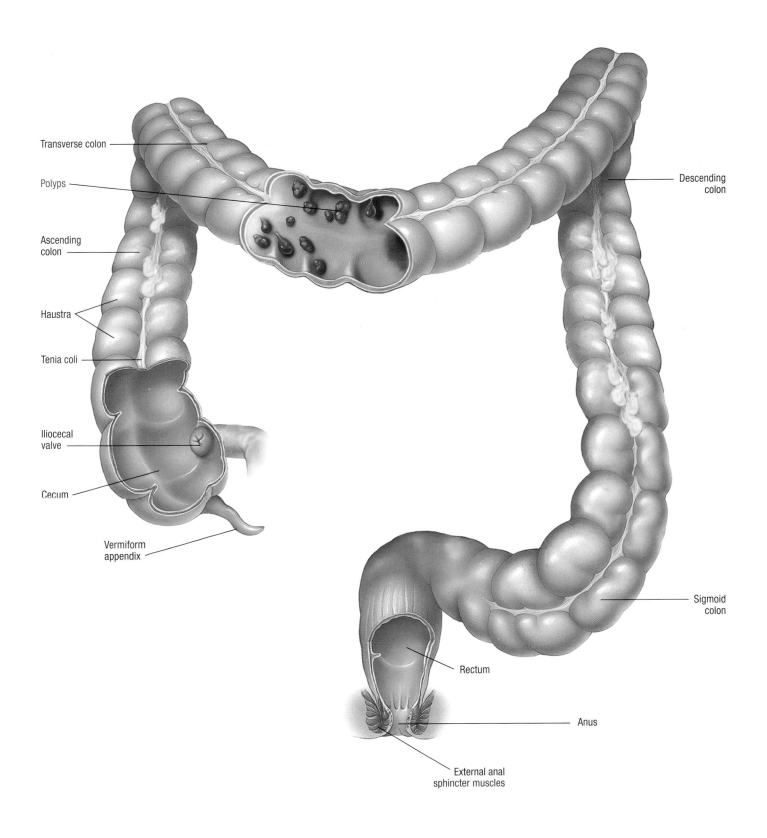

Transverse colon

Polyps

Ascending colon

Haustra

Tenia coli

Iliocecal valve

Cecum

Vermiform appendix

Descending colon

Sigmoid colon

Rectum

Anus

External anal sphincter muscles

COLORECTAL CANCER

Colorectal cancer is the second most common visceral malignant neoplasm in the United States and Europe. It tends to progress slowly and remains localized for a long time. Incidence is equally distributed between men and women. It's potentially curable in about 90% of patients if early diagnosis allows resection before nodal involvement.

Causes
Unknown.
Risk factors:
- Intake of excessive saturated animal fat
- Other diseases of the digestive tract
- Age (over 40)
- History of ulcerative colitis (average interval before onset of cancer is 11 to 17 years)
- Familial polyposis (cancer almost always develops by age 50).

Pathophysiology
Most lesions of the large bowel are moderately differentiated adenocarcinomas. These tumors tend to grow slowly and remain asymptomatic for long periods of time. Tumors in the sigmoid and descending colon grow circumferentially and constrict the intestinal lumen. At diagnosis, tumors in the ascending colon are usually large and are palpable on physical examination.

Signs and symptoms
- Changes in bowel habits, such as bleeding, pain, anemia, and anorexia
- Symptoms of local obstruction
- Symptoms of direct extension to adjacent organs (bladder, prostate, ureters, vagina, sacrum)
- Symptoms from distant metastasis (usually liver).

Signs specific to site of obstruction:
- Right colon:
- black, tarry stools; anemia
- abdominal aching or pressure; dull cramps
- weakness, fatigue, exertional dyspnea
- weight loss
- Left colon:
- rectal bleeding; dark or bright red blood or mucus in stools
- abdominal fullness or cramping
- rectal pressure
- obstipation
- diarrhea
- ribbon- or pencil-shaped stools
- pain relieved by flatus or bowel movement.

Diagnostic tests
- Fecal occult blood
- Digital rectal examination (can detect almost 15% of tumors)
- Proctoscopy or sigmoidoscopy
- Colonoscopy
- Tumor biopsy
- Barium X-ray, using dual contrast with air
- Computed tomography scan
- Carcinoembryonic antigen (not specific or sensitive enough for early diagnosis; helpful in monitoring for metastasis or recurrence).

Treatment
- Surgery to remove tumor plus adjacent tissues and any lymph nodes that may contain cancer cells
- Chemotherapy for patients with metastasis, residual disease, or a recurrent inoperable tumor
- Radiation therapy for tumor mass reduction, done before or after surgery or combined with chemotherapy.

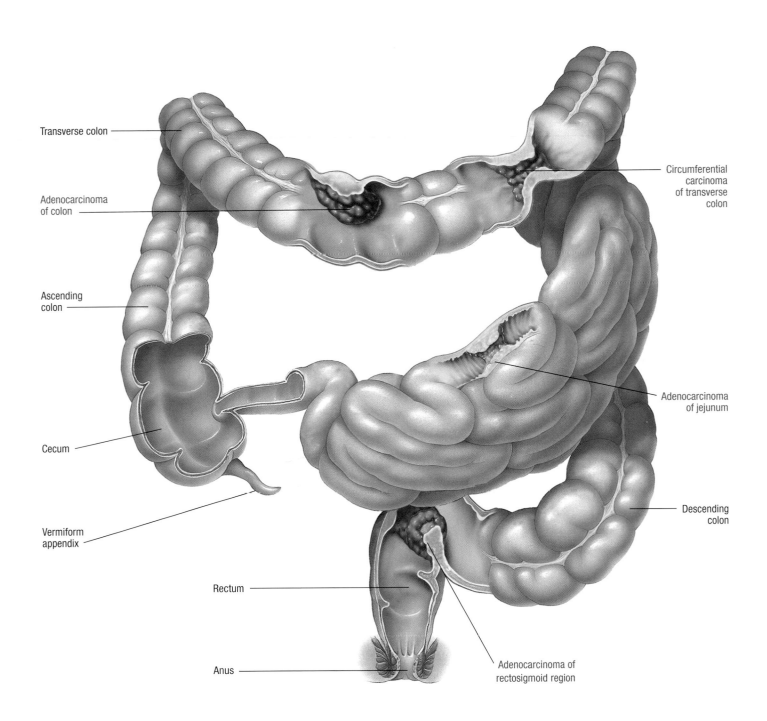

Transverse colon

Adenocarcinoma of colon

Ascending colon

Cecum

Vermiform appendix

Rectum

Anus

Circumferential carcinoma of transverse colon

Adenocarcinoma of jejunum

Descending colon

Adenocarcinoma of rectosigmoid region

CROHN'S DISEASE

Crohn's disease, also known as *regional enteritis* or *granulomatous colitis*, is inflammation of any part of the GI tract (usually the terminal ileum), extending through all layers of the intestinal wall. It may also involve regional lymph nodes and the mesentery.

 AGE ALERT
Crohn's disease is most prevalent in adults ages 20 to 40.

Causes

Unknown.

Possible contributing conditions:
- Lymphatic obstruction
- Allergies, immune disorders
- Infection
- Genetic predisposition.

Pathophysiology

Whatever the cause of Crohn's disease, inflammation spreads slowly and progressively. Enlarged lymph nodes block lymph flow in the submucosa. Lymphatic obstruction leads to edema, mucosal ulceration and fissures, abscesses, and sometimes granulomas. Mucosal ulcerations are called "skipping lesions" because they are not continuous, as in ulcerative colitis.

Oval, elevated patches of closely packed lymph follicles — called Peyer's patches — develop in the lining of the small intestine. Subsequent fibrosis thickens the bowel wall and causes stenosis, or narrowing of the lumen. The serous membrane becomes inflamed (serositis), inflamed bowel loops adhere to other diseased or normal loops, and diseased bowel segments become interspersed with healthy ones. Finally, diseased parts of the bowel become thicker, narrower, and shorter.

Signs and symptoms

- Steady, colicky pain in right lower quadrant
- Cramping, tenderness
- Weight loss
- Diarrhea, steatorrhea, bloody stools
- Low-grade fever.

Diagnostic tests

- Fecal occult blood
- Small-bowel X-ray, barium enema
- Sigmoidoscopy, colonoscopy
- Biopsy
- Blood tests, including white blood cell count, hemoglobin, erythrocyte sedimentation rate, electrolytes.

Treatment

- Corticosteroids, immunosuppressants
- Sulfasalazine
- Metronidazole
- Antidiarrheals (not in patients with significant bowel obstruction)
- Narcotic analgesics
- Stress reduction and reduced physical activity
- Vitamin supplements
- Avoidance of fruits and vegetables; high-fiber, spicy, or fatty foods; dairy products; carbonated or caffeine-containing beverages; foods or liquids that stimulate intestinal activity
- Surgery, if necessary.

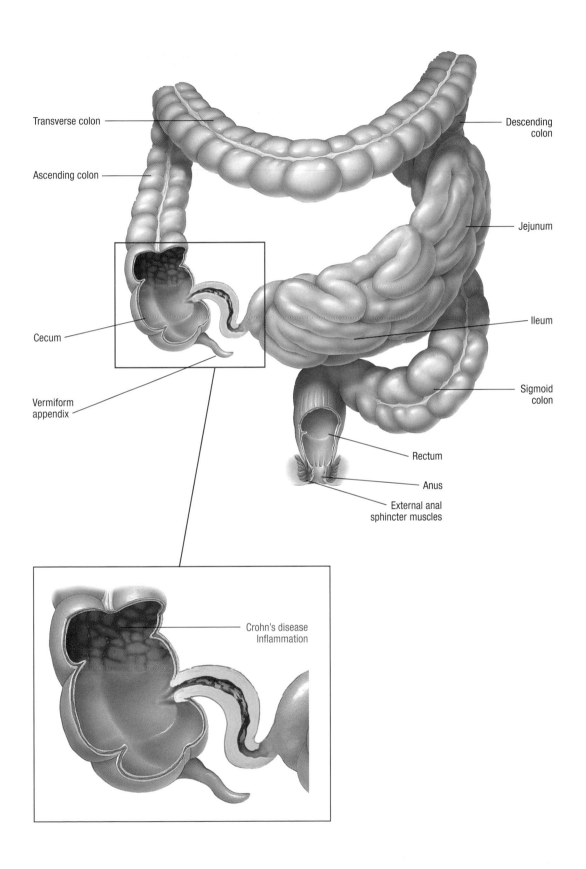

Transverse colon

Ascending colon

Cecum

Vermiform appendix

Descending colon

Jejunum

Ileum

Sigmoid colon

Rectum

Anus

External anal sphincter muscles

Crohn's disease Inflammation

DIVERTICULAR DISEASE

In diverticular disease, bulging pouches (diverticula) in the GI wall push the mucosal lining through the surrounding muscle. Although the most common site for diverticula is in the sigmoid colon, they may develop anywhere, from the proximal end of the pharynx to the anus. Common sites include the duodenum, near the pancreatic border or the ampulla of Vater, and the jejunum.

Diverticular disease of the stomach is rare and is usually a precursor of peptic or neoplastic disease. Diverticular disease of the ileum (Meckel's diverticulum) is the most common congenital anomaly of the GI tract.

Diverticular disease has two clinical forms:
• diverticulosis – diverticula present but asymptomatic
• diverticulitis – inflamed diverticula; may cause potentially fatal obstruction, infection, hemorrhage.

 AGE ALERT
Diverticular disease is most prevalent in men over age 40 and persons who eat a low-fiber diet. More than half of patients older than 50 years have colonic diverticula.

Causes
• Exact cause unknown
• Diminished colonic motility and increased intraluminal pressure
• Defects in colon wall strength.

Pathophysiology
Diverticula probably result from high intraluminal pressure on an area of weakness in the GI wall where blood vessels enter. Diet may be a contributing factor, because insufficient fiber reduces fecal residue, narrows the bowel lumen, and leads to high intra-abdominal pressure during defecation.

In *diverticulitis*, undigested food and bacteria accumulate in the diverticular sac. This hard mass cuts off the blood supply to the thin walls of the sac, making them more susceptible to attack by colonic bacteria. Inflammation follows and may lead to perforation, abscess, peritonitis, obstruction, or hemorrhage. Occasionally, the inflamed colon segment adheres to the bladder or other organs and causes a fistula.

Signs and symptoms
Diverticulosis:
• Asymptomatic.
  Mild diverticulitis:
• Moderate left lower abdominal pain
• Low-grade fever
• Leukocytosis
• Nausea and vomiting.
  Severe diverticulitis:
• Nausea and vomiting
• Left lower quadrant pain; abdominal rigidity
• High fever, chills, hypotension, shock
• Microscopic to massive hemorrhage.
  Chronic diverticulitis:
• Constipation, ribbon-like stools, intermittent diarrhea, abdominal distention
• Abdominal rigidity and pain, diminished or absent bowel sounds, nausea, and vomiting.

Diagnostic tests
• Upper GI series
• Barium enema
• Biopsy
• Blood studies, including erythrocyte sedimentation rate.

Treatment
• Liquid or bland diet, stool softeners, occasional doses of mineral oil
• Meperidine
• Antispasmodics
• Antibiotics
• Exercise
• Colon resection with removal of involved segment
• Temporary colostomy if necessary
• Blood transfusions if necessary
• High-residue diet after pain has subsided.

DIVERTICULOSIS OF COLON

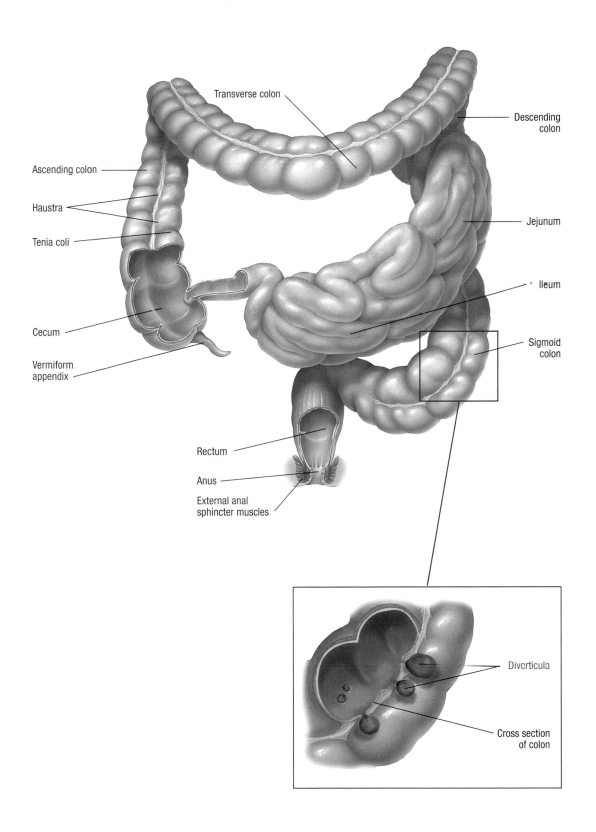

Transverse colon

Descending colon

Ascending colon

Haustra

Tenia coli

Jejunum

Ileum

Cecum

Sigmoid colon

Vermiform appendix

Rectum

Anus

External anal sphincter muscles

Diverticula

Cross section of colon

ESOPHAGEAL CANCER

Esophageal cancer is nearly always fatal. This disease occurs worldwide, but incidence varies geographically. It's most common in Japan, China, the Middle East, and parts of South Africa. Common sites of distant metastasis include the liver and lungs.

 AGE ALERT
Esophageal cancer most commonly develops in men over age 60.

Causes
Unknown.
Predisposing factors:
- Chronic irritation by heavy smoking and excessive use of alcohol
- Stasis-induced inflammation
- Nutritional deficiency
- Diets high in nitrosoamines.

Pathophysiology
Esophageal cancer includes two types of malignant tumors: squamous cell carcinoma and adenocarcinoma. Most esophageal cancers are poorly differentiated squamous cell carcinomas. Adenocarcinomas are less frequent and are contained to the lower third of the esophagus. Esophageal tumors are usually fungating and infiltrating.

Signs and symptoms
- Dysphagia and weight loss (most common)
- Esophageal obstruction
- Pain
- Hoarseness, coughing
- Cachexia.
  Complications of metastases:
- Tracheoesophageal fistulas
- Mediastinitis
- Aortic perforation.

Diagnostic tests
- X-ray, barium swallow, motility studies
- Endoscopic examination
- Punch and brush biopsies
- Exfoliative cytology.

Treatment
- Usually multimodal
- Resection to maintain a passageway for food
- Palliative treatments:
- feeding gastrostomy and chemotherapy
- insertion of a prosthetic tube and chemotherapy.

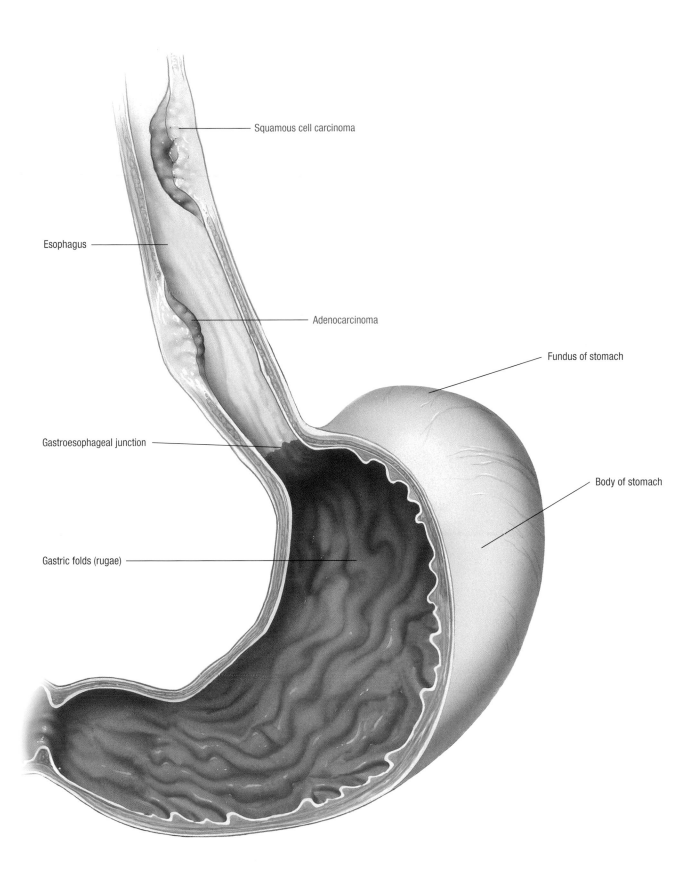

Squamous cell carcinoma

Esophagus

Adenocarcinoma

Fundus of stomach

Gastroesophageal junction

Body of stomach

Gastric folds (rugae)

GASTRIC CANCER

Gastric carcinoma is common throughout the world and affects all races; however, mortality is highest in Japan, Iceland, Chile, and Austria. In the United States, the incidence has decreased by 50% over the past 25 years and the resulting death rate is one-third of what it was 30 years ago.

 AGE ALERT
Incidence of gastric cancer is highest in men over age 40.

Causes
Unknown; commonly associated with atrophic gastritis.
Predisposing factors:
- Tobacco smoke
- Asbestos exposure
- High alcohol intake
- Intake of smoked, pickled, or salt-preserved foods
- Type A blood
- *Heliocobacter pylori* infection (distal gastric cancer).

Pathophysiology
According to gross appearance, gastric carcinoma can be classified as polypoid, ulcerating, ulcerating and infiltrating, or diffuse. The parts of the stomach affected by gastric carcinoma, listed in order of decreasing frequency, are the pylorus and antrum, the lesser curvature, the cardia, the body of the stomach, and the greater curvature. Gastric carcinoma infiltrates rapidly to regional lymph nodes, omentum, liver, and lungs.

Signs and symptoms
Early clues:
- Chronic dyspepsia, epigastric discomfort.
  Later clues:
- Weight loss, anorexia
- Dysphagia, feeling of fullness after eating
- Anemia, fatigue
- Coffee-ground emesis.

Diagnostic tests
- Reinvestigation of persistent or recurring GI changes and complaints
- Blood, stool, and gastric-fluid studies to rule out conditions producing similar symptoms
- Barium X-rays with fluoroscopy
- Fiber-optic gastroscopy and photography
- Studies to rule out specific organ metastases, such as computed tomography scans, magnetic resonance imaging, chest X-rays, liver and bone scans, and liver biopsy.

Treatment
- Excision of lesion with appropriate margins (possible in over one-third of patients) by subtotal or total gastrectomy or gastrojejunostomy
- Palliative surgery
- Radiation therapy with chemotherapy for patients with unresectable or partially resectable disease
- Antispasmodics, antacids for GI distress.

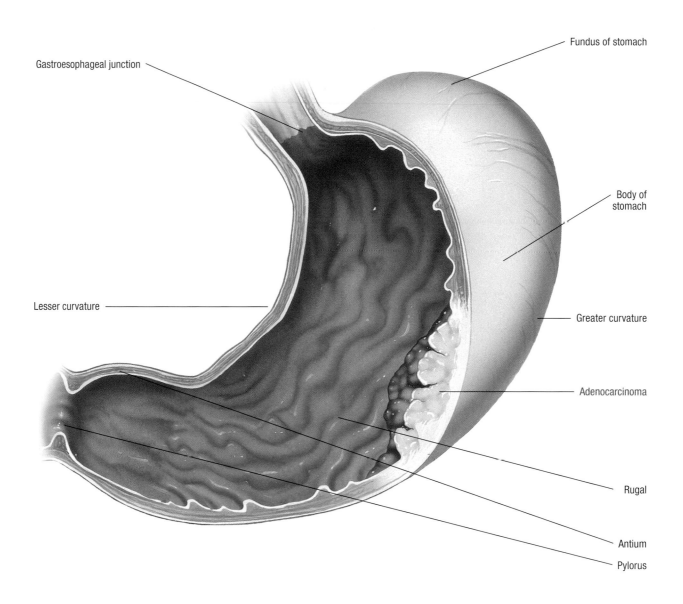

Fundus of stomach

Gastroesophageal junction

Body of stomach

Lesser curvature

Greater curvature

Adenocarcinoma

Rugal

Antium

Pylorus

GASTRITIS

Gastritis, an inflammation of the gastric mucosa, may be acute or chronic. *Acute gastritis* produces mucosal reddening, edema, hemorrhage, and erosion; this benign, self-limiting disease is usually a response to local irritants. *Chronic gastritis* is common among elderly persons and those with pernicious anemia. It's characterized by progressive cell atrophy and commonly occurs as chronic atrophic gastritis (inflammation of all stomach mucosal layers and reduced numbers of chief and parietal cells). Acute or chronic gastritis can occur at any age.

Causes
Acute gastritis:
● Habitually ingested irritants, such as hot peppers, alcohol
● Drugs, such as aspirin, other nonsteroidal anti-inflammatory agents, cytotoxic agents, caffeine, corticosteroids, antimetabolites, phenylbutazone
● Poisons, such as DDT, ammonia, mercury, carbon tetrachloride, corrosive substances
● Bacterial endotoxins, such as staphylococci, *Escherichia coli*, salmonella.
   Nonerosive chronic gastritis:
● *Helicobacter pylori* infection.

Pathophysiology
Gastritis is an inflammation of the lining of the stomach. As mucus membranes become more eroded, gastric juices, containing pepsin and acid, come into contact with the erosion and an ulcer forms.

Acute gastritis leading to stress ulcers also may develop in acute illnesses, especially when the patient has had major traumatic injuries; burns; severe infection; hepatic, renal, or respiratory failure; or major surgery.

Chronic gastritis may be associated with peptic ulcer disease or gastrostomy, both of which cause chronic reflux of pancreatic secretions, bile, and bile acids from the duodenum into the stomach. Recurring exposure to irritating substances, such as drugs, alcohol, cigarette smoke, or environmental agents, may also lead to chronic gastritis. Chronic gastritis may occur in patients with pernicious anemia, renal disease, or diabetes mellitus.

Pernicious anemia is often associated with atrophic gastritis, a chronic inflammation of the stomach resulting from degeneration of the gastric mucosa. In pernicious anemia, the stomach can no longer secrete intrinsic factor, which is needed for vitamin B_{12} absorption.

Signs and symptoms
Acute gastritis:
● Rapid onset after exposure to offending substance; symptoms lasting from a few hours to a few days
● Epigastric discomfort, indigestion
● Cramping
● Anorexia; nausea, vomiting
● Hematemesis.
   Chronic gastritis:
● Similar to acute form
● Mild epigastric discomfort
● Vague complaints, such as an intolerance of spicy or fatty foods or slight pain relieved by eating.
   Chronic atrophic gastritis:
● May be asymptomatic.

Diagnostic tests
● Gastroscopy (contraindicated after ingestion of a corrosive agent)
● Laboratory analyses for occult blood in vomitus or stools (or both)
● Hemoglobin levels and hematocrit.

Treatment
● Elimination of the cause
● Antacids; histamine antagonists
● Blood replacement
● Iced saline lavage, possibly with norepinephrine
● Angiography with vasopressin
● Surgery — vagotomy, pyloroplasty, partial or total gastrectomy.

CLINICAL TIP
Simply avoiding aspirin and spicy foods may relieve chronic gastritis.

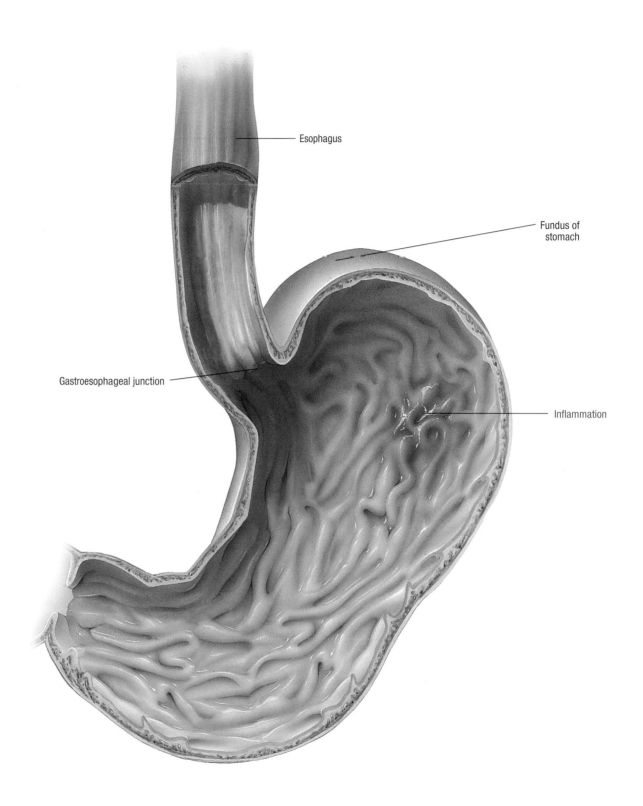

Esophagus

Fundus of stomach

Gastroesophageal junction

Inflammation

GASTROESOPHAGEAL REFLUX DISEASE

Popularly known as heartburn, gastroesophageal reflux disease (GERD) refers to backflow of gastric or duodenal contents or both into the esophagus and past the lower esophageal sphincter (LES), without associated belching or vomiting. The reflux of gastric contents causes acute epigastric pain, usually after a meal. The pain may radiate to the chest or arms. It commonly occurs in pregnant or obese persons. Lying down after a meal also contributes to reflux.

Causes
- Weak esophageal sphincter
- Increased abdominal pressure, as in obesity or pregnancy
- Hiatal hernia
- Medications, such as morphine, meperidine, diazepam, calcium channel blockers, anticholinergic agents
- Food (eating lowers LES pressure)
- Alcohol, cigarette smoke
- Nasogastric intubation for longer than 4 days.

Pathophysiology
Normally, the LES maintains enough pressure around the lower end of the esophagus to close it and prevent reflux. Typically, the sphincter relaxes after each swallow to allow food into the stomach. In GERD, the sphincter does not remain closed (usually due to deficient LES pressure or pressure within the stomach exceeding LES pressure) and stomach contents flow into the esophagus. The high acidity of the stomach contents causes pain and irritation in the esophagus, and stricture or ulceration can occur. If the gastric contents enter the throat and are aspirated, chronic pulmonary disease may result.

Signs and symptoms
- Burning epigastric pain, possibly radiating to arms and chest, usually after a meal or when lying down
- Feeling of fluid accumulation in the throat without a sour or bitter taste
- Dyspepsia.

Diagnostic tests
- Esophageal acidity monitoring to evaluate LES competence
- Acid perfusion test
- Esophagoscopy
- Barium swallow, upper GI series
- Esophageal manometry.

Treatment
- Frequent, small meals; avoidance of eating just before going to bed
- Sitting up during and after meals; sleeping with head of bed elevated
- Increased fluid intake
- Antacids, histamine-2-receptor antagonists
- Proton pump inhibitors
- Smoking cessation; reduction or cessation of alcohol intake
- Surgery if hiatal hernia is the cause or patient has refractory symptoms.

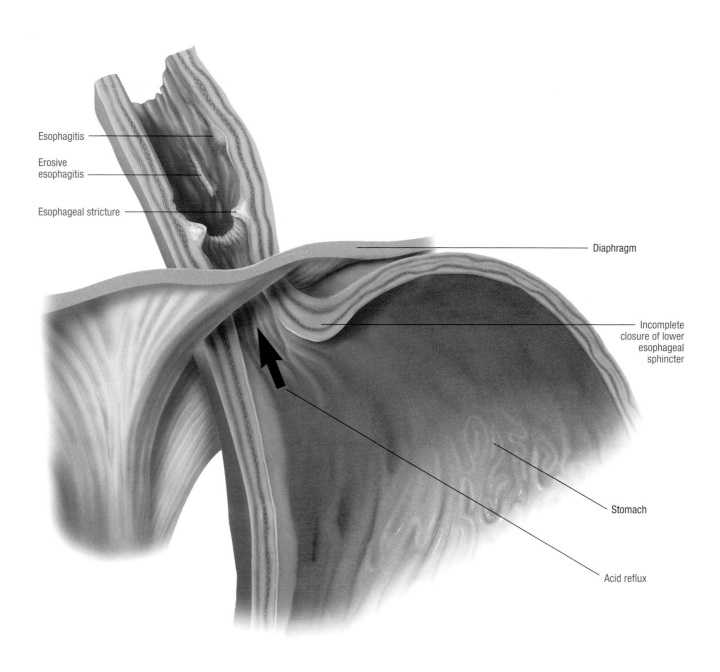

Esophagitis

Erosive esophagitis

Esophageal stricture

Diaphragm

Incomplete closure of lower esophageal sphincter

Stomach

Acid reflux

Hemorrhoids

Hemorrhoids are varicosities in the superior or inferior hemorrhoidal venous plexus. Dilation and enlargement of the plexus of superior hemorrhoidal veins above the dentate line cause internal hemorrhoids. Enlargement of the plexus of inferior hemorrhoidal veins below the dentate line causes external hemorrhoids, which may protrude from the rectum. Hemorrhoids occur in both sexes.

 AGE ALERT
Incidence is generally highest between ages 20 and 50.

Causes
- Straining at defecation, constipation, low-fiber diet
- Pregnancy
- Obesity
- Prolonged sitting.
  Predisposing factors:
- Hepatic disease, such as amebic abscesses, or hepatitis
- Alcoholism
- Anorectal infections.

Pathophysiology
Hemorrhoids result from activities that increase intravenous pressure, causing distention and engorgement. Hemorrhoids are classified according to severity, as follows:
- *First-degree*: confined to the anal canal
- *Second-degree*: prolapse during straining but reduce spontaneously
- *Third-degree*: prolapse and require manual reduction after each bowel movement
- *Fourth-degree*: irreducible.

Signs and symptoms
- Bright red blood on outside of the stool or on toilet tissue
- Painless, intermittent bleeding during defecation
- Anal itching, vague anal discomfort
- Prolapse of rectal mucosa
- Pain
- Secondary anemia.

Diagnostic tests
- Anoscopy
- Flexible sigmoidoscopy.

Treatment
- High-fiber diet, increased fluid intake, bulking agents
- Avoidance of straining
- Local anesthetic agents, hydrocortisone cream, suppositories
- Warm sitz baths
- Injection sclerotherapy or rubber band ligation
- Hemorrhoidectomy.

INTERNAL AND EXTERNAL HEMORRHOIDS

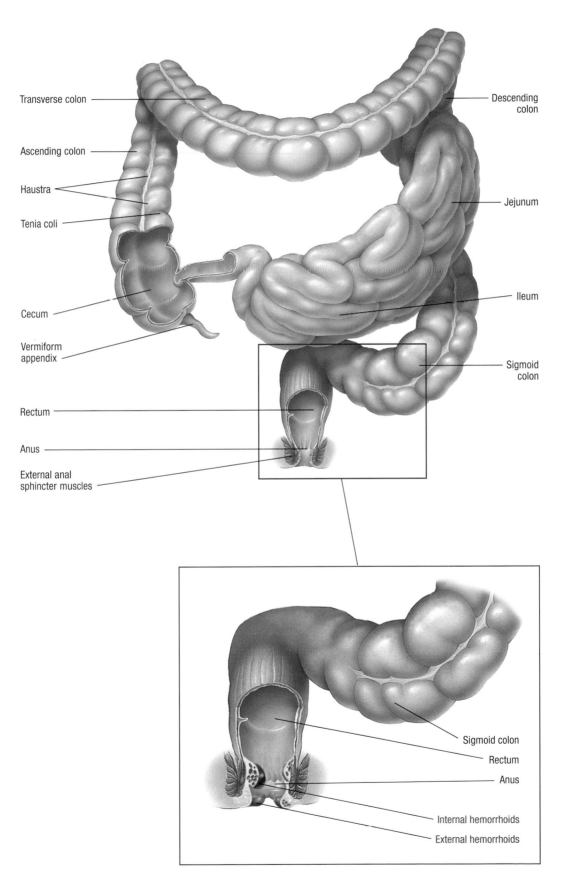

Transverse colon

Ascending colon

Haustra

Tenia coli

Cecum

Vermiform appendix

Rectum

Anus

External anal sphincter muscles

Descending colon

Jejunum

Ileum

Sigmoid colon

Sigmoid colon

Rectum

Anus

Internal hemorrhoids

External hemorrhoids

HEPATITIS

Nonviral hepatitis is an inflammation of the liver that usually re-sults from exposure to certain chemicals or drugs. Most pa-tients recover from this illness, although a few develop fulmi-nating hepatitis, hepatic failure, or cirrhosis.

Viral hepatitis is a common infection, resulting in hepatic cell destruction, necrosis, and autolysis. In most patients, hepatic cells eventually regenerate with little or no residual damage. However, old age and serious underlying disorders make com-plications more likely. The prognosis is poor if edema and he-patic encephalopathy develop.

Types of hepatitis

Five major forms of viral hepatitis are currently recognized:
- *Type A* (infectious or short-incubation hepatitis): most com-mon among children and young adults; transmitted by fecal contamination of food, water, or poorly cooked shellfish
- *Type B* (serum or long-incubation hepatitis): most common among people infected with the HIV-positive population; rou-tine screening of donor blood for the hepatitis B surface anti-gen has reduced the incidence of posttransfusion cases, but transmission by needles shared among drug abusers remains a major problem
- *Type C:* accounts for about 20% of all viral hepatitis cases and for most posttransfusion cases
- *Type D* (delta hepatitis): responsible for about 50% of all cases of fulminant hepatitis, which has a high mortality. Developing in 1% of patients with viral hepatitis, fulminant he-patitis causes unremitting liver failure with encephalopathy. It progresses to coma and commonly leads to death within 2 weeks. In the United States, type D occurs only in people who are frequently exposed to blood and blood products, such as I.V. drug users and hemophilia patients.
- *Type E* (formerly grouped with types C and D under the name non-A, non-B hepatitis): occurs primarily among pa-tients who have recently returned from an endemic area (such as India, Africa, Asia, or Central America); more common in young adults; more severe in pregnant women.

Causes

Nonviral:
- Hepatotoxic chemicals, such as carbon tetrachloride, trichloroethylene, vinyl chloride
- Hepatotoxic drugs, such as acetaminophen
- Poisonous mushrooms.
  Viral:
- Infection by hepatitis virus A, B, C, D, or E.

Pathophysiology

Nonviral:
After exposure to a hepatotoxin, hepatic cellular necrosis, scar-ring, Kupffer cell hyperplasia, and infiltration by mononuclear phagocytes occur with varying severity. Alcohol, anoxia, and preexisting liver disease exacerbate the effects of some toxins.

Drug-induced hepatitis may begin with a hypersensitivity reaction unique to the individual, unlike toxic hepatitis, which appears to affect all exposed people indiscriminately. Symp-toms usually manifest after 2 to 5 weeks of therapy.

Viral:
Hepatic damage is usually similar in all types of viral hepatitis, but extent of cell injury or necrosis varies.

The virus causes hepatocyte injury and death, either by di-rectly killing the cells or by activating inflammatory and im-mune reactions. The inflammatory and immune reactions, in turn, injure or destroy hepatocytes by lysing the infected or neighboring cells. Later, direct antibody attack against the viral antigens causes further destruction of the infected cells. Edema and swelling of the interstitium lead to collapse of cap-illaries, decreased blood flow, tissue hypoxia, scarring, and fi-brosis. Complications include chronic persistent hepatitis (which may prolong recovery up to 8 months), chronic active hepatitis, cirrhosis, hepatic failure and death, and primary he-patocellular carcinoma.

Signs and symptoms

Nonviral:
- Anorexia, nausea, vomiting
- Jaundice, dark urine, clay-colored stool
- Hepatomegaly
- Possible abdominal pain
- Pruritus.
  Viral, prodromal phase:
- Easy fatigue, generalized malaise, anorexia, mild weight loss
- Arthralgia, myalgia
- Nausea, vomiting, changes in senses of taste and smell
- Fever
- Right upper quadrant tenderness
- Dark-colored urine, clay-colored stools.
  Icteric phase:
- Jaundice
- Worsening of prodromal symptoms
- Pruritus
- Abdominal pain or tenderness.
  Recovery:
- Symptoms subside and appetite returns.

Diagnostic tests

- Hepatitis profile
- Liver enzymes
- Total and direct bilirubin
- White blood cell and eosinophil counts
- Prothrombin time
- Liver biopsy.

Treatment

Nonviral:
- Lavage, catharsis, or hyperventilation, depending on the route of exposure — as soon as possible after exposure
- Acetylcysteine as antidote for acetaminophen poisoning
- Corticosteroids.
  Viral:
- Rest to minimize energy demands
- Avoidance of alcohol or other hepatotoxic drugs
- Small, high-calorie meals
- Parenteral nutrition if patient can't eat.

EFFECT OF HEPATITIS ON LIVER APPEARANCE

Normal liver

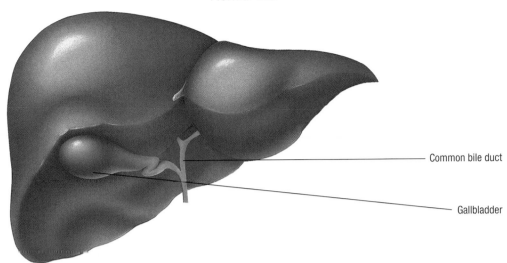

Common bile duct

Gallbladder

Nonviral hepatitis

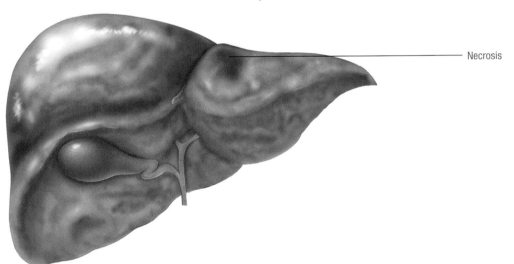

Necrosis

Viral hepatitis

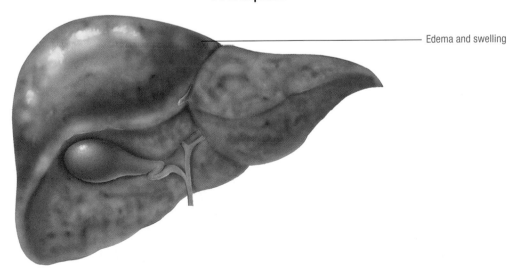

Edema and swelling

HIATAL HERNIA

Hiatal hernia is a defect in the diaphragm that permits a portion of the stomach to pass through the diaphragmatic opening into the chest. Hiatal hernia is the most common problem of the diaphragm affecting the alimentary canal. Treatment can prevent complications such as strangulation of the herniated intrathoracic portion of the stomach.

Causes
- Esophageal carcinoma
- Kyphoscoliosis
- Trauma
- Congenital diaphragm malformations.
    Contributing factors:
- Aging, obesity, trauma.

Pathophysiology
Hernias typically result when an organ protrudes through an abnormal opening in the muscle wall of the cavity that surrounds it. In hiatal hernias, a portion of the stomach protrudes through the diaphragm.

Three types of hiatal hernia can occur: sliding, paraesophageal (rolling), or mixed, which include features of both. In a sliding hernia, both the stomach and the gastroesophageal junction slip up into the chest, so the gastroesophageal junction is above the diaphragmatic hiatus. In paraesophageal hernia, a part of the greater curvature of the stomach rolls through the diaphragmatic defect.

Signs and symptoms
Sliding with competent lower esophageal sphincter (LES):
- No reflux or symptoms.
    Sliding with incompetent LES:
- Pyrosis
  - onset 1 to 4 hours after eating
  - aggravated by reclining, belching, increased intra-abdominal pressure
- Retrosternal or substernal pain.
    Paraesophageal hernia:
- Produces no symptoms; usually found incidentally on X-ray or when testing for occult blood.

Diagnostic tests
- Chest X-ray
- Barium study
- Endoscopy and biopsy
- Esophageal motility and pH studies
- Acid perfusion (Bernstein) test
- Complete blood count, stool guaiac test to detect GI bleeding
- Analysis of gastric contents for blood.

Treatment
- Restrict activities that raise intra-abdominal pressure (coughing, straining, bending)
- Pharmacologic agents: antiemetics, stool softeners, cough suppressants, antacids, and cholinergics
- Diet modifications: small, frequent, bland meals; not eating 2 hours prior to lying down; weight-loss programs
- Surgical repair.

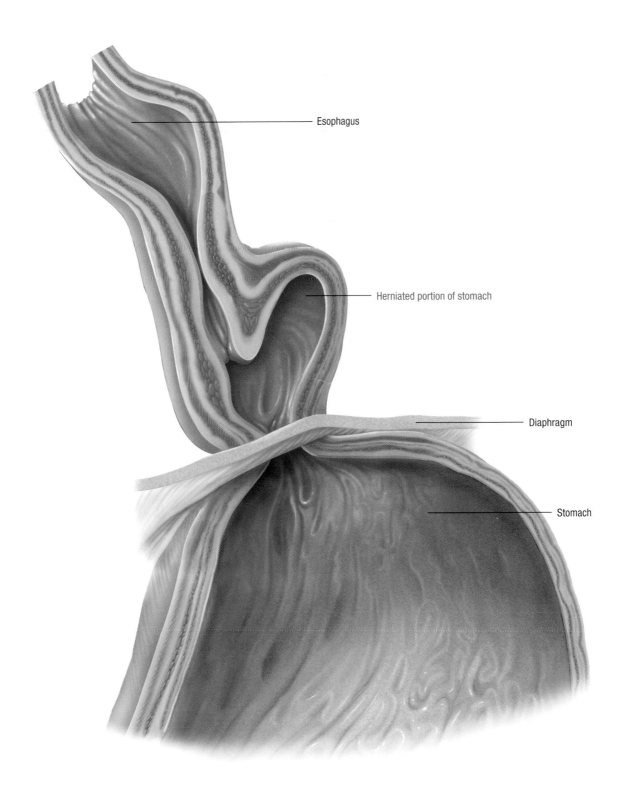

Esophagus

Herniated portion of stomach

Diaphragm

Stomach

Hirschsprung's disease

Hirschsprung's disease, also called congenital megacolon or congenital aganglionic megacolon, is a congenital disorder of the large intestine, characterized by absence or marked reduction of parasympathetic ganglion cells in the colorectal wall. Hirschsprung's disease appears to be a familial, congenital defect, occurring in 1 in 5,000 to 1 in 8,000 live births. It's up to seven times more common in males than in females (although the aganglionic segment is usually shorter in males) and is most prevalent in whites. Total aganglionosis affects both sexes equally. Females with Hirschsprung's disease are at higher risk for having affected children. This disease usually coexists with other congenital anomalies, particularly trisomy 21 and anomalies of the urinary tract such as megaloureter.

 CLINICAL TIP
Without prompt treatment, an infant with colonic obstruction may die within 24 hours from enterocolitis that leads to severe diarrhea and hypovolemic shock. With prompt treatment, prognosis is good.

Cause
Familial congenital defect.

Pathophysiology
In Hirschsprung's disease, parasympathetic ganglion cells in the colorectal wall are absent or markedly reduced in number. The aganglionic bowel segment contracts without the reciprocal relaxation needed to propel feces forward. Impaired intestinal motility causes severe, intractable constipation. Colonic obstruction can ensue, dilating the bowel and occluding surrounding blood and lymphatic vessels. The ensuing mucosal edema, ischemia, and infarction draw large amounts of fluid into the bowel, causing copious amounts of liquid stool. Continued infarction and destruction of the mucosa lead to infection and sepsis.

Signs and symptoms
In newborns:
- Failure to pass meconium within 24 to 48 hours
- Bile-stained or fecal vomitus
- Constipation, overflow diarrhea
- Abdominal distention
- Dehydration, feeding difficulties, and failure to thrive.
  In children:
- Intractable constipation
- Large protuberant abdomen, easily palpated fecal masses
- Wasted extremities (in severe cases)
- Loss of subcutaneous tissue (in severe cases).
  In adults (rare):
- Abdominal distention
- Chronic intermittent constipation.
  Complications:
- Bowel perforation, electrolyte imbalances, nutritional deficiencies, enterocolitis, hypovolemic shock, sepsis.

Diagnostic tests
- Rectal biopsy
- Barium enema
- Rectal manometry
- Upright plain abdominal X-rays.

Treatment
- Corrective surgery
- Daily colonic lavage
- Temporary colostomy or ileostomy.

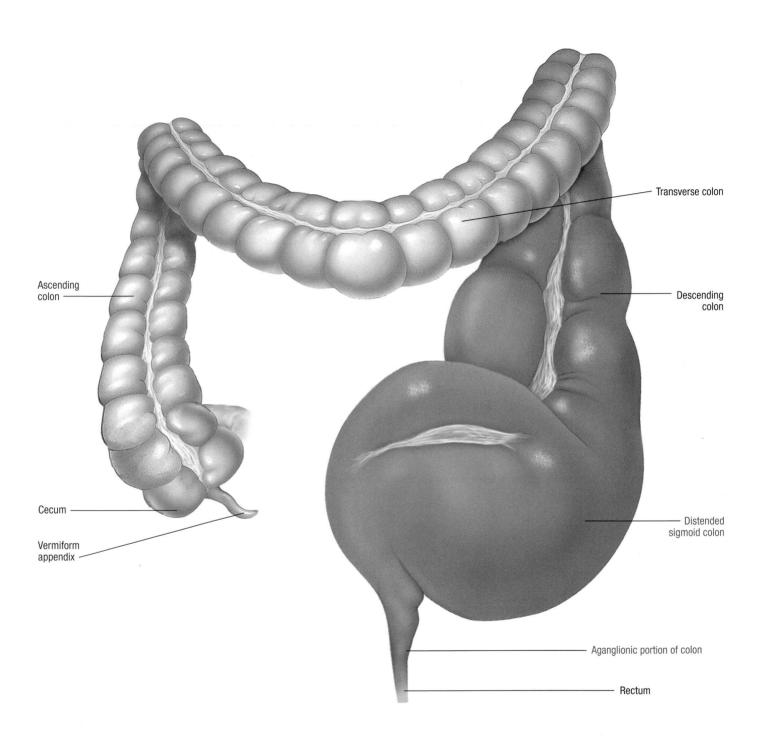

Transverse colon

Ascending
colon

Descending
colon

Cecum

Distended
sigmoid colon

Vermiform
appendix

Aganglionic portion of colon

Rectum

INGUINAL HERNIA

A hernia occurs when part of an internal organ protrudes through an abnormal opening in the wall of the cavity that surrounds it. Most hernias occur in the abdominal cavity. Although many kinds of abdominal hernias are possible, inguinal hernias (also called ruptures) are most common. Inguinal hernias may be direct or indirect. Indirect are more common; they may develop at any age, are three times more common in males, and are especially prevalent in infants.

Causes
- *Indirect:* weakness in fascial margin of internal inguinal ring.
- *Direct:* a weakness in fascial floor of inguinal canal.

Pathophysiology
In an inguinal hernia, the large or small intestine, omentum, or bladder protrudes into the inguinal canal. Hernias can be *reduced* (if the hernia can be manipulated back into place with relative ease), *incarcerated* (if the hernia can't be reduced because adhesions have formed, obstructing the intestinal flow), or *strangulated* (part of the herniated intestine becomes twisted or edematous, seriously interfering with normal blood flow and peristalsis, and possibly leading to intestinal obstruction and necrosis). In an infant, an inguinal hernia commonly coexists with an undescended testicle or a hydrocele.

Signs and symptoms
Reduced or incarcerated hernia:
- Lump over the herniated area; present when the patient stands or strains; absent when the patient is supine
- Sharp, steady groin pain when tension is applied to herniated contents; fades when the hernia is reduced.
  Strangulated hernia:
- Severe pain.
  Partial bowel obstruction:
- Anorexia
- Vomiting
- Pain and tenderness in groin
- Irreducible mass
- Diminished bowel sounds.

Complete bowel obstruction:
- Shock
- High fever
- Absent bowel sounds
- Bloody stools.

CLINICAL TIP
To detect a hernia in a male patient:
- Ask the patient to stand with his ipsilateral leg slightly flexed and his weight resting on the other leg.
- Insert an index finger into the lower part of the scrotum and invaginate the scrotal skin so the finger can advance through the external inguinal ring to the internal ring.
- Tell the patient to cough. If you feel pressure against the fingertip, an indirect hernia exists; pressure felt against the side of the finger indicates that a direct hernia exists.

Diagnostic tests
For suspected bowel obstruction:
- X-ray
- White blood cell count (may be elevated).

Treatment
Temporary measures:
- Reduction and a truss.
  In infants and otherwise healthy adults:
- Herniorrhaphy.
  For incarcerated or necrotic hernia:
- Possibly, bowel resection.

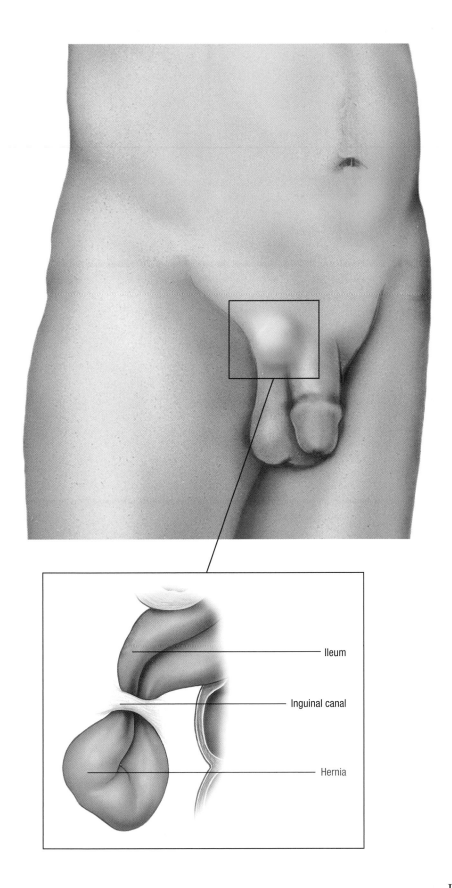

Ileum

Inguinal canal

Hernia

IRRITABLE BOWEL SYNDROME

Also referred to as spastic colon or spastic colitis, irritable bowel syndrome (IBS) is marked by chronic symptoms of abdominal pain, alternating constipation and diarrhea, excess flatus, a sense of incomplete evacuation, and abdominal distention. IBS is a common, stress-related disorder. About 20% of patients never seek medical attention for this benign condition that has no anatomical abnormality or inflammatory component. It's twice as common in women as in men.

Causes
- Psychological stress (most common)
- Ingested irritants (coffee, raw fruit, or vegetables)
- Lactose intolerance
- Abuse of laxatives
- Hormonal changes (menstruation).

Pathophysiology
IBS appears to reflect motor disturbances of the entire colon in response to stimuli. Some muscles of the small bowel are particularly sensitive to motor abnormalities and distention; others are particularly sensitive to certain foods and drugs. The patient may be hypersensitive to the hormones gastrin and cholecystokinin. The pain of IBS seems to be caused by abnormally strong contractions of the intestinal smooth muscle as it reacts to distention, irritants, or stress.

Signs and symptoms
- Crampy lower abdominal pain, occurring during the day and relieved by defecation or passage of flatus
- Pain that intensifies 1 to 2 hours after a meal
- Constipation alternating with diarrhea, with one dominant
- Passage of mucus through the rectum
- Abdominal distention and bloating.

Diagnostic tests
- Stool analysis for ova, parasites, bacteria, and blood
- Lactose tolerance test
- Barium enema
- Sigmoidoscopy, colonoscopy
- Rectal biopsy.

Treatment
- Stress management measures, including counseling or mild antianxiety agents
- Identification and avoidance of food irritants
- Application of heat to abdomen
- Bulking agents
- Antispasmodics (dicyclomine, hyoscyamine sulfate)
- Possible, loperamide
- Bowel training (if cause is chronic laxative abuse) to regain muscle control.

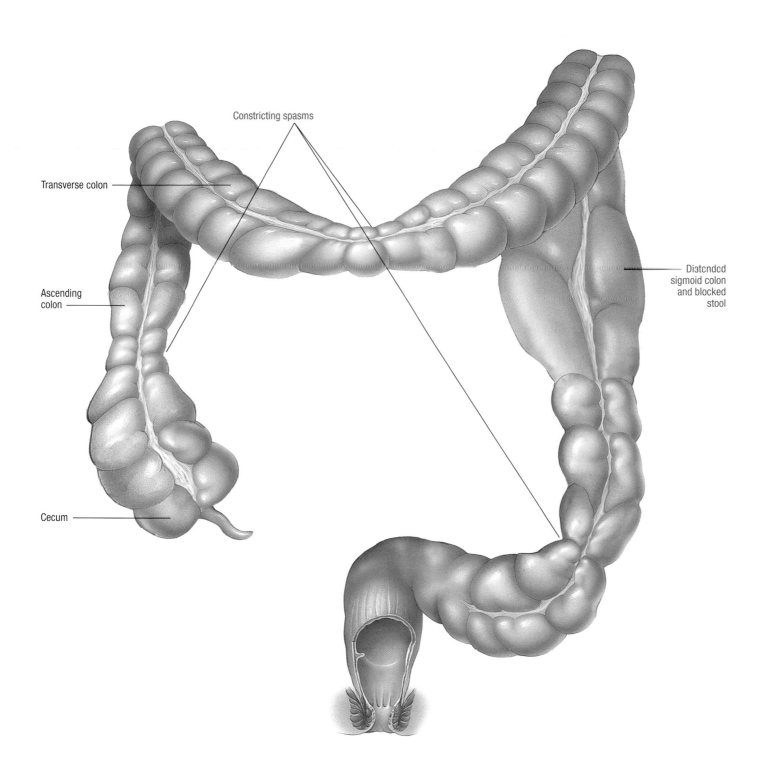

Constricting spasms

Transverse colon

Ascending
colon

Cecum

Distended
sigmoid colon
and blocked
stool

LIVER CANCER

Liver cancer, also known as primary or metastatic hepatic carcinoma, is a rare form of cancer in the United States. It is rapidly fatal, usually within 6 months, from GI hemorrhage, progressive cachexia, liver failure, or metastasis.

AGE ALERT
Liver cancer is most prevalent in men (particularly over age 60), and incidence increases with age.

It is common for patients with hepatomas also to have cirrhosis. (Hepatomas are 40 times more likely to develop in a cirrhotic liver than in a normal one.) Whether cirrhosis is a premalignant state or alcohol and malnutrition predispose the liver to develop hepatomas is still unclear. Other risk factors are exposure to the hepatitis C or hepatitis B virus.

CLINICAL TIP
The liver is one of the most common sites of metastasis from other primary cancers, particularly those of the colon, rectum, stomach, pancreas, esophagus, lung, breast, or melanoma. In the United States, metastatic carcinoma is over 20 times more common than primary carcinoma and, after cirrhosis, is the leading cause of death related to liver disease. Liver metastasis may appear as a solitary lesion, the first sign of recurrence after a remission.

Causes
- Immediate cause unknown
- Possibly congenital in children.
  Possible causes in adults:
- Environmental exposure to carcinogens
- Androgens
- Oral estrogens
- Cirrhosis.

Pathophysiology
Most primary liver tumors (90%) originate in the parenchymal cells and are *hepatomas* (hepatocellular carcinoma, primary lower-cell carcinoma). Primary tumors that originate in the intrahepatic bile ducts are known as *cholangiomas* (cholangiocarcinoma, cholangiocellular carcinoma). Rarer tumors include a mixed-cell type, Kupffer cell sarcoma, and hepatoblastomas (which occur almost exclusively in children and are usually resectable and curable).

Signs and symptoms
- Mass or enlargement in right upper quadrant
- Tender, nodular liver on palpation
- Severe epigastric or right upper quadrant pain
- Bruit, hum, or rubbing sound if tumor is large
- Weight loss, weakness, anorexia, fever.

Diagnostic tests
Confirming test:
- Needle or open biopsy.
  May provide useful information:
- Aspartate aminotransferase, alanine aminotransferase, alkaline phosphatase, lactic dehydrogenase, bilirubin
- Alpha-fetoprotein
- Chest X-ray
- Liver scan
- Arteriography
- Electrolyte studies.

Treatment
- Resection if cancer is in early stage; few hepatic tumors are resectable
- Liver transplantation for a small subset of patients
- Palliative measures:
- radiation therapy, chemotherapy
- controlling signs and symptoms of encephalopathy
- caring for transhepatic catheters
- hospice.

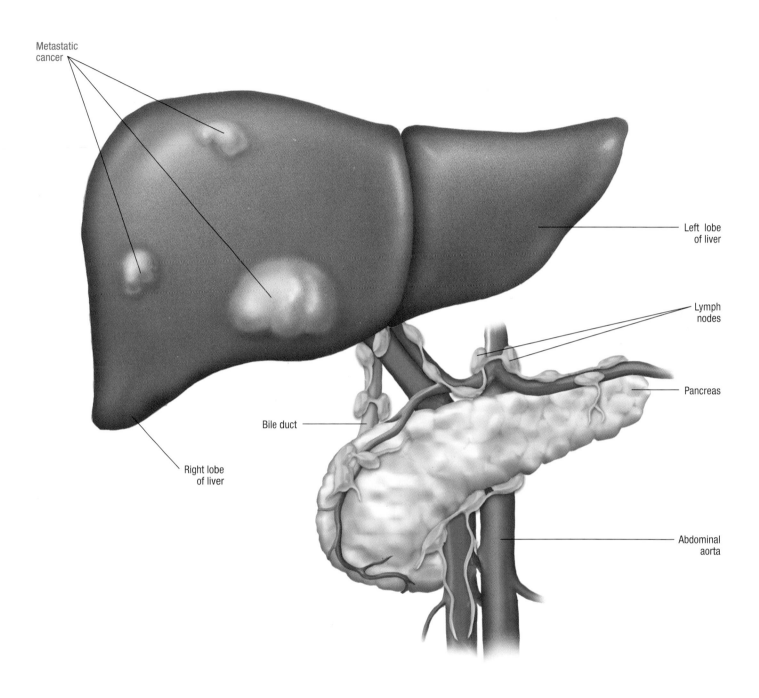

Metastatic cancer

Left lobe of liver

Lymph nodes

Pancreas

Bile duct

Right lobe of liver

Abdominal aorta

LIVER FAILURE

Any liver disease can end in organ failure. The liver performs over 100 separate functions in the body. When it fails, a complex syndrome involving the impairment of many different organs and body functions ensues. The only cure for liver failure is liver transplantation.

Causes
- Viral or nonviral hepatitis
- Cirrhosis
- Liver cancer.

Pathophysiology
Manifestations of liver failure include hepatic encephalopathy and hepatorenal syndrome.

Hepatic encephalopathy, a set of central nervous system disorders, results when the liver can no longer detoxify the blood. Liver dysfunction and collateral vessels that shunt blood around the liver to the systemic circulation permit toxins absorbed from the GI tract to circulate freely to the brain. Ammonia, a byproduct of protein metabolism, is one of the main toxins causing hepatic encephalopathy. The normal liver transforms ammonia to urea, which the kidneys excrete. When the liver fails, ammonia is delivered to the brain. Short-chain fatty acids, serotonin, tryptophan, and false neurotransmitters may also accumulate in the blood and contribute to hepatic encephalopathy.

Hepatorenal syndrome is renal failure concurrent with liver disease. The kidneys appear to be normal but abruptly cease functioning. Blood volume expands, hydrogen ions accumulate, and electrolyte disturbances ensue. It is most common in patients with alcoholic cirrhosis or fulminating hepatitis. The cause may be the accumulation of vasoactive substances that cause inappropriate constriction of renal arterioles, leading to decreased glomerular filtration and oliguria. The vasoconstriction may also be a compensatory response to portal hypertension and the pooling of blood in the splenic circulation.

Signs and symptoms
- Jaundice
- Abdominal pain or tenderness
- Nausea, anorexia, weight loss
- Fetor hepaticus
- Fatigue
- Pruritus
- Oliguria
- Splenomegaly
- Ascites, peripheral edema
- Varices of esophagus, rectum, abdominal wall
- Bleeding tendencies from thrombocytopenia (secondary to blood accumulation in the spleen), prolonged prothrombin time (from the impaired production of coagulation factors), petechiae
- Amenorrhea, gynecomastia.
    Complications:
- Variceal bleeding
- GI hemorrhage
- Coma
- Death.

Diagnostic tests
- Aspartate aminotransferase, alanine aminotransferase, alkaline phosphatase, bilirubin
- Complete blood count, bleeding and clotting times, ammonia levels, glucose levels
- Urine osmolarity.

Treatment
- Liver transplantation
- Low-protein, high-carbohydrate diet
- Lactulose.
    For ascites:
- Salt restriction, potassium-sparing diuretics, potassium supplements
- Eliminating alcohol intake
- Paracentesis, shunt placement.
    For portal hypertension:
- Shunt placement between the portal vein and another systemic vein.
    For variceal bleeding:
- Vasoconstrictor drugs
- Balloon tamponade
- Surgery
- Vitamin K.

SIGNS OF LIVER FAILURE

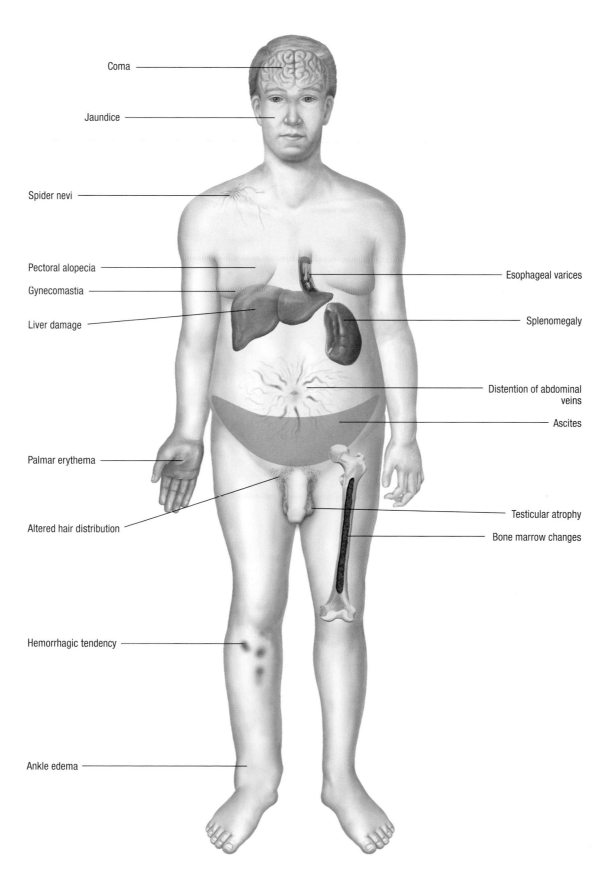

Coma

Jaundice

Spider nevi

Pectoral alopecia

Gynecomastia

Liver damage

Palmar erythema

Altered hair distribution

Hemorrhagic tendency

Ankle edema

Esophageal varices

Splenomegaly

Distention of abdominal veins

Ascites

Testicular atrophy

Bone marrow changes

PANCREATIC CANCER

Pancreatic cancer occurs primarily in the head of the organ and progresses to death within a year of diagnosis. Rarer tumors are those of the body and tail of the pancreas and islet cell tumors.

 AGE ALERT
The incidence of pancreatic cancer increases with age, peaking between ages 60 and 70.

Causes
- Inhalation or absorption of carcinogens, which are excreted by the pancreas:
  - cigarette smoke
  - food additives
  - industrial chemicals, such as beta-naphthalene, benzidine, and urea.
    Predisposing factors:
- Chronic pancreatitis (may be early manifestation of disease)
- Diabetes mellitus (may be early manifestation of disease)
- Chronic alcohol abuse.

Pathophysiology
Most pancreatic tumors are adenocarcinomas that arise in the head of the pancreas. The two main tissue types are cylinder-cell and large, fatty, granular-cell tumors. Cancers of the pancreas progress insidiously and most have metastasized before diagnosis. Cancer cells may invade the stomach, duodenum, major blood vessels, bile duct, colon, spleen, and kidney, as well as the lymph nodes.

Signs and symptoms
- Weight loss, anorexia, fatigue
- Pruritus, skin lesions (usually on the legs)
- Abdominal or low back pain
- Jaundice
- Diarrhea
- Fever
- Hyperglycemia, glucose intolerance.

Diagnostic tests
Definitive diagnosis:
- Laparotomy with biopsy.
  Other tests:
- Ultrasonography, computed tomography scan, magnetic resonance imaging
- Angiography
- Endoscopic retrograde cholangiopancreatography.
  Laboratory tests:
- Serum bilirubin, liver enzymes
- Prothrombin time
- Plasma insulin immunoassay, fasting blood glucose
- Fecal occult blood.

Treatment
- Seldom successful because disease is usually metastatic at diagnosis
- Surgery: total pancreatectomy, cholecystojejunostomy, choledochoduodenostomy, choledochojejunostomy, pancreatoduodenectomy or Whipple's procedure, gastrojejunostomy
- Possibly, radiation therapy and chemotherapy.

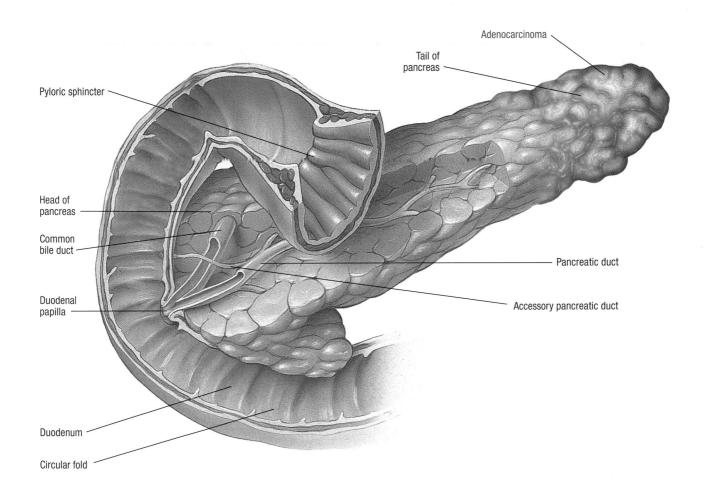

Adenocarcinoma

Tail of
pancreas

Pyloric sphincter

Head of
pancreas

Common
bile duct

Pancreatic duct

Accessory pancreatic duct

Duodenal
papilla

Duodenum

Circular fold

PANCREATITIS

Pancreatitis, inflammation of the pancreas, occurs in acute and chronic forms and may be due to edema, necrosis, or hemorrhage. In men, this disease is commonly associated with alcoholism, trauma, or peptic ulcer and carries a poor prognosis. In women, it's associated with biliary tract disease and has a good prognosis. Mortality in pancreatitis with necrosis and hemorrhage is as high as 60%.

Causes
- Biliary tract disease
- Alcoholism
- Abnormal organ structure
- Metabolic or endocrine disorders, such as high cholesterol levels or overactive thyroid
- Pancreatic cysts or tumors
- Penetrating peptic ulcers
- Blunt trauma, surgical trauma
- Drugs, such as glucocorticoids, sulfonamides, thiazides, oral contraceptives, nonsteroidal anti-inflammatory drugs
- Kidney failure or transplantation
- Endoscopic examination of bile ducts and pancreas.

Pathophysiology
Acute pancreatitis occurs in two forms: edematous (interstitial) and necrotizing. *Edematous* pancreatitis causes fluid accumulation and swelling. *Necrotizing* pancreatitis causes cell death and tissue damage. In both types, inappropriate activation of enzymes causes tissue damage.

Normally, the acini in the pancreas secrete enzymes in an inactive form. Two theories suggest why enzymes become prematurely activated:
- A toxic agent such as alcohol may alter the way the pancreas secretes enzymes. Alcohol probably increases pancreatic secretion, alters the metabolism of the acinar cells, and encourages duct obstruction by causing pancreatic secretory proteins to precipitate.
- *Autodigestion* may occur when duodenal contents containing activated enzymes reflux into the pancreatic duct, activating other enzymes and setting up a cycle of more pancreatic damage.

In chronic pancreatitis, persistent inflammation produces irreversible changes in the structure and function of the pancreas. It sometimes follows an episode of acute pancreatitis. Protein precipitates block the pancreatic duct and eventually harden or calcify. Structural changes lead to fibrosis and atrophy of the glands. Growths called pseudocysts contain pancreatic enzymes and tissue debris. An abscess results if pseudocysts become infected.

CLINICAL TIP
If pancreatitis damages the islets of Langerhans, diabetes mellitus may result. Sudden severe pancreatitis causes massive hemorrhage and total destruction of the pancreas, manifested as diabetic acidosis, shock, or coma.

Signs and symptoms
- Pain
- Mottled skin
- Tachycardia
- Low-grade fever
- Cold, sweaty extremities
- Restlessness
- In a severe attack: persistent vomiting, abdominal distention, diminished bowel activity, crackles at lung bases, left pleural effusion
- Extreme malaise (in chronic pancreatitis).

CLINICAL TIP
Complications of untreated disease include massive hemorrhage/shock, pseudocyst, biliary and duodenal obstruction, portal and splenic vein thrombosis, diabetes mellitus, and respiratory failure.

Diagnostic tests
- Serum amylase, lipase, bilirubin, calcium
- Blood and urine glucose
- White blood cell count
- Stool lipids and trypsin
- Computed tomography scan, ultrasonography
- Endoscopic retrograde cholangiopancreatography.

Treatment
- Nothing by mouth; I.V. fluids, protein, and electrolytes
- Blood transfusions
- Nasogastric suctioning
- Pain medication
- Antacids, histamine antagonists
- Antibiotics
- Anticholinergics
- Insulin
- Surgical drainage
- Laparotomy if biliary tract obstruction causes acute pancreatitis.

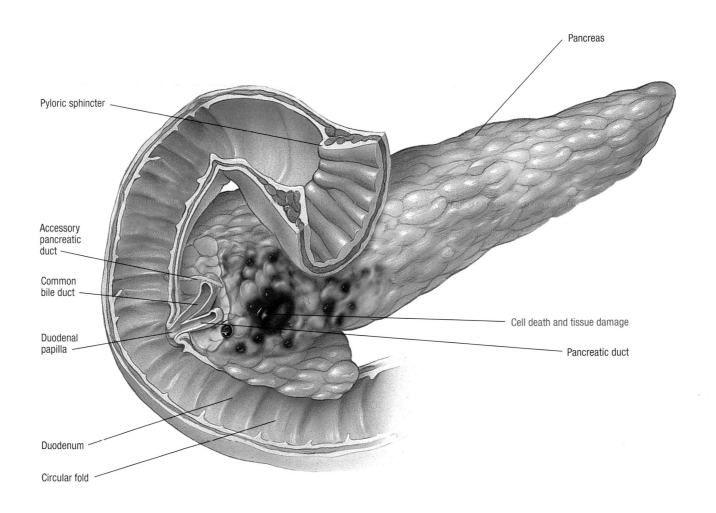

Pancreas

Pyloric sphincter

Accessory
pancreatic
duct

Common
bile duct

Duodenal
papilla

Cell death and tissue damage

Pancreatic duct

Duodenum

Circular fold

PERITONITIS

Peritonitis is an acute or chronic inflammation of the peritoneum, the membrane that lines the abdominal cavity and covers the visceral organs. Inflammation may extend throughout the peritoneum or may be localized as an abscess. Peritonitis commonly decreases intestinal motility and causes intestinal distention with gas. With antibiotics, mortality is now 10%, and it is usually due to bowel obstruction.

Causes

Bacterial inflammation:
- Appendicitis, diverticulitis
- Peptic ulcer, ulcerative colitis
- Volvulus, strangulated obstruction
- Abdominal neoplasm
- Penetrating trauma, such as a stab wound.
  Chemical inflammation:
- Rupture of a fallopian tube or the bladder
- Perforation of a gastric ulcer
- Released pancreatic enzymes.

Pathophysiology

Although the GI tract normally contains bacteria, the peritoneum is sterile. When bacteria or chemical irritants invade the peritoneum due to inflammation and perforation of the GI tract, peritonitis is the result. In both chemical and bacterial inflammation, accumulated fluids containing protein and electrolytes make the transparent peritoneum opaque, red, inflamed, and edematous. Because the peritoneal cavity is so resistant to contamination, infection is commonly localized as an abscess.

Signs and symptoms

- Sudden, severe, and diffuse abdominal pain that tends to intensify and localize in the area of the underlying disorder, such as right lower quadrant in appendicitis
- Acutely tender, distended, rigid abdomen; rebound tenderness

- Pallor, excessive sweating, cold skin
- Absent or diminished bowel sounds
- Nausea, vomiting, abdominal rigidity
- Signs and symptoms of dehydration (oliguria, thirst, dry swollen tongue, and pinched skin)
- Temperature of 103° F (39.4° C) or higher
- Shoulder pain.

CLINICAL TIP

Abdominal distention and resulting upward displacement of the diaphragm may decrease respiratory capacity. Typically, the patient with peritonitis tends to breathe shallowly and move as little as possible to minimize pain. He may lie on his back, with knees flexed, to relax abdominal muscles.

Diagnostic tests
- Abdominal and chest X-rays
- White blood cell count
- Paracentesis
- Laparotomy.

Treatment

Emergency treatment:
- Nothing by mouth — to slow peristalsis and prevent perforation
- Massive antibiotic therapy, usually cefoxitin with an aminoglycoside or penicillin G and clindamycin with an aminoglycoside, depending on the infecting organisms
- Parenteral fluids and electrolytes.
  When peritonitis results from perforation:
- Surgery as soon possible to eliminate the source of infection by evacuating the spilled contents and inserting drains.

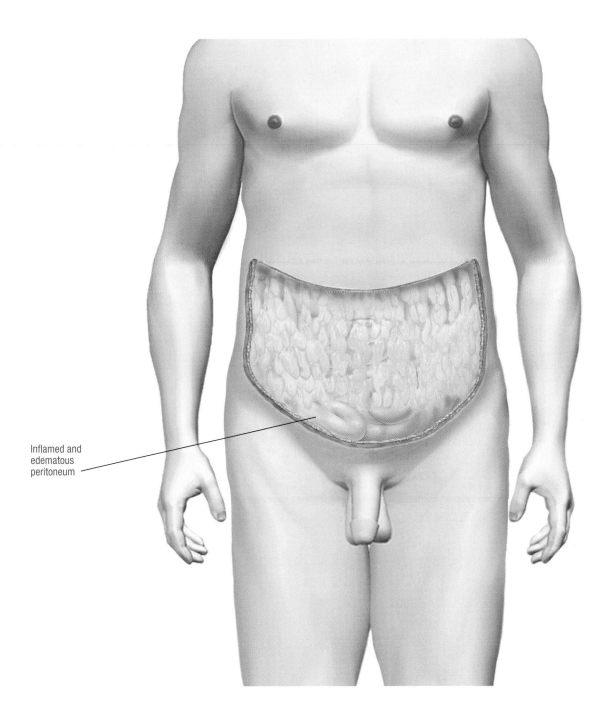

Inflamed and
edematous
peritoneum

ULCERATIVE COLITIS

Ulcerative colitis is a continuous inflammatory disease that affects the mucosa of the colon and rectum. It invariably begins in the rectum and sigmoid colon, and commonly extends upward into the entire colon, rarely affecting the small intestine, except for the terminal ileum. Ulcerative colitis produces edema (leading to mucosal friability) and ulcerations. Severity ranges from a mild, localized disorder to a fulminant disease that may cause a perforated colon, progressing to potentially fatal peritonitis and toxemia. The disease cycles between exacerbation and remission.

AGE ALERT
Ulcerative colitis occurs primarily in young adults, especially women. Onset of symptoms seems to peak between ages 15 and 30 and between ages 55 and 65.

Causes
- Unknown
- May be related to abnormal immune response to food or bacteria, such as *Escherichia coli*.

Pathophysiology
Ulcerative colitis usually begins as inflammation in the base of the mucosal layer of the large intestine. The colon's mucosal surface becomes dark, red, and velvety. Inflammation leads to erosions that coalesce and form ulcers. The mucosa becomes diffusely ulcerated, with hemorrhage, congestion, edema, and exudative inflammation. Abscesses in the mucosa drain purulent pus, become necrotic, and ulcerate. Sloughing causes bloody, mucus filled stools. As abscesses heal, scarring and thickening may appear in the bowel's inner muscle layer. As granulation tissue replaces the muscle layer, the colon narrows, shortens, and loses its characteristic pouches (hatral folds).

Signs and symptoms
- Recurrent bloody diarrhea, often containing pus and mucus (hallmark sign)
- Abdominal cramping, fecal urgency
- Weight loss
- Weakness.

CLINICAL TIP
Complications may include perforated colon, toxic megacolon, liver disease, stricture formation, colon cancer, anemia, or arthritis.

Diagnostic tests
- Sigmoidoscopy
- Colonoscopy and biopsy
- Barium enema
- Stool specimen analysis for blood, pus, mucus
- Electrolytes, albumin, white blood cell count, hemoglobin, prothrombin time, erythrocyte sedimentation rate.

Treatment
- Corticotropin and adrenal corticosteroids
- Sulfasalazine
- Antidiarrheals
- Iron supplements
- Liquid nutritional supplements.
  For severe disease:
- Total parenteral nutrition and nothing by mouth
- I.V. hydration
- Proctocolectomy with ileostomy.

MUCOSAL CHANGES IN ULCERATIVE COLITIS

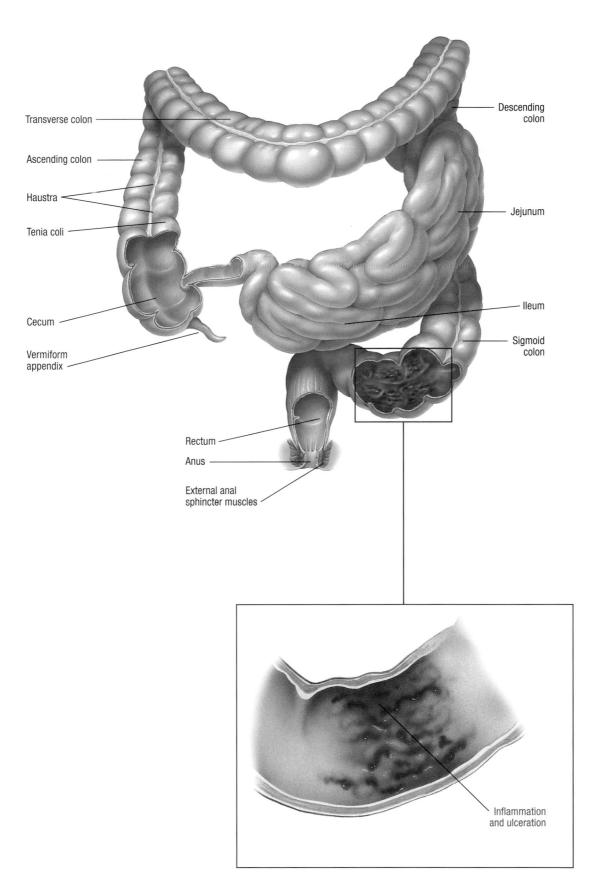

Transverse colon

Ascending colon

Haustra

Tenia coli

Cecum

Vermiform
appendix

Rectum

Anus

External anal
sphincter muscles

Descending
colon

Jejunum

Ileum

Sigmoid
colon

Inflammation
and ulceration

ULCERS

Ulcers, circumscribed lesions in the mucosal membrane extending below the epithelium, can develop in the lower esophagus, stomach, pylorus, duodenum, or jejunum. Although erosions are often referred to as ulcers, erosions are breaks in the mucosal membranes that do not extend below the epithelium. Ulcers may be acute or chronic in nature. Acute ulcers are usually multiple and superficial. Chronic ulcers are identified by scar tissue at their base.

AGE ALERT
Gastric ulcers are most common in middle-aged and elderly men, especially in chronic users of nonsteroidal anti-inflammatory drugs (NSAIDs), alcohol, or tobacco.

Causes
● *Helicobacter pylori* infection
● NSAIDs
● Inadequate protection of mucus membrane
● Pathologic hypersecretory disorders.
   Predisposing factors include:
● Blood type (gastric ulcers and type A; duodenal ulcers and type O)
● Other genetic factors
● Exposure to irritants, such as alcohol, coffee, tobacco
● Emotional stress
● Physical trauma and normal aging.

Pathophysiology
Although the stomach contains acidic secretions that can digest substances, intrinsic defenses protect the gastric mucosal membrane from injury. A thick, tenacious layer of gastric mucus protects the stomach from autodigestion, mechanical trauma, and chemical trauma. Prostaglandins provide another line of defense. Gastric ulcers may be a result of destruction of the mucosal barrier.

The duodenum is protected from ulceration by the function of Brunner's glands. These glands produce a viscid, mucoid, alkaline secretion that neutralizes the acid chyme. Duodenal ulcers appear to result from excessive acid production in the duodenum.

H. pylori release a toxin that destroys the gastric and duodenal mucosa, reducing the epithelium's resistance to acid digestion and causing gastritis and ulcer disease.

Salicylates and other NSAIDs inhibit the secretion of prostaglandins (substances that block ulceration). Certain illnesses, such as pancreatitis, hepatic disease, Crohn's disease, preexisting gastritis, and Zollinger-Ellison syndrome, also contribute to ulceration.

Signs and symptoms
Gastric ulcer:
● Pain that worsens with eating
● Nausea and anorexia.
   Duodenal ulcer:
● Epigastric pain that's gnawing and dull; similar to hunger
● Pain relieved by food or antacids, but usually recurring 2 to 4 hours after ingestion.

CLINICAL TIP
Complications may occur and include hemorrhage, shock, gastric perforation, and gastric outlet obstruction.

Diagnostic tests
● Barium swallow or upper GI and small bowel series
● Endoscopy
● Fecal occult blood
● White blood cell count
● Gastric secretory studies
● Carbon-13 urea breath test.

Treatment
● Physical and emotional rest
● For *H. pylori* infection: tetracycline, metronidazole, or clarithromycin; ranitidine, bismuth citrate, bismuth salicylate, or a proton pump inhibitor
● Misoprostol (a prostaglandin analogue)
● Antacids
● Avoidance of caffeine, tobacco, and alcohol
● Anticholinergic drugs
● Histamine$_2$ antagonists
● Sucralfate
● Dietary therapy: small frequent meals and avoidance of eating before bedtime.

Erosion — Penetration of only the superficial layer

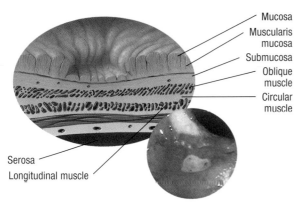

Mucosa
Muscularis mucosa
Submucosa
Oblique muscle
Circular muscle
Serosa
Longitudinal muscle

Acute ulcer — Penetration into muscle layer

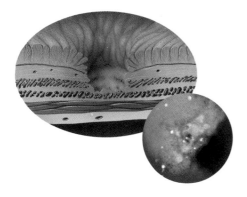

Perforating ulcer — Penetration of wall

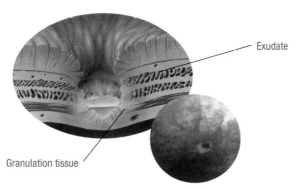

Exudate
Granulation tissue

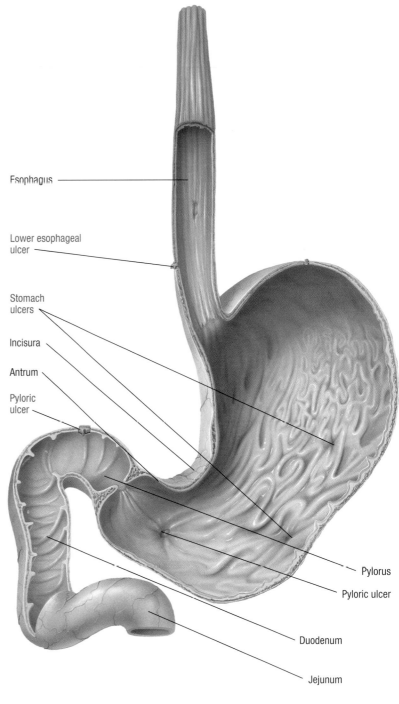

Esophagus

Lower esophageal ulcer

Stomach ulcers

Incisura

Antrum

Pyloric ulcer

Pylorus

Pyloric ulcer

Duodenum

Jejunum

BONE TUMORS

Primary malignant bone tumors (also called sarcomas of the bone and bone cancer) are rare, constituting less than 1% of all malignant tumors. Most bone tumors are secondary, caused by seeding from a primary site.

 AGE ALERT
Primary malignant bone tumors are more common in males, especially in children and adolescents, although some types do occur in persons between ages 35 and 60.

Causes
Unknown.
   Suggested mechanisms:
● Rapid bone growth — children and young adults with primary bone tumors are much taller than average
● Heredity
● Trauma
● Excessive radiotherapy.

Pathophysiology
Bone tumors may originate in osseous or nonosseous tissue. *Osseous* bone tumors arise from the bony structure itself and include osteogenic sarcoma (the most common), parosteal osteogenic sarcoma, chondrosarcoma, and malignant giant cell tumor. Together they make up 60% of all malignant bone tumors. *Nonosseous* tumors arise from hematopoietic, vascular, or neural tissues and include Ewing's sarcoma, fibrosarcoma, and chordoma. Osteogenic and Ewing's sarcomas are the most common bone tumors in childhood.

Signs and symptoms
● Bone pain (most common indication of primary malignant bone tumors); characteristics include:
 – greater intensity at night
 – usually associated with movement
 – dull and usually localized
 – may be referred from hip or spine and result in weakness or a limp
● Mass or tumor
● Pathologic fractures
● Cachexia, fever, impaired mobility in later stages.

Diagnostic tests
● Biopsy by incision or aspiration
● X-ray
● Radioisotope bone scan
● Computed tomography scan
● Serum alkaline phosphatase level.

Treatment
● Excision of tumor with a 3″ (7.6 cm) margin
● Preoperative chemotherapy
● Postoperative chemotherapy
● Radical surgery, such as hemipelvectomy or interscapulothoracic amputation, if necessary (seldom)
● Intensive chemotherapy.

TYPES OF BONE TUMORS

Giant cell tumor

Chondroblastoma

Osteogenic sarcoma

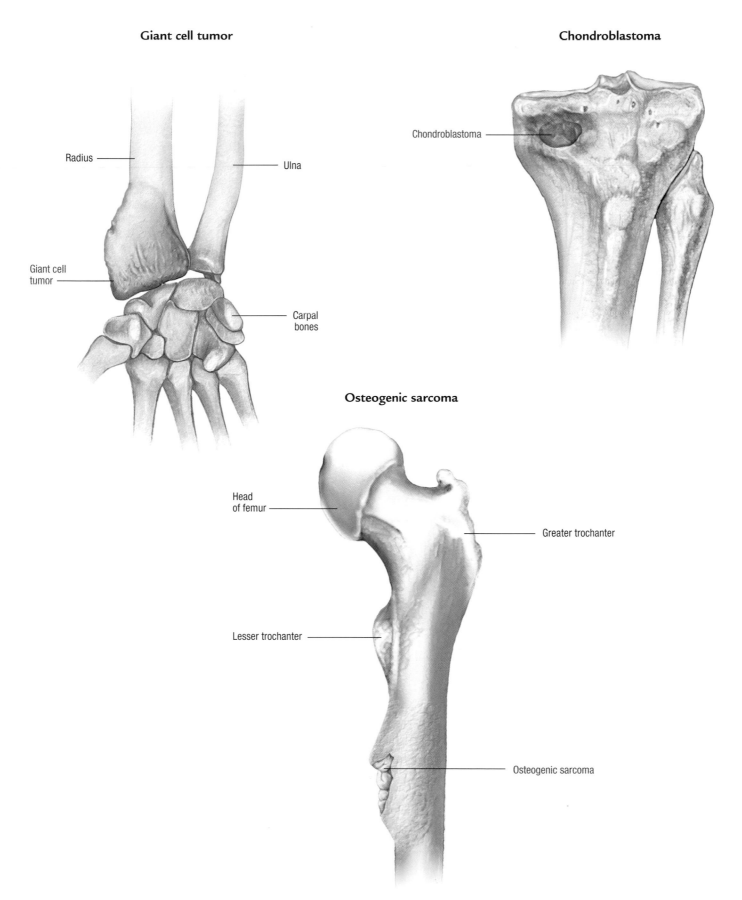

Radius

Ulna

Chondroblastoma

Giant cell tumor

Carpal bones

Head of femur

Greater trochanter

Lesser trochanter

Osteogenic sarcoma

BURSITIS

Bursitis is a painful inflammation of one or more of the bursae — closed sacs lubricated with small amounts of synovial fluid that facilitate the motion of muscles and tendons over bony prominences. Bursitis usually occurs in the subdeltoid, olecranon, trochanteric, calcaneal, or prepatellar bursae.

Causes
- Recurring trauma that stresses or presses a joint
- Inflammatory joint disease, such as rheumatoid arthritis or gout
- Chronic bursitis — repeated attacks of acute bursitis, trauma, or infection
- Septic bursitis — wound infection; bacterial invasion of overlying skin.

Pathophysiology
The role of the bursa is to act as a cushion and allow the tendon to move over bone as it contracts and relaxes. It is a fibrous sac lined with synovial fluid. Bursitis is an inflammation of the bursa. The inflammation leads to excessive production of fluid in the sac, which becomes distended and presses on sensory nerve endings, causing pain.

Signs and symptoms
- Irritation
- Inflammation
- Sudden or gradual onset of pain and limited movement.
  Site-specific:
- Subdeltoid bursa — limited arm abduction
- Prepatellar bursa — so-called "housemaid's knee"; pain when climbing stairs
- Hip bursa — pain when climbing, squatting, crossing legs.

Diagnostic tests
Bursitis often occurs concurrently with tendinitis, and the two may be difficult to distinguish as discrete problems. X-rays are usually normal in the early stages. In calcific bursitis, they may show calcium deposits.

Treatment
- Resting joint by immobilization with a sling, splint, or cast
- Application of cold or heat
- Ultrasonography
- Mixture of a corticosteroid and an anesthetic such as lidocaine injected into bursal sac for immediate pain relief
- Nonsteroidal anti-inflammatory drugs until patient is free of pain and able to perform range-of-motion exercises easily
- Short-term analgesics, such as propoxyphene, codeine, acetaminophen with codeine, and, occasionally, oxycodone
- For chronic bursitis, lifestyle changes to prevent recurring joint irritation.

Hip

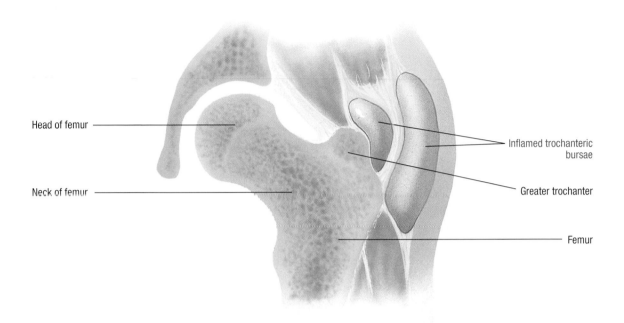

Head of femur

Neck of femur

Inflamed trochanteric bursae

Greater trochanter

Femur

Knee

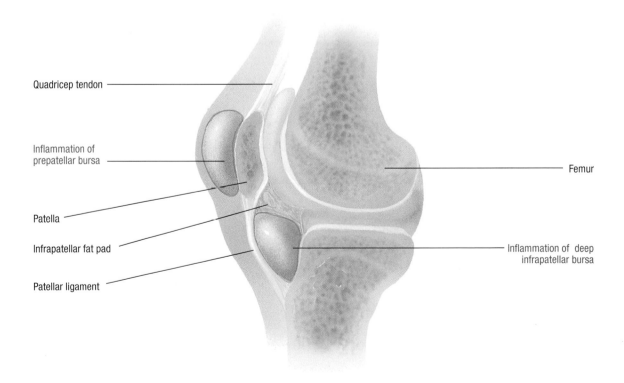

Quadricep tendon

Inflammation of prepatellar bursa

Patella

Infrapatellar fat pad

Patellar ligament

Femur

Inflammation of deep infrapatellar bursa

CARPAL TUNNEL SYNDROME

Carpal tunnel syndrome, a form of repetitive stress injury, is the most common of the nerve entrapment syndromes.

AGE ALERT
Carpal tunnel injury usually occurs in women between ages 30 and 60 and poses a serious occupational health problem.

Assembly-line workers and packers and people who repeatedly use poorly designed tools are most likely to develop this disorder. Computer keyboard and mouse users are also frequently affected. Any strenuous use of the hands — sustained grasping, twisting, or flexing — aggravates this condition.

Causes

Mostly idiopathic, or may result from:
- repetitive stress injury
- rheumatoid arthritis
- flexor tenosynovitis (often associated with rheumatic disease)
- nerve compression
- pregnancy
- multiple myeloma
- diabetes mellitus
- acromegaly
- hypothyroidism
- amyloidosis
- obesity
- benign tumor
- other conditions that increase fluid pressure in the wrist, including alterations in the endocrine or immune systems
- wrist dislocation or sprain, including Colles' fracture followed by edema.

Pathophysiology

The carpal bones and the transverse carpal ligament form the carpal tunnel. Inflammation or fibrosis of the tendon sheaths that pass through the carpal tunnel often cause edema and compression of the median nerve. This compression neuropathy causes sensory and motor changes in the median distribution of the hand, initially impairing sensory transmission to the thumb, index finger, second finger, and inner aspect of the third finger.

Signs and symptoms
- Weakness, pain, burning, numbness, or tingling in one or both hands
- Paresthesia in thumb, forefinger, middle finger, and half of the fourth finger
- Inability to clench fist
- Pain extending to forearm and, in severe cases, to shoulder
- Pain usually relieved by shaking or rubbing hands vigorously or dangling arms
- Symptoms typically worse at night and in the morning (Vasodilation, stasis, and prolonged wrist flexion during sleep may contribute to compression of the carpal tunnel.)
- Possibly, atrophic nails
- Dry, shiny skin

Diagnostic tests
- Electromyography — median-nerve motor conduction delay of more than 5 milliseconds
- Tests to identify underlying disease.

CLINICAL TIP
The following tests provide rapid diagnosis of carpal tunnel syndrome:
- Tinel's sign — tingling over the median nerve on light percussion
- Phalen's wrist-flexion test — holding the forearms vertically and allowing both hands to drop into complete flexion at the wrists for 1 minute reproduces symptoms of carpal tunnel syndrome
- Compression test — blood pressure cuff inflated above systolic pressure on the forearm for 1 to 2 minutes provokes pain and paresthesia along the distribution of the median nerve.

Treatment
- Conservative treatment — resting the hands by splinting the wrists in neutral extension for 1 to 2 weeks, along with gentle daily range-of-motion exercises
- Nonsteroidal anti-inflammatory drugs for symptomatic relief
- Injection of the carpal tunnel with hydrocortisone and lidocaine
- Correction of any underlying disorder
- Surgical decompression of the nerve by resecting the entire transverse carpal tunnel ligament or by using endoscopic surgical techniques
- Possibly, neurolysis (freeing of the nerve fibers)
- Change of occupation if a definite link has been established between the patient's occupation and the development of repetitive stress injury.

Cross section of normal wrist

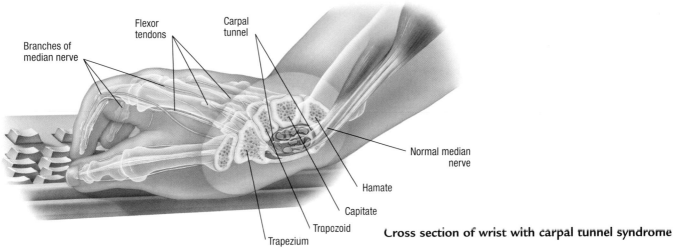

Branches of median nerve

Flexor tendons

Carpal tunnel

Normal median nerve

Hamate

Capitate

Trapozoid

Trapezium

Cross section of wrist with carpal tunnel syndrome

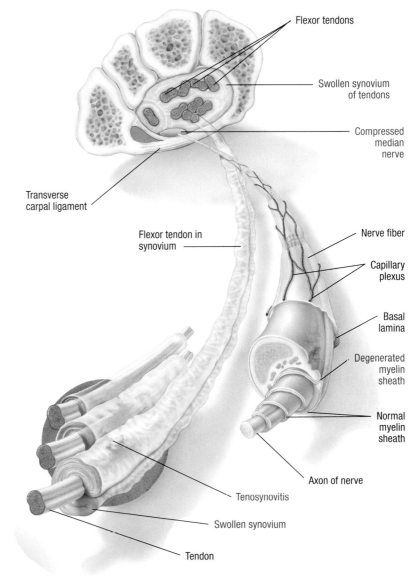

Flexor tendons

Swollen synovium of tendons

Compressed median nerve

Transverse carpal ligament

Flexor tendon in synovium

Nerve fiber

Capillary plexus

Basal lamina

Degenerated myelin sheath

Normal myelin sheath

Axon of nerve

Tenosynovitis

Swollen synovium

Tendon

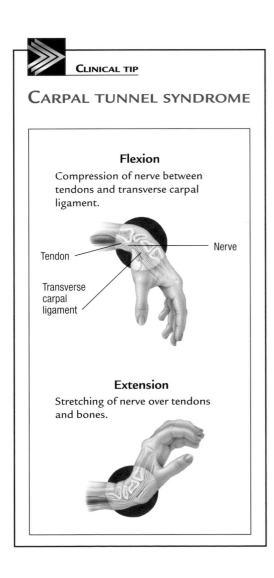

▶▶▶ **CLINICAL TIP**

CARPAL TUNNEL SYNDROME

Flexion

Compression of nerve between tendons and transverse carpal ligament.

Tendon

Nerve

Transverse carpal ligament

Extension

Stretching of nerve over tendons and bones.

DEVELOPMENTAL DYSPLASIA OF THE HIP

Developmental dysplasia of the hip (DDH) is an abnormal development or dislocation of the hip joint present from birth.

 AGE ALERT
It is the most common disorder affecting the hip joints of children younger than age 3. About 85% of affected infants are females.

DDH can be unilateral or bilateral. It affects the left hip more often (67%) than the right. This abnormality occurs in three degrees of severity:
● dislocatable — hip positioned normally but manipulation can cause dislocation
● subluxatable — femoral head rides on edge of acetabulum
● dislocated — femoral head totally outside the acetabulum.

Causes
Unknown.
Risk factors:
● Breech delivery (malposition in utero; DDH 10 times more common than after cephalic delivery)
● Elevated maternal relaxin
● Large neonates and twins (more common).

Pathophysiology
The precise cause of DDH is unknown, although it is thought to be related to trauma during birth, malposition in utero, or maternal hormonal factors. For example, the hormone relaxin, secreted by the corpus luteum during pregnancy, causes relaxation of pubic symphysis and cervical dilation; excessive levels may promote relaxation of the joint ligaments, predisposing the infant to DDH. It is commonly associated with torticollis (20%) and metatarsus adductus (10%).

Signs and symptoms
● In newborns: no gross deformity or pain
● Complete dysplasia: hip rides above the acetabulum, causing the level of the knees to be uneven
● Limited abduction on the dislocated side as the growing child begins to walk
● Swaying from side to side ("duck waddle").

Diagnostic tests
● X-ray
● Sonography
● Magnetic resonance imaging.
Femoral dysplasia:
● X-rays to demonstrate location of femoral head and shallow acetabulum (and to monitor disease or treatment progress).

Treatment
Infants younger than age 3 months:
● Reduce dislocation — gentle manipulation
● Maintain reduction — splint-brace or harness worn for 2 to 3 months to hold the hips in flexed and abducted position
● Tighten and stabilize joint capsule in correct alignment — night splint for another month.
Beginning at ages 3 months to 2 years:
● Try to reduce dislocation — gradual abduction of the hips with bilateral skin traction (in infant); or skeletal traction (in child who is walking)
● Maintain immobilization — Bryant's traction or divarication traction for 2 to 3 weeks (with both extremities in traction, even if only one is affected); for children weighing less than 35 lb (16 kg)
● If traction fails — gentle closed reduction under general anesthesia to further abduct the hips, followed by spica cast for 4 to 6 months
● If closed treatment fails — open reduction and immobilization in spica cast for an average of 6 months or surgical division and realignment of bone (osteotomy).
Beginning at ages 2 to 5:
● Skeletal traction and subcutaneous adductor tenotomy (surgical cutting of the tendon)
● Osteotomy.
Delayed until after age 5:
● Restoration of satisfactory hip function is rare.

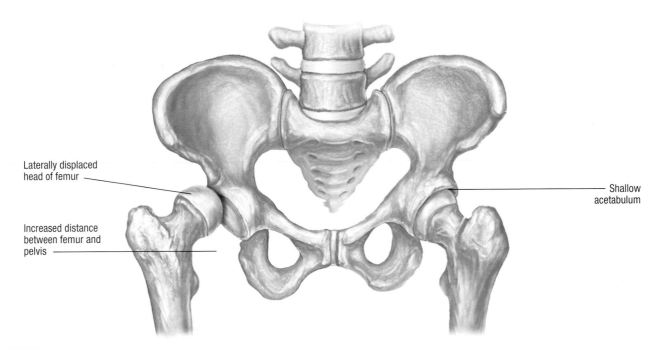

Laterally displaced head of femur

Increased distance between femur and pelvis

Shallow acetabulum

CLINICAL TIP

DIAGNOSING DDH

Observations during physical examination of the relaxed child that strongly suggest DDH include:
- Ortolani's test — elevation and abduction of the femur with the infant supine relocates a dislocated hip
- Barlow's test — adduction and depression of the femur dislocates a *dislocatable hip*; click or jerk is felt as the femoral head moves over the acetabular rim
- skin folds over the thighs — an extra fold on affected side when the child with *subluxation* or *dislocation* is lying supine, also apparent when the child lies prone
- buttock fold — higher on the affected side when the child is lying prone (also restricted abduction of the affected hip)
- Galeazzi's sign — when knees are flexed and feet together, the knee on the affected side appears lower

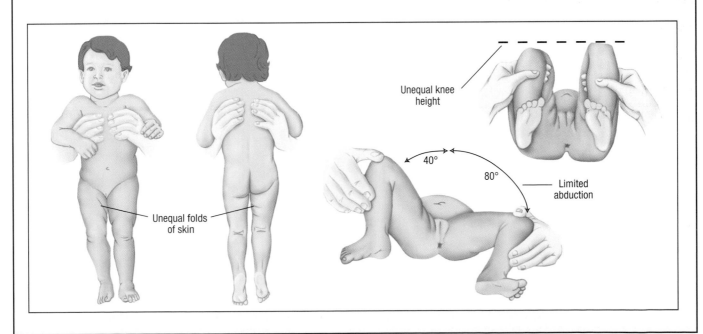

Unequal knee height

40°

80°

Limited abduction

Unequal folds of skin

FRACTURES

When a force exceeds the compressive or tensile strength of the bone, a fracture will occur. An estimated 25% of the population has traumatic musculoskeletal injury each year, and a significant number of these involve fractures. The prognosis varies with the extent of disability or deformity, amount of tissue and vascular damage, adequacy of reduction and immobilization, and patient's age, health, and nutritional status.

 AGE ALERT
Children's bones usually heal rapidly and without deformity. However, epiphyseal plate fractures in children are likely to cause deformity because they interfere with normal bone growth. In the elderly, underlying systemic illness, impaired circulation, or poor nutrition may cause slow or poor healing.

Causes
- Falls, motor vehicle accidents, sports
- Drugs that impair judgment or mobility
- Young age (immaturity of bone)
- Bone tumors
- Metabolic illnesses (such as hypoparathyroidism or hyperparathyroidism)
- Medications that cause iatrogenic osteoporosis, such as corticosteroids.

 AGE ALERT
The highest incidence of fractures occurs in young males between ages 15 and 24 (tibia, clavicle, and distal humerus); these fractures are usually the result of trauma. In the elderly, fractures of proximal femur, proximal humerus, vertebrae, distal radius, or pelvis are often associated with osteoporosis.

Pathophysiology
A fracture disrupts the periosteum and blood vessels in the cortex, marrow, and surrounding soft tissue. A hematoma forms between the broken ends of the bone and beneath the periosteum, and granulation tissue eventually replaces the hematoma.

Damage to bone tissue triggers an intense inflammatory response in which cells from surrounding soft tissue and the marrow cavity invade the fracture area, and blood flow to the entire bone increases. Osteoblasts in the periosteum, endosteum, and marrow produce osteoid (collagenous, young bone that has not yet calcified, also called callus). The osteoid hardens along the outer surface of the shaft and over the broken ends of the bone. Osteoclasts reabsorb material from previously formed bones and osteoblasts to rebuild bone. Osteoblasts then transform into osteocytes (mature bone cells).

Signs and symptoms
- Deformity
- Swelling, muscle spasm, tenderness
- Ecchymosis
- Impaired sensation distal to fracture site
- Limited range of motion
- Crepitus or clicking sounds on movement.

Diagnostic tests
X-rays are used to confirm the diagnosis and, after treatment, to confirm alignment.

Treatment
Emergency treatment for arm or leg fractures:
- Splinting the limb above and below the suspected fracture
- Applying a cold pack and elevating the limb.
  For severe fractures that cause blood loss:
- Direct pressure to control bleeding
- Fluid replacement as soon as possible.
  Closed reduction:
- Local anesthetic, analgesic, muscle relaxant or a sedative
- Manual manipulation.
  Open reduction if closed reduction is impossible or unsuccessful:
- Prophylactic tetanus immunization and antibiotics
- Surgery:
- thorough wound debridement
- immobilization by rods, plates, screws, or external fixation device.

FRACTURES OF THE ELBOW

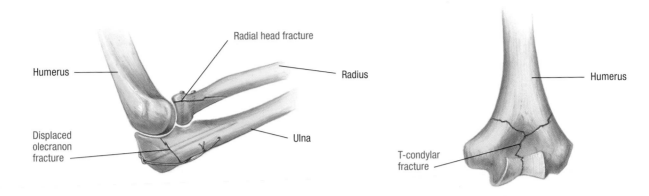

Humerus

Radial head fracture

Radius

Displaced olecranon fracture

Ulna

Humerus

T-condylar fracture

FRACTURES OF THE HAND AND WRIST

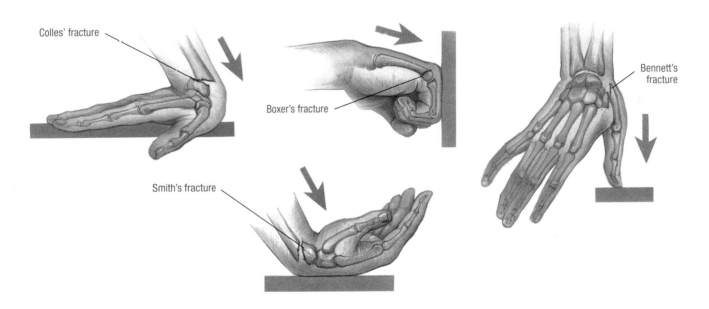

Colles' fracture

Boxer's fracture

Bennett's fracture

Smith's fracture

FRACTURES OF THE HIP

FRACTURES OF THE FOOT AND ANKLE

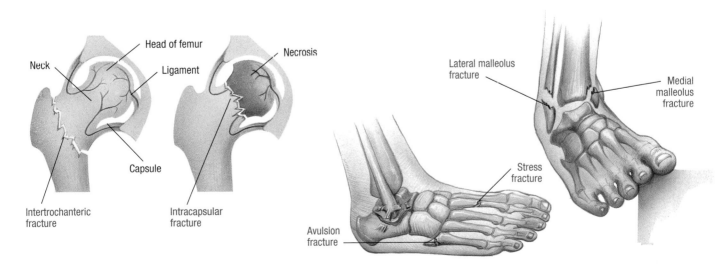

Neck

Head of femur

Ligament

Necrosis

Capsule

Intertrochanteric fracture

Intracapsular fracture

Lateral malleolus fracture

Medial malleolus fracture

Stress fracture

Avulsion fracture

GOUT

Primary gout is a metabolic disease marked by urate deposits that cause painfully arthritic joints. Secondary gout develops during the course of another disease. Gouty arthritis most commonly affects the foot, especially the great toe, ankle, or midfoot, but it may affect any joint. Gout follows an intermittent course, and patients may be completely free of symptoms for years between attacks. The prognosis is good with treatment. However, renal-tubular damage by aggregates of urate crystals may result in progressively poorer excretion of uric acid and chronic renal dysfunction.

AGE ALERT
Primary gout usually occurs in men after age 30 (95% of cases) and in postmenopausal women; secondary gout occurs in the elderly.

Causes

Primary gout:
• Possibly genetic defect in purine metabolism, causing overproduction of uric acid (hyperuricemia), retention of uric acid, or both.

  Secondary gout:
• Obesity, diabetes mellitus, hypertension, sickle cell anemia, renal disease
• Drug therapy, especially hydrochlorothiazide or pyrazinamide, which decrease excretion of urate (ionic form of uric acid).

Pathophysiology

When uric acid becomes supersaturated in blood and other body fluids, it crystallizes and forms tophi — accumulations of urate salts in connective tissue throughout the body. The presence of the crystals triggers an acute inflammatory response in which neutrophils begin to ingest the crystals. Tissue damage begins when the neutrophils release their lysosomes, which not only damage the tissues, but also perpetuate the inflammation.

In asymptomatic gout, serum urate levels rise but don't crystallize or produce symptoms. As the disease progresses, it may cause hypertension or urate kidney stones.

The first acute attack strikes suddenly and peaks quickly. Although it generally involves only one or a few joints, this initial attack is extremely painful. Affected joints appear hot, tender, inflamed, and dusky red or cyanotic. The metatarsophalangeal joint of the great toe usually becomes inflamed first (podagra), then the instep, ankle, heel, knee, or wrist joints. Sometimes a low-grade fever is present.

Mild acute attacks often subside quickly but tend to recur at irregular intervals. Severe attacks may persist for days or weeks. *Intercritical periods* are the symptom-free intervals between gout attacks. Most patients have a second attack within 6 months to 2 years.

Some attacks, common when gout goes untreated, tend to be longer and more severe than initial attacks. Such attacks are polyarticular, invariably affecting joints in the feet and legs, and sometimes accompanied by fever. A *migratory attack* sequentially strikes various joints and the Achilles' tendon and is associated with either subdeltoid or olecranon bursitis.

Eventually, *chronic polyarticular gout* sets in. Persistent painful polyarthritis, with large tophi in cartilages, synovial membranes, tendons, and soft tissue, mark this final, unremitting stage of the disease. Tophi form in fingers, hands, knees, feet, ulnar sides of the forearms, pinnae of the ears, Achilles' tendons and, rarely, in internal organs, such as the kidneys and myocardium. The skin over the tophus may ulcerate and release a chalky, white exudate that consists primarily of uric acid crystals.

Signs and symptoms

• Joint pain, redness, swelling
• Tophi in great toe, ankle, pinna of ear
• Elevated skin temperature.

Diagnostic tests

• Needle aspiration of synovial fluid or biopsy of tophi
• Serum uric acid
• 24-hour urine uric acid
• X-rays.

Treatment

Acute gout:
• Immobilization and protection of the inflamed, painful joints; local application of heat or cold
• Increased fluid intake to prevent kidney stone formation
• Colchicine (oral or I.V.) to inhibit phagocytosis of uric acid crystals by neutrophils (doesn't affect uric acid level)
• Nonsteroidal anti-inflammatory drugs for pain and inflammation.

  Chronic gout:
• Allopurinol to suppress uric acid formation or control uric acid levels, preventing further attacks (use cautiously in renal failure)
• Colchicine to prevent recurrent acute attacks until uric acid level subsides (doesn't affect uric acid level)
• Uricosuric agents (probenecid or sulfinpyrazone) to promote uric acid excretion and inhibit uric acid accumulation (of limited value in patients with renal impairment)
• Avoidance of alcohol and purine-rich foods (shellfish, liver, sardines, anchovies) that increase urate levels.

GOUTY ARTHRITIS OF THE KNEE

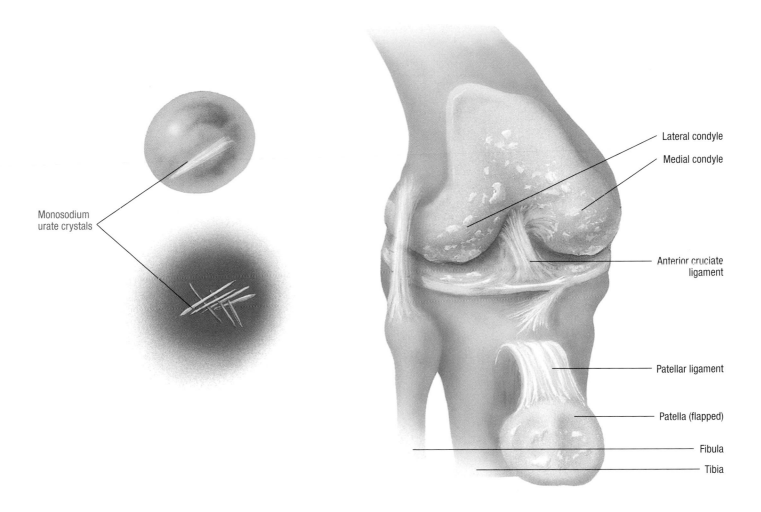

Monosodium urate crystals

Lateral condyle

Medial condyle

Anterior cruciate ligament

Patellar ligament

Patella (flapped)

Fibula

Tibia

GOUT OF THE FOOT

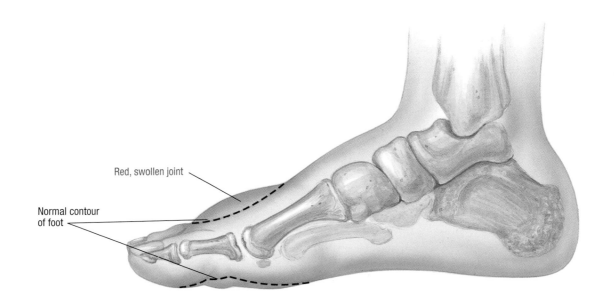

Red, swollen joint

Normal contour of foot

MUSCULAR DYSTROPHY

Muscular dystrophy is a group of congenital disorders characterized by progressive symmetric wasting of skeletal muscles without neural or sensory defects. Paradoxically, some wasted muscles tend to enlarge (pseudohypertrophy) because connective tissue and fat replace muscle tissue, giving a false impression of increased muscle mass. The prognosis varies with the form of disease. The four main types of muscular dystrophy are:

• *Duchenne,* or *pseudohypertrophic* (50% of all cases): strikes during early childhood, is usually fatal during the second decade of life, and affects 13 to 33 per 100,000 persons, mostly males
• *Becker's,* or *benign pseudohypertrophic* (milder form of Duchenne): becomes apparent between ages 5 and 15 years, is usually fatal by age 50, and affects 1 to 3 per 100,000 persons, mostly males
• *Facioscapulohumeral (Landouzy-Dejerine)* and *limb-girdle:* usually manifest in second to fourth decades of live, don't shorten life expectancy and affect both sexes equally.

CLINICAL TIP
Possible complications of Duchenne muscular dystrophy are:
• weakened cardiac and respiratory muscles leading to tachycardia, electrocardiographic abnormalities, and pulmonary complications
• sudden heart failure, respiratory failure, infection.

Causes
Genetic mechanisms, typically causing an enzymatic or metabolic defect:
• Duchenne or Becker dystrophy — X-linked recessive disorders; mapped to the Xp21 locus for the muscle protein dystrophin, which is essential for maintaining muscle cell membrane; muscle cells deteriorate or die without it
• Limb-girdle dystrophy — autosomal recessive disorder
• Facioscapulohumeral dystrophy — autosomal dominant disorder.

Pathophysiology
Abnormally permeable cell membranes allow leakage of a variety of muscle enzymes, particularly creatine kinase. The metabolic defect that causes the muscle cells to die is present from fetal life onward. The absence of progressive muscle wasting at birth suggests that other factors compound the effect of dystrophin deficiency. The specific trigger is unknown, but phagocytosis of the muscle cells by inflammatory cells causes scarring and loss of muscle function.

As the disease progresses, skeletal muscle becomes almost totally replaced by fat and connective tissue. The skeleton eventually becomes deformed, causing progressive immobility.

Cardiac muscle and smooth muscle of the GI tract often become fibrotic. The brain exhibits no consistent structural abnormalities.

Signs and symptoms
Duchenne (pseudohypertrophic):
• Insidious onset between ages 3 and 5
• Initial effects on legs, pelvis, shoulders:
– enlarged, firm calf muscles
– waddling gait, toe-walking, and lumbar lordosis
– difficulty climbing stairs
– frequent falls
– positive Gower's sign — patient stands from a sitting position by "walking" hands up legs to compensate for pelvic and trunk weakness.
Becker's (benign pseudohypertrophic):
• Similar to those of Duchenne type but with slower progression.
Facioscapulohumeral (Landouzy-Dejerine):
• Weak face, shoulder, and upper arm muscles (initial sign):
– pendulous lip and absent nasolabial fold
– abnormal facial movements; absence of facial movements when laughing or crying
– masklike expression
• Inability to raise arms above head.
Limb-girdle:
• Weakness in upper arms and pelvis (initial sign)
• Lumbar lordosis, protruding abdomen
• Winging of scapulae
• Waddling gait, poor balance
• Inability to raise arms.

Diagnostic tests
• Electromyography
• Muscle biopsy
• Immunologic and molecular biological assays.

Treatment
Supportive only:
• Coughing and deep-breathing exercises
• Diaphragmatic breathing
• Teaching parents to recognize early signs of respiratory complications
• Orthopedic appliances, physical therapy
• Surgery to correct contractures
• Adequate fluid intake, increased dietary bulk, and stool softener
• Low-calorie, high-protein, high-fiber diet.

MUSCLES AFFECTED IN DIFFERENT TYPES OF MUSCULAR DYSTROPHY

Duchenne

Limb-girdle

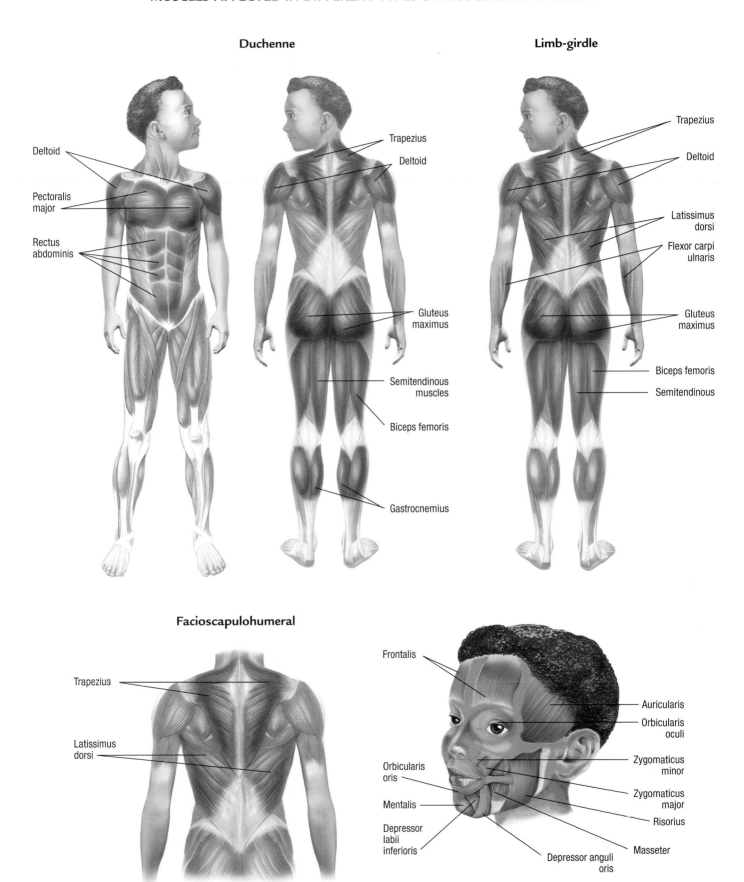

Deltoid

Pectoralis major

Rectus abdominis

Trapezius

Deltoid

Gluteus maximus

Semitendinous muscles

Biceps femoris

Gastrocnemius

Trapezius

Deltoid

Latissimus dorsi

Flexor carpi ulnaris

Gluteus maximus

Biceps femoris

Semitendinous

Facioscapulohumeral

Trapezius

Latissimus dorsi

Frontalis

Orbicularis oris

Mentalis

Depressor labii inferioris

Depressor anguli oris

Auricularis

Orbicularis oculi

Zygomaticus minor

Zygomaticus major

Risorius

Masseter

OSTEOARTHRITIS

Osteoarthritis, the most common form of arthritis, is a chronic condition caused by deterioration of joint cartilage. It usually affects weight-bearing joints (knees, feet, hips, lumbar vertebrae). Osteoarthritis is widespread (affecting more than 60 million persons in the United States) and is more common in women. Typically, its earliest symptoms manifest in middle age and progress. Osteoarthritis may be secondary to the wear and tear of aging (idiopathic) or to some abnormal initiating event.

Osteoarthritis is the most common cause of disability in the U.S. Disability depends on the site and severity of involvement and can range from minor limitation of finger movement to severe disability in persons with hip or knee involvement. The rate of progression varies, and joints may remain stable for years in an early stage of deterioration.

Causes

Idiopathic — contributing factors:
- Metabolic — endocrine disorders such as hyperparathyroidism
- Genetic — decreased collagen synthesis
- Chemical — drugs that stimulate collagen-digesting enzymes in synovial membranes, such as corticosteroids
- Mechanical factors — repeated stress.
  Secondary — identifiable predisposing event:
- Trauma (most common)
- Congenital deformity
- Obesity, poor posture
- Occupational stress.

Pathophysiology

Osteoarthritis occurs in synovial joints. The joint cartilage deteriorates, and reactive new bone forms at the margins and subchondral areas of the joints. The degeneration results from damage to the chondrocytes. Cartilage softens with age, narrowing the joint space. Mechanical injury erodes articular cartilage, leaving the underlying bone unprotected. This causes sclerosis, or thickening and hardening of the bone underneath the cartilage.

Cartilage particles irritate the synovial lining, which becomes fibrotic and limits joint movement. Synovial fluid may be forced into defects in the bone, causing cysts. New bone, called osteophyte (bone spur), forms at joint margins as the articular cartilage erodes, causing gross alteration of the bony contours and enlargement of the joint.

Signs and symptoms
- Deep, aching joint pain
- Stiffness in the morning and after exercise (relieved by rest)
- Crepitus, or grating of the joint during motion
- Heberden's nodes (bony enlargements of distal interphalangeal joints)
- Altered gait from contractures
- Decreased range of motion
- Joint enlargement
- Localized headaches (may be direct result of cervical spine arthritis)
- Bouchard's nodes (bony enlargement of proximal interphalangeal joint).

Diagnostic tests
- Erythrocyte sedimentation rate
- X-ray
- Arthroscopy.

Treatment
- Weight loss to reduce stress on the joint
- Balanced rest and exercise
- Medications, including aspirin and other nonsteroidal anti-inflammatory drugs; propoxyphene, acetaminophen, glucosamine
- Support or stabilization of joint with crutches, braces, cane, walker, cervical collar, or traction
- Intra-articular injections of corticosteroids (every 4 to 6 months) to try to delay node formation in fingers.
  Surgical treatment, for severe disability or uncontrollable pain:
- Arthroplasty — partial or total replacement of joint with prosthetic appliance
- Arthrodesis or laminectomy — fusion of bones, primarily in spine
- Osteoplasty — scraping and lavage of deteriorated bone
- Osteotomy — changing alignment of bone to relieve stress on joint.

JOINTS AFFECTED BY OSTEOARTHRITIS

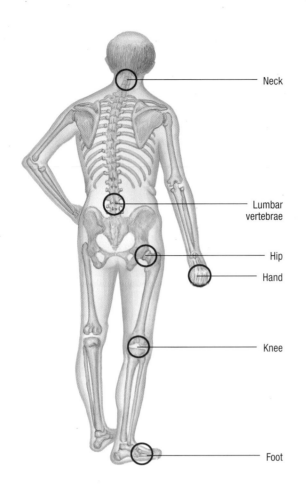

- Neck
- Lumbar vertebrae
- Hip
- Hand
- Knee
- Foot

Hand

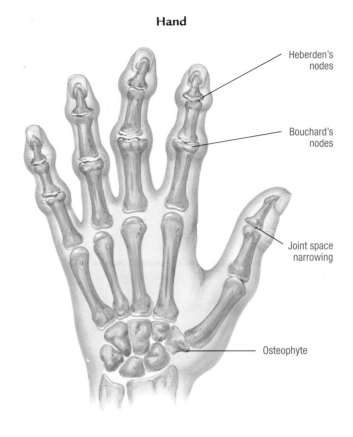

- Heberden's nodes
- Bouchard's nodes
- Joint space narrowing
- Osteophyte

Right knee

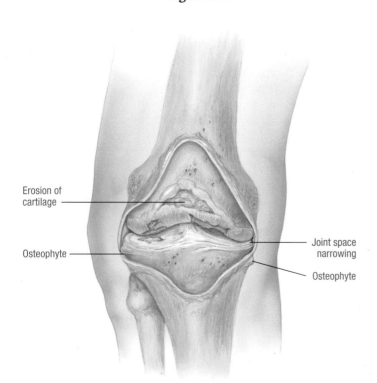

- Erosion of cartilage
- Osteophyte
- Joint space narrowing
- Osteophyte

Hip

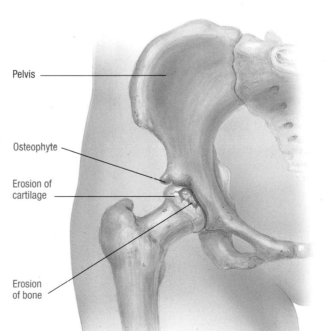

- Pelvis
- Osteophyte
- Erosion of cartilage
- Erosion of bone

OSTEOMYELITIS

Osteomyelitis is a bone infection characterized by progressive inflammatory destruction after formation of new bone. It may be chronic or acute. It commonly results from a combination of local trauma — usually trivial but causing a hematoma — and an acute infection originating elsewhere in the body. Although osteomyelitis usually remains localized, it can spread through the bone to the marrow, cortex, and periosteum. Possible consequences include amputation of an arm or leg when resistant chronic osteomyelitis causes severe, unrelenting pain and decreased function due to weakened bone cortex. Acute osteomyelitis is usually a blood-borne disease and most commonly affects rapidly growing children. Draining sinus tracts and widespread lesions characterize chronic osteomyelitis, which is rare.

 AGE ALERT
Osteomyelitis occurs more often in children (especially boys) than in adults — usually as a complication of an acute localized infection. The most common sites in children are the distal femur and the proximal tibia, humerus, and radius. The most common sites in adults are the pelvis and vertebrae, generally after surgery or trauma.

Incidence of osteomyelitis is declining, except in drug abusers. With prompt treatment, prognosis is good for acute osteomyelitis but remains poor for chronic osteomyelitis.

Causes
- *Staphylococcus aureus* (most common)
- *Streptococcus pyogenes*
- *Pneumococcus species*
- *Pseudomonas aeruginosa*
- *Escherichia coli*
- *Proteus vulgaris*
- *Pasteurella multocida* (part of normal mouth flora in cats and dogs).

Pathophysiology
Typically, a pathogen finds a culture site in a hematoma after recent trauma or in a weakened area, such as the site of local infection (for example, furunculosis), and travels through the bloodstream to the metaphysis, the section of a long bone that is continuous with the epiphysis plates, where the blood flows into sinusoids.

Signs and symptoms
- Sudden pain and tenderness in the affected bone
- Swelling, restricted movement of surrounding soft tissues
- Chronic infection presenting intermittently for years, flaring after minor trauma or persisting as drainage of pus from a pocket in a sinus tract.

Diagnostic tests
- White blood cell count, erythrocyte sedimentation rate
- Blood cultures
- X-ray — may not show bone involvement until disease has been active for 2 to 3 weeks
- Bone scan, magnetic resonance imaging.

Treatment
- Immobilization of affected body part by cast, traction, or bed rest
- Supportive measures, such as analgesics for pain and I.V. fluids to maintain hydration
- Incision, drainage, and culture of an abscess or sinus tract.
  Acute infection:
- Systemic antibiotics
- Intracavitary instillation through closed-system continuous irrigation with low intermittent suction
- Limited irrigation; blood drainage system with suction (Hemovac)
- Packed, wet, antibiotic-soaked dressings.
  Chronic osteomyelitis:
- Surgery to remove dead bone and promote drainage (prognosis remains poor even after surgery)
- Hyperbaric oxygen
- Skin, bone, and muscle grafts.

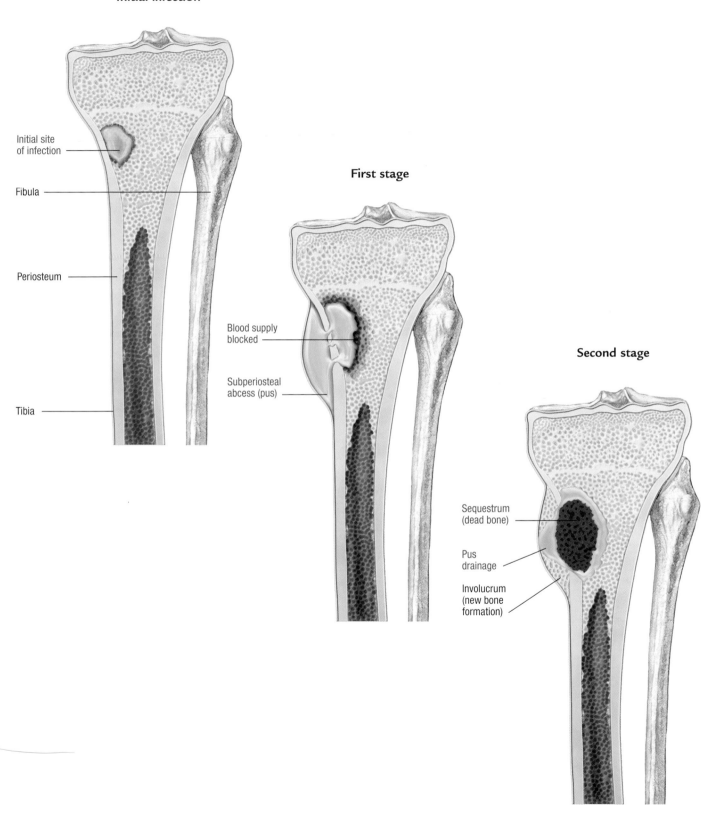

Initial infection

Initial site
of infection

Fibula

Periosteum

Tibia

First stage

Blood supply
blocked

Subperiosteal
abcess (pus)

Second stage

Sequestrum
(dead bone)

Pus
drainage

Involucrum
(new bone
formation)

OSTEOPOROSIS

Osteoporosis is a metabolic bone disorder in which the rate of bone resorption accelerates while the rate of bone formation slows, causing a loss of bone mass. Bones affected by this disease lose calcium and phosphate salts and become porous, brittle, and abnormally vulnerable to fractures. Osteoporosis may be primary or secondary to an underlying disease, such as Cushing syndrome or hyperthyroidism. It primarily affects the weight-bearing vertebrae. Only when the condition is advanced or severe, as in secondary disease, do similar changes occur in the skull, ribs, and long bones. Often, the femoral heads and pelvic acetabula are selectively affected.

AGE ALERT
Primary osteoporosis is often called senile or postmenopausal osteoporosis because it most commonly develops in postmenopausal women.

Causes

Primary osteoporosis:
- Unknown.
- Contributory factors include:
- mild but prolonged negative calcium balance
- declining gonadal and adrenal function
- relative or progressive estrogen deficiency
- sedentary lifestyle.

   Secondary osteoporosis:
- Prolonged therapy with corticosteroids, heparin, anticonvulsants
- Total immobilization or disuse of a bone (as in hemiplegia)
- Alcoholism, malnutrition, malabsorption, scurvy
- Lactose intolerance
- Endocrine disorders such as hyperthyroidism, hyperparathyroidism, Cushing syndrome, diabetes mellitus
- Osteogenesis imperfecta
- Sudeck's atrophy (localized to hands and feet).

Pathophysiology

In normal bone, the rates of bone formation and resorption are constant; replacement follows resorption immediately, and the amount of bone replaced equals the amount of bone resorbed. The endocrine system maintains plasma and bone calcium and phosphate balance. Estrogen also supports normal bone metabolism by stimulating osteoblastic activity and limiting the osteoclastic-stimulating effects of parathyroid hormones. Osteoporosis develops when new bone formation falls behind resorption. For example, heparin promotes bone resorption by inhibiting collagen synthesis or enhancing collagen breakdown. Elevated levels of cortisone, either endogenous or exogenous, inhibit gastrointestinal absorption of calcium.

CLINICAL TIP
When the rate of bone resorption exceeds that of bone formation, the bone becomes less dense. Men have approximately 30% greater bone mass than women, which may explain why osteoporosis develops later in men.

Signs and symptoms
- Typically, asymptomatic until a fracture occurs
- Spontaneous fractures or those involving minimal trauma to vertebrae, distal radius, or femoral neck
- Progressive deformity — kyphosis, loss of height
- Decreased exercise tolerance.

Diagnostic tests
- Serial height measurements
- Dual- or single-photon absorptiometry
- X-ray
- Computed tomography scan
- Serum calcium, phosphorus, alkaline phosphatase, parathyroid hormone.

Treatment

Early prevention to control bone loss, prevent fractures, control pain:
- Limited alcohol and tobacco use, balanced diet
- Early mobilization after surgery, trauma, or illness
- Identification and treatment of risk factors
- Physical therapy emphasizing regular, moderate weight-bearing exercise
- Supportive devices, such as a back brace
- Prompt, effective treatment of underlying disorder to prevent secondary osteoporosis.

   Pharmacotherapy:
- Hormone replacement therapy to slow bone loss
- Analgesics and local heat to relieve pain
- Calcium and vitamin D supplements
- Calcitonin, biophosphonates, or fluoride.

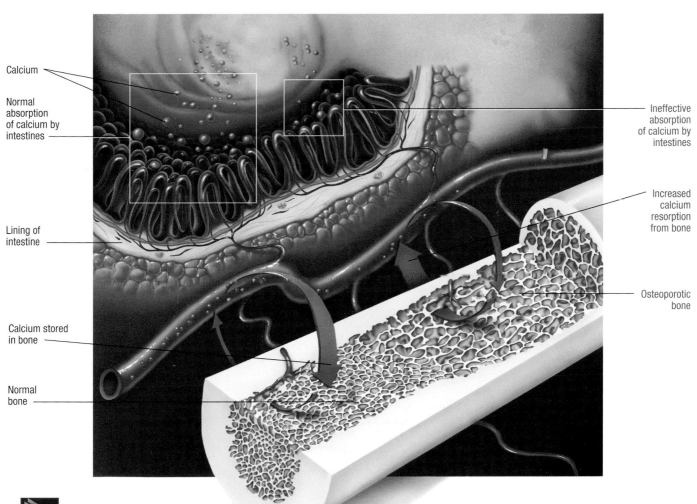

Calcium

Normal absorption of calcium by intestines

Lining of intestine

Calcium stored in bone

Normal bone

Ineffective absorption of calcium by intestines

Increased calcium resorption from bone

Osteoporotic bone

 CLINICAL TIP

OSTEOPOROSIS

Dorsal kyphosis, or dowager's hump, often results from fractures to the front of the vertebral body. These wedge-shaped injuries are commonly associated with age-related osteoporosis.

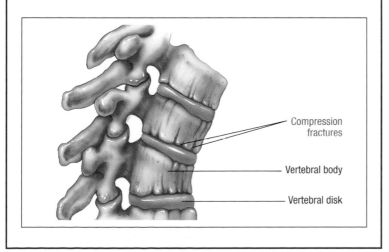

Compression fractures

Vertebral body

Vertebral disk

SCOLIOSIS

Scoliosis is a lateral curvature of the thoracic, lumbar, or thoracolumbar spine. The curve may be convex to the right (more common in thoracic curves) or to the left (more common in lumbar curves). Rotation of the vertebral column around its axis may cause rib cage deformity. Scoliosis may be associated with kyphosis (humpback) and lordosis (swayback).

 AGE ALERT
About 2% to 3% of adolescents have scoliosis. In general, the greater the magnitude of the curve and the younger the child at the time of diagnosis, the greater the risk for progression of the spinal abnormality. Optimal treatment usually achieves favorable outcome.

Scoliosis may be functional, a reversible deformity, or structural (fixed deformity of spinal column). The most common curve in functional or structural scoliosis arises in the thoracic segment, with convexity to the right. As the spine curves laterally, compensatory curves (S curves) with convexity to the left develop in the cervical and lumbar segments to maintain body balance.

Idiopathic scoliosis, the most common type of structural scoliosis, varies according to age at onset, as follows:
• infantile — affects mostly male infants between birth and age 3; left thoracic and right lumbar curves
• juvenile — affects both sexes between ages 4 and 10; no typical curvature
• adolescent — generally affects girls between age 10 and skeletal maturity; no typical curvature.

Causes

Functional:
• Poor posture
• Uneven leg length.
    Structural:
• Congenital — wedge vertebrae, fused ribs or vertebrae, hemivertebrae
• Paralytic or musculoskeletal — asymmetric paralysis of trunk muscles due to polio, cerebral palsy, or muscular dystrophy
• Idiopathic — most common; appears in a previously straight spine during the growing years; may be transmitted as an autosomal dominant or multifactorial trait.

Pathophysiology

Differential stress on vertebral bone causes an imbalance of osteoblastic activity; thus, the curve progresses rapidly during adolescent growth spurt. Without treatment, the imbalance continues into adulthood. A lateral curve continues to progress at the rate of 1 degree a year even after skeletal maturity.

Signs and symptoms

• Backache
• Fatigue
• Dyspnea.
    Subtle signs:
• Uneven hemlines or pant legs that appear unequal in length
• Apparent discrepancy in hip height.
    Physical examination:
• Unequal shoulder heights, elbow levels, and heights of iliac crests
• Asymmetric thoracic cage and misalignment of the spinal vertebrae when patient bends forward
• Asymmetric paraspinal muscles, rounded on the convex side of the curve and flattened on the concave side
• Asymmetric gait.

Diagnostic tests

• Anterior, posterior, and lateral spinal X-rays, taken with the patient standing upright and bending
• Scoliosiometry to measure the angle of trunk rotation.

Treatment

Mild scoliosis (less than 25 degrees):
• Observation — X-rays to monitor curve, examination every 3 months
• Exercise to strengthen torso muscles and prevent curve progression.
    Moderate scoliosis (30 to 50 degrees):
• Spinal exercises and a brace (may halt progression but doesn't correct established curvature); braces can be adjusted as the patient grows and worn until bone growth is complete
• Alternative therapy using transcutaneous electrical nerve stimulation.
    Severe scoliosis (50 degrees or more):
• Surgery — supportive instrumentation; spinal fusion in severe cases.

NORMAL AND ABNORMAL CURVATURES OF THE SPINE

Normal

Scoliosis

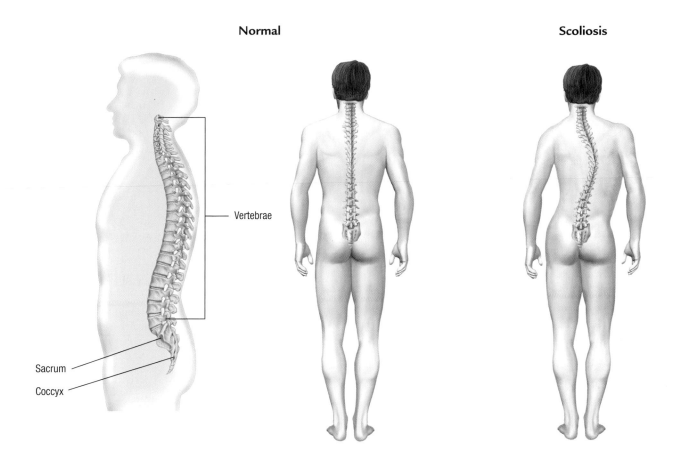

Vertebrae

Sacrum

Coccyx

LORDOSIS

CAUSES OF KYPHOSIS

Absence of a corner or flattening by compression

Incomplete vertebral segmentation

Absence of a vertebra (T12)

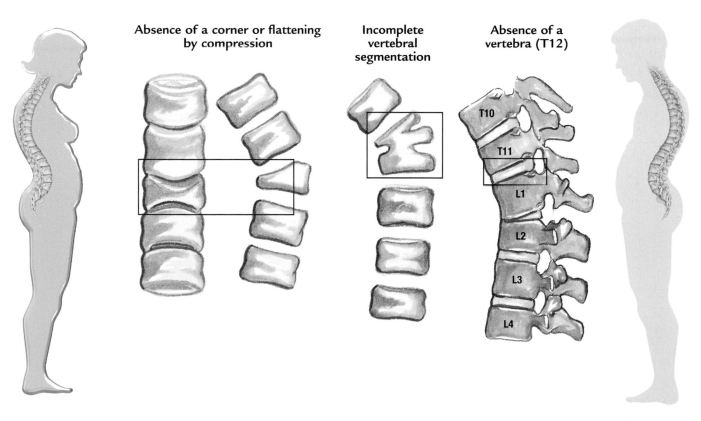

T10

T11

L1

L2

L3

L4

SPRAINS

A sprain is a complete or incomplete tear of the supporting ligaments surrounding a joint when a joint is forced beyond its normal range of motion. Joint dislocations and fractures may accompany a severe sprain. The ankle is the most commonly sprained joint. Finger, wrist, knee, and shoulder sprains are also common.

Causes
- Falls
- Motor vehicle accidents
- Sports injuries.

Pathophysiology
A ligament may tear either at any point along the ligament itself or at its attachment to bone (with or without avulsion of bone). Bleeding and formation of hematoma are followed by formation of an inflammatory exudate and development of granulation tissue. Collagen formation begins 4 to 5 days after the injury, eventually organizing fibers parallel to the lines of stress. However, swelling, stretching or impinging on nerves or vessels around the joint may cause neurovascular compromise. Further reorganization results in eventual strengthening of the damaged ligament, although persistent laxity may result in chronic joint instability.

Signs and symptoms
- Localized pain (especially during joint movement) and tenderness
- Swelling and warmth
- Progressive loss of motion
- Ecchymosis.

 CLINICAL TIP

Sprains are graded according to the degree of swelling and instability:
Grade I: stable, minimal swelling
Grade II: moderate instability and swelling
Grade III: gross instability, extensive swelling and ecchymosis.

Diagnostic tests
- Stress radiography
- Magnetic resonance imaging
- Arthrography (rarely used).

Treatment
- Elevate the joint above the level of the heart for 48 to 72 hours (immediately after the injury)
- Intermittent ice packs for 12 to 48 hours
- Immobilizer or splint during acute phase (up to 1 week)
- Nonsteroidal anti-inflammatory drugs and analgesics
- Early range-of-motion exercise as tolerated
- Acute surgical repair if indicated — notably, for ulnar collateral ligament of thumb, multiple ligament injuries of the knee or elbow due to dislocation
- Late surgical reconstruction if indicated for chronic instability of shoulder, knee, ankle.

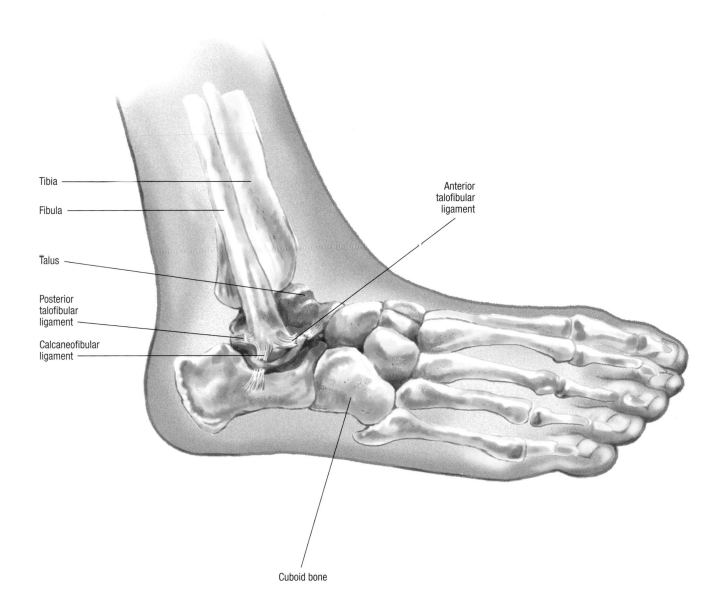

Tibia

Fibula

Talus

Posterior talofibular ligament

Calcaneofibular ligament

Anterior talofibular ligament

Cuboid bone

STRAINS

A strain is an injury to a muscle-tendon unit. Sudden forceful contraction of a muscle under stretch overloads its tensile strength resulting in failure at the muscle-tendon junction. Muscles that cross two joints are most susceptible to strain. These include the hamstrings, rectus femoris of the thigh, gastrocnemius of the calf, and biceps brachialis of the upper arm.

Causes
- Sudden or unanticipated muscle contraction due to falling, sprinting, throwing, or other forceful activity
- Inadequate warm-ups and conditioning
- Degenerative changes in muscle-tendon units secondary to aging, or anabolic steroid use.

Pathophysiology
Bleeding into the muscle and surrounding tissue occurs when a muscle is torn. When a tendon or muscle is torn, an inflammatory exudate develops between the torn ends. Granulation tissue grows inward from the surrounding soft tissue and cartilage. Collagen formation begins 4 to 5 days after the injury, eventually organizing fibers parallel to the lines of stress. With the aid of vascular fibrous tissue, the new tissue eventually fuses with surrounding tissues. As further reorganization takes place, the new tendon or muscle separates from the surrounding tissue and eventually becomes strong enough to withstand normal muscle strain.

If a muscle is chronically strained, calcium may deposit in the muscle, limiting movement by causing stiffness, and muscle fatigue.

Signs and symptoms
- Pain
- Inflammation
- Erythema
- Ecchymosis
- Elevated skin temperature.

Diagnostic tests
- X-ray
- Stress radiography
- Muscle biopsy (rarely done).

Treatment
- Compression wrap
- Elevating injured part above the level of the heart
- Analgesics
- Application of ice for up to 48 hours, then application of heat
- Surgery to suture tendon or muscle ends in close approximation.

  Chronic strains:
- Treatment usually unnecessary
- Heat, nonsteroidal anti-inflammatory drugs, analgesic muscle relaxants to relieve discomfort.

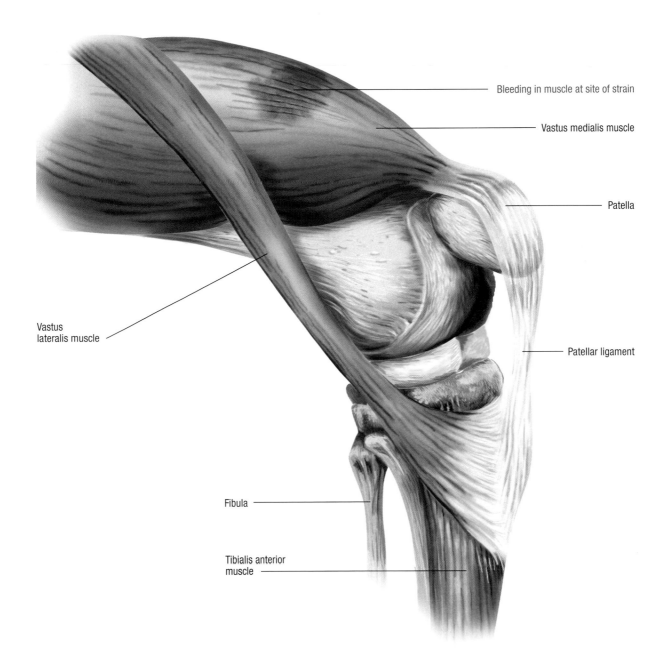

Bleeding in muscle at site of strain

Vastus medialis muscle

Patella

Vastus
lateralis muscle

Patellar ligament

Fibula

Tibialis anterior
muscle

TENDINITIS

Tendinitis is a painful inflammation of tendons and of tendon-muscle attachments to bone, especially in the shoulder rotator cuff, Achilles' tendon, or hamstring.

Causes
- Overuse, such as strain during sports activity
- Other musculoskeletal disorder, such as rheumatic diseases, congenital defects
- Postural misalignment.

Pathophysiology
A tendon is a band of dense fibrous connective tissue that attaches muscle to bone. Tendons are extremely strong, flexible, and inelastic. Tendinitis is an inflammation of the tendon, usually resulting from a strain.

AGE ALERT
Common forms of tendinitis in adolescents (both males and females) are patellar tendinitis associated with inflammation of the tibial apophysis (Osgood-Schlatter disease) and Achilles' tendinitis at the calcaneal apophysis (Sever's disease).

Signs and symptoms
- Restricted range of motion
- Localized pain (most severe at night; commonly interferes with sleep)
- Swelling

- Calcific tendinitis:
- proximal weakness (due to calcium deposits in the tendon)
- calcium erosion into adjacent bursae (acute calcific bursitis)
- Normal X-rays at first; later, bony fragments, osteophyte sclerosis, or calcium deposits.

Diagnostic tests
- X-ray
- Arthrography
- Computed tomography scan
- Magnetic resonance imaging.

Treatment
- Rest — immobilization with a sling, splint, or cast
- Systemic analgesics
- Application of cold or heat
- Injection of a corticosteroid and an anesthetic such as lidocaine into tendon sheath
- Oral nonsteroidal anti-inflammatory drugs until patient is free of pain and able to perform range-of-motion exercises easily
- Surgical debridement of degenerative tendon or excision of calcific deposits may be needed.

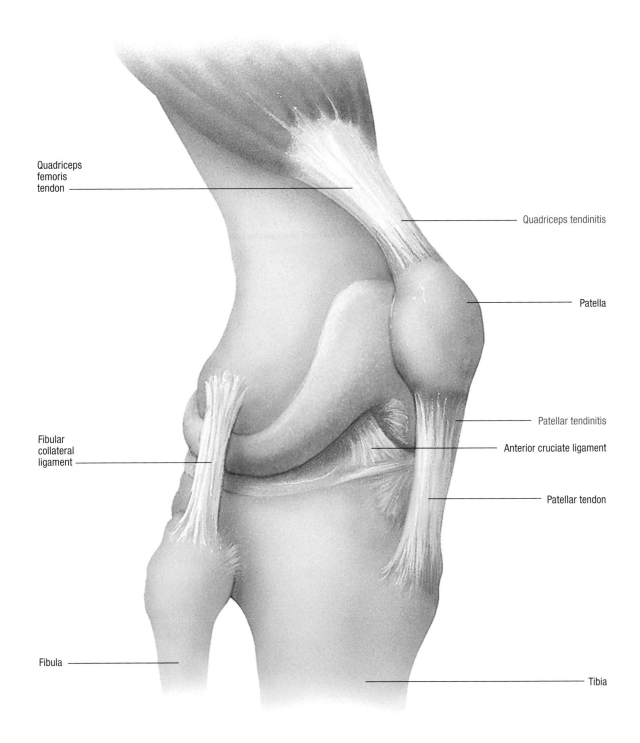

Quadriceps femoris tendon

Quadriceps tendinitis

Patella

Patellar tendinitis

Anterior cruciate ligament

Fibular collateral ligament

Patellar tendon

Fibula

Tibia

APLASTIC ANEMIA

Aplastic, or hypoplastic, anemias result from injury to or destruction of stem cells in bone marrow or the bone marrow matrix, causing pancytopenia (anemia, leukopenia, and thrombocytopenia) and bone marrow hypoplasia. Although commonly used interchangeably with other terms for bone marrow failure, *aplastic anemia* properly refers to pancytopenia resulting from the decreased functional capacity of a hypoplastic, fatty bone marrow.

These disorders generally produce fatal bleeding or infection, especially when they are idiopathic or caused by chloramphenicol or infectious hepatitis.

Causes
- Congenital
- Autoimmune reactions, or other severe disease (especially hepatitis)
- Radiation (about half of such anemias)
- Drugs (antibiotics, anticonvulsants)
- Toxic agents (such as benzene or chloramphenicol).

 AGE ALERT
Two identified forms of aplastic anemia are congenital — hypoplastic or Blackfan-Diamond anemia (develops between ages 2 and 3 months); and Fanconi syndrome (develops between birth and age 10).

Pathophysiology
Aplastic anemia usually develops when damaged or destroyed stem cells inhibit blood cell production. Less commonly, damage to bone marrow microvasculature creates an unfavorable environment for cell growth and maturation.

Signs and symptoms
- Progressive weakness and fatigue, shortness of breath, headache, pallor and, ultimately, tachycardia and heart failure
- Ecchymosis, petechiae, and hemorrhage, especially from the mucous membranes (nose, gums, rectum, vagina) or into the retina or central nervous system
- Infection (fever, oral and rectal ulcers, sore throat) without characteristic inflammation due to neutropenia (neutrophil deficiency).

Diagnostic tests
- Complete blood count
- Serum iron studies
- Bone marrow biopsy.

Treatment
- Packed red blood cell (RBC) or platelet transfusion; experimental histocompatibility locus antigen-matched leukocyte transfusions
- Bone marrow transplantation (treatment of choice for anemia due to severe aplasia and for patients who need constant RBC transfusions)
- Special measures to prevent infection, such as avoidance of exposure to communicable diseases, diligent handwashing
- Specific antibiotics for infection — not given prophylactically because they encourage resistant strains of organisms
- Respiratory support with oxygen for patients with low hemoglobin levels
- Corticosteroids to suppress autoimmune disease; marrow-stimulating agents, such as androgens (controversial); antilymphocyte globulin (experimental); colony-stimulating factors to encourage growth of specific cellular components.

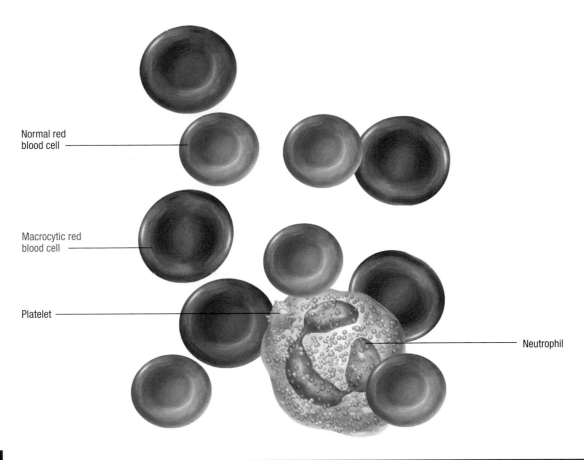

Normal red blood cell

Macrocytic red blood cell

Platelet

Neutrophil

CLINICAL TIP

BONE MARROW ASPIRATION AND BIOPSY

Bone marrow aspiration and biopsy provides the only definitive diagnosis of aplastic anemia. The usual sites are the sternum and the iliac crest.

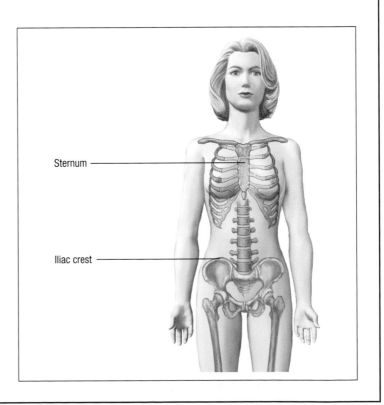

Sternum

Iliac crest

DISSEMINATED INTRAVASCULAR COAGULATION

Disseminated intravascular coagulation (DIC) occurs as a complication of diseases and conditions that accelerate clotting. It causes small blood vessel occlusion, organ necrosis, depletion of circulating clotting factors and platelets, activation of the fibrinolytic system, and consequent severe hemorrhage. Clotting in the microcirculation usually affects the kidneys and extremities but may occur in the brain, lungs, pituitary and adrenal glands, and GI mucosa. DIC, also called *consumption coagulopathy* or *defibrination syndrome,* is generally an acute condition but may be chronic in cancer patients (Trousseau's syndrome). Prognosis depends on early detection and treatment, the severity of the hemorrhage, and treatment of the underlying disease.

Causes

The etiology of DIC remains unclear. However, in many patients, the triggering mechanisms may be the entrance of foreign protein into the circulation and vascular endothelial injury.

DIC may result from:
- Infections — gram-negative or gram-positive septicemia; viral, fungal, rickettsial, protozoal infection (malaria)
- Obstetric complications — abruptio placentae, amniotic fluid embolism, retained dead fetus, septic abortion, eclampsia
- Neoplasia — acute leukemia, metastatic carcinoma, especially adenocarcinoma
- Necrosis — extensive burns or trauma, brain tissue destruction, transplant rejection, hepatic necrosis.

Other causes include heatstroke, shock, poisonous snakebite, cirrhosis, fat embolism, incompatible blood transfusion, cardiac arrest, surgery necessitating cardiopulmonary bypass, giant hemangioma, severe venous thrombosis, and purpura fulminans.

It's not clear why such disorders lead to DIC; nor is it certain that they lead to it through a common mechanism. In many patients, the triggering mechanisms may be the entrance of foreign protein into the circulation and vascular endothelial injury.

Pathophysiology

Regardless of how DIC begins, the typical accelerated clotting results in generalized activation of prothrombin and a consequent excess of thrombin. The thrombin converts fibrinogen to fibrin, producing fibrin clots in the microcirculation. This process uses huge amounts of coagulation factors (especially fibrinogen, prothrombin, platelets, and factors V and VIII), causing hypofibrinogenemia, hypoprothrombinemia, thrombocytopenia, and deficiencies in factors V and VIII. Circulating thrombin also activates the fibrinolytic system, which dissolves fibrin clots into fibrin degradation products. Hemorrhage may be mostly the result of the anticoagulant activity of fibrin degradation products as well as depletion of plasma coagulation factors.

Signs and symptoms

- Abnormal bleeding:
- cutaneous oozing of serum, bleeding from surgical or I.V. sites, bleeding from the GI tract
- petechiae or blood blisters (purpura), epistaxis, hemoptysis
- Cyanosis; cold, mottled fingers and toes
- Severe muscle, back, abdominal, and chest pain
- Nausea and vomiting (may be a manifestation of GI bleeding)
- Shock
- Confusion
- Dyspnea
- Oliguria
- Hematuria.

Diagnostic tests

- Complete blood count, red blood cell (RBC) morphology, platelet count
- Prothrombin time, partial thromboplastin time
- Fibrin monomers, fibrinogen fibrin split products, D-dimer (an asymmetrical carbon compound fragment formed in the presence of fibrin split products)
- Factors V and VIII.

Treatment

- Prompt recognition and treatment of underlying disorder
- Blood, fresh frozen plasma, platelet or packed RBC transfusions to support hemostasis in active bleeding
- Heparin in early stages to prevent microclotting and as a last resort in hemorrhage (controversial in acute DIC after sepsis).

NORMAL CLOTTING PROCESS

Blood vessel walls

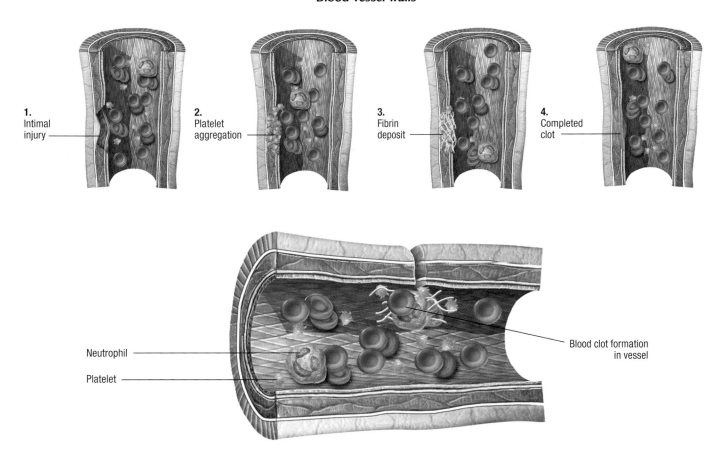

1. Intimal injury

2. Platelet aggregation

3. Fibrin deposit

4. Completed clot

Neutrophil

Platelet

Blood clot formation in vessel

UNDERSTANDING DIC

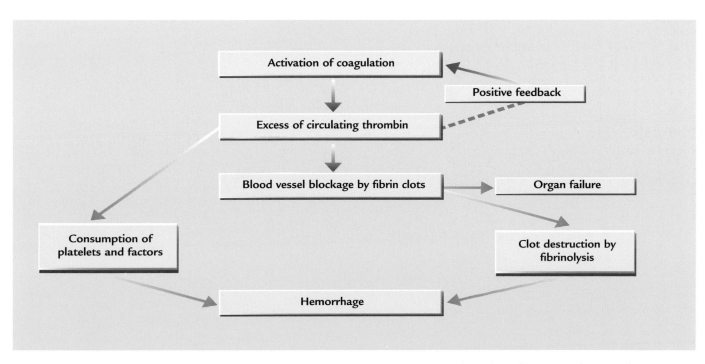

Activation of coagulation

Positive feedback

Excess of circulating thrombin

Blood vessel blockage by fibrin clots → Organ failure

Consumption of platelets and factors

Clot destruction by fibrinolysis

Hemorrhage

HEMOPHILIA

Hemophilia, a hereditary bleeding disorder, results from a deficiency of specific clotting factors. The severity of bleeding and the prognosis vary with the degree of deficiency, or nonfunction,, and the site of bleeding. Hemophilia occurs in 20 of 100,000 male births.

Hemophilia A (classic hemophilia) results from a deficiency of factor VIII. More common than type B, it affects more than 80% of all hemophiliacs and is the most common X-linked genetic disease. Hemophilia B (*Christmas disease*) affects approximately 15% of all hemophiliacs and results from a deficiency of factor IX.

Advances in treatment have greatly improved the prognosis for hemophiliacs, many of whom live normal life spans. Surgical procedures can be done safely at special treatment centers under the guidance of a hematologist.

Causes

Hemophilia types A and B: X-linked recessive genetic traits.

Pathophysiology

Hemophilia is an X-linked recessive genetic disease causing abnormal bleeding because of specific clotting factor malfunction. Factors VIII and IX are components of the intrinsic clotting pathway; factor IX is an essential factor and factor VIII is a critical cofactor that accelerates the activation of factor X by several thousandfold. Excessive bleeding occurs when these clotting factors are reduced by more than 75%. A deficiency or nonfunction of factor VIII causes hemophilia A, and a deficiency or nonfunction of factor IX causes hemophilia B.

Hemophilia may be severe, moderate, or mild, depending on the degree of activation of clotting factors. Patients with severe disease have no detectable factor VIII or factor IX activity. Moderately afflicted patients have 1% to 4% of normal clotting activity, and mildly afflicted patients have 5% to 25% of normal clotting activity.

A patient with hemophilia forms a platelet plug at a bleeding site, but clotting factor deficiency impairs the ability to form a stable fibrin clot. Bleeding occurs primarily into large joints, especially after trauma or surgery. Delayed bleeding is more common than immediate hemorrhage. Spontaneous intracranial bleeding may be fatal.

Signs and symptoms

Abnormal bleeding, severity depending on degree of factor deficiency:
- Mild — prolonged bleeding after major trauma or surgery
- Severe — spontaneous bleeding, severe bleeding after minor trauma.

  Site-specific symptoms:
- Pain, swelling, extreme tenderness, possibly, permanent deformity due to bleeding into joints and muscles
- Peripheral neuropathy, pain, paresthesia, muscle atrophy due to bleeding near peripheral nerves
- Ischemia, gangrene due to impaired blood flow through a major vessel distal to bleeding
- Shock and death.

Diagnostic tests

Hemophilia A:
- Factor VIII assay
- Partial thromboplastin time, prothrombin time, bleeding time, platelet count and function.

  Hemophilia B:
- Factor IX and VIII assays
- Baseline coagulation studies, as in hemophilia A.

Treatment

Factor replacement with cryoprecipitate, factor VIII or IX, fresh frozen plasma:
- Mild hemophilia A: I.V. or intranasal desmopressin (DDAVP) to manage bleeding episodes
- Moderate to severe hemophilia A: factor VIII concentrate
- Hemophilia B: factor IX concentrate
- Both types of hemophilia: careful management and factor replacement before and after surgery.

Normal   **Hemophilia**

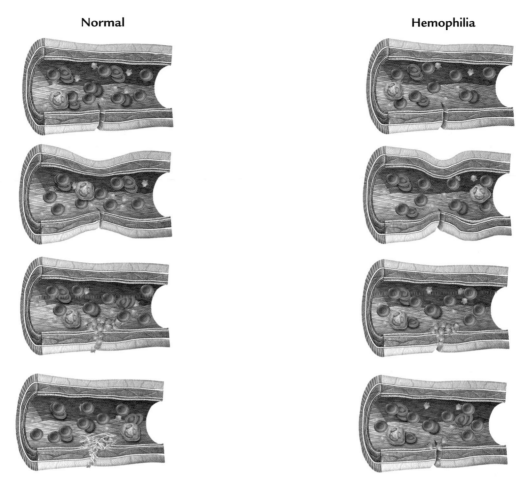

 CLINICAL TIP

X-LINKED RECESSIVE INHERITANCE

The diagram shows the children of a normal parent and a parent with a recessive gene on the X chromosome (shown by an open dot). All daughters of an affected male will be carriers. The son of a female carreier may inherit a recessive gene on the X chromosome and be affected by the disease. Unaffected sons can't transmit the disorder.

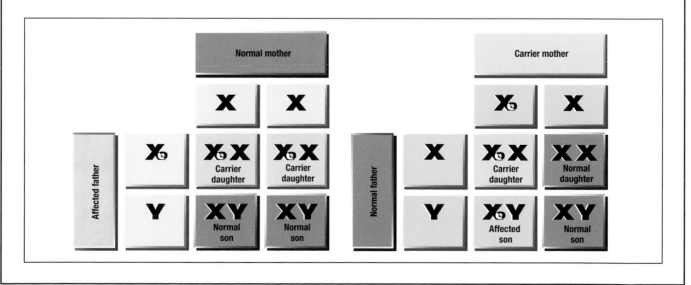

HODGKIN'S DISEASE

Hodgkin's disease is a neoplastic disease characterized by painless, progressive enlargement of lymph nodes, spleen, and other lymphoid tissue resulting from proliferation of lymphocytes, histiocytes, eosinophils, and Reed-Sternberg giant cells. Untreated, Hodgkin's disease follows a variable but relentlessly progressive and ultimately fatal course. With immediate and aggressive treatment, Hodgkin's disease may be curable in up to 80% of affected persons.

Causes

Unknown; viral etiology suspected; Epstein-Barr virus is a leading candidate.

 AGE ALERT
The disease is most common in young adults, and more common in males than in females. Incidence peaks in two age-groups: ages 15 to 38 and after age 50 — except in Japan, where it occurs exclusively among people over age 50.

Pathophysiology

Hodgkin's disease is characterized by proliferation of a tumor in which only a small proportion of the cells are malignant and most are normal lymphocytes. The characteristic malignant cells — called Reed-Sternberg cells — are most likely multinucleated, giant-cell mutations of the T-lymphocyte. Infiltration of the nodes with eosinophils and plasma cells is associated with lymph node necrosis and fibrosis.

Signs and symptoms

- Painless swelling of one cervical lymph node (sometimes an axillary, mediastinal, or inguinal node)
- Respiratory symptoms if mediastinum is initially involved (rare)
- Pruritus — mild at first and becoming acute as disease progresses.
  In older patients, nonspecific early signs:
- Persistent fever, night sweats
- Fatigue, malaise.
  In later stages:
- Rapid enlargement of lymph nodes, causing pain and obstruction
- Systemic manifestations, including enlargement of retroperitoneal nodes and nodular infiltrations of the spleen, the liver, and bones
- Edema of face and neck, progressive anemia, jaundice, nerve pain, increasing susceptibility to infection.

Diagnostic tests

- Lymph node biopsy for Reed-Sternberg cells, fibrosis, necrosis
- Bone marrow, liver, mediastinal, spleen biopsies
- Complete blood count
- Routine chest X-ray
- Abdominal computed tomography scan, lung scan, bone scan
- Lymphangiography.

Treatment

- Chemotherapy, radiation, or both, appropriate to stage of the disease — based on histologic interpretation and clinical staging
- Concomitant antiemetics, sedatives, or antidiarrheals to combat adverse GI effects
- After relapse — remission and potential cure with high dose chemotherapy and autologous stem cell transplantation.

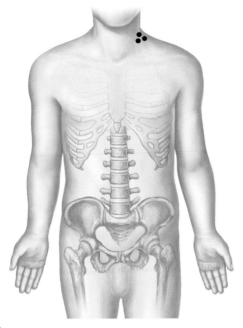

Stage I
- Involvement of single lymph node region
  or
- Involvement of single extralymphatic site (stage I$_E$)

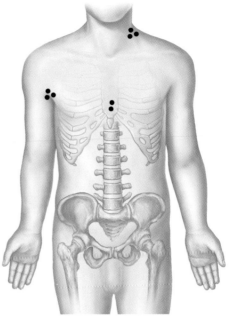

Stage II
- Involvement of 2 or more lymph node regions on same side of diaphragm
- May include localized extralymphatic involvement on same side of diaphragm (stage II$_E$)

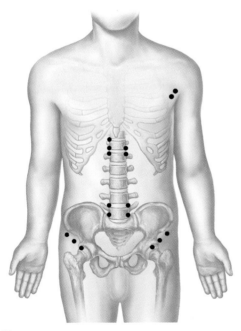

Stage III
- Involvement of lymph node regions on both sides of diaphragm
- May include involvement of spleen (stage III$_S$) or localized extranodal disease (stage III$_E$)
- Hodgkin's disease Stage III$_1$: disease limited to upper abdomen — spleen, splenic hilar, celiac, or portohepatic nodes
- Hodgkin's disease Stage III$_2$: disease limited to lower abdomen — periaortic, pelvic, or inguinal nodes

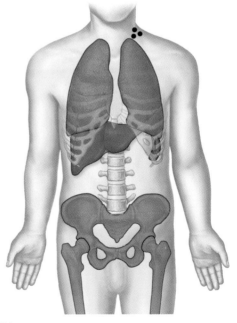

Stage IV
- Diffuse extralymphatic disease (for example, in liver, bone marrow, lung, skin)

IRON DEFICIENCY ANEMIA

Iron deficiency anemia is a disorder of oxygen transport in which hemoglobin synthesis is deficient. The most common hematologic disease worldwide, iron deficiency anemia affects 10% to 30% of the adult population of the United States. The prognosis after replacement therapy is favorable.

AGE ALERT
Iron deficiency anemia occurs most commonly in premenopausal women, infants (particularly premature or low-birth-weight infants), children, and adolescents (especially girls).

Causes
● Inadequate dietary intake of iron (less than 1 to 2 mg/day), as in prolonged nonsupplemented breast-feeding or bottle-feeding of infants; or during periods of stress, such as rapid growth, in children and adolescents
● Iron malabsorption, as in chronic diarrhea, partial or total gastrectomy, or malabsorption syndromes, such as celiac disease and pernicious anemia
● Blood loss:
– drug-induced GI bleeding (anticoagulants, aspirin, steroids)
– heavy menses; hemorrhage from trauma, peptic ulcers, cancer, varices
● Pregnancy, which diverts maternal iron to fetus for erythropoiesis
● Intravascular hemolysis-induced hemoglobinuria or paroxysmal nocturnal hemoglobinuria
● Mechanical trauma by prosthetic heart valve or vena cava filters.

Pathophysiology
Iron deficiency anemia occurs when the supply of iron is inadequate for optimal formation of red blood cells (RBCs); the result is small (microcytic) cells with pale color (hypochromic) on staining. Body stores of iron, including plasma iron, become depleted, and the concentration of serum transferrin, which binds with and transports iron, decreases. Insufficient iron stores lead to a depleted RBC mass with low hemoglobin concentration and consequent impaired oxygen-carrying capacity.

Signs and symptoms
● None or only symptoms of an underlying condition
● Dyspnea on exertion, fatigue, listlessness, pallor, inability to concentrate, irritability, headache, and a susceptibility to infection
● Increased cardiac output and tachycardia
● Coarsely ridged, spoon-shaped (koilonychia), brittle, and thin nails
● Sore, red, and burning tongue; sore, dry skin in corners of mouth.

Diagnostic tests
● Hemoglobin and hematocrit
● Serum iron, iron-binding capacity, serum ferritin
● RBC count, mean corpuscular hemoglobin
● Iron stores by specific staining
● Bone marrow assay for precursor cells
● Tests to exclude other causes of anemia, such as thalassemia minor, cancer, and chronic inflammatory, hepatic, or renal disease.

Treatment
● Oral iron or iron and ascorbic acid combination (enhances iron absorption)
● Parenteral iron (for patient noncompliant with oral dose, needing more iron than can be given orally, with malabsorption preventing adequate iron absorption, or for a maximum rate of hemoglobin regeneration). Requires careful administration; side effects include anaphylaxis.

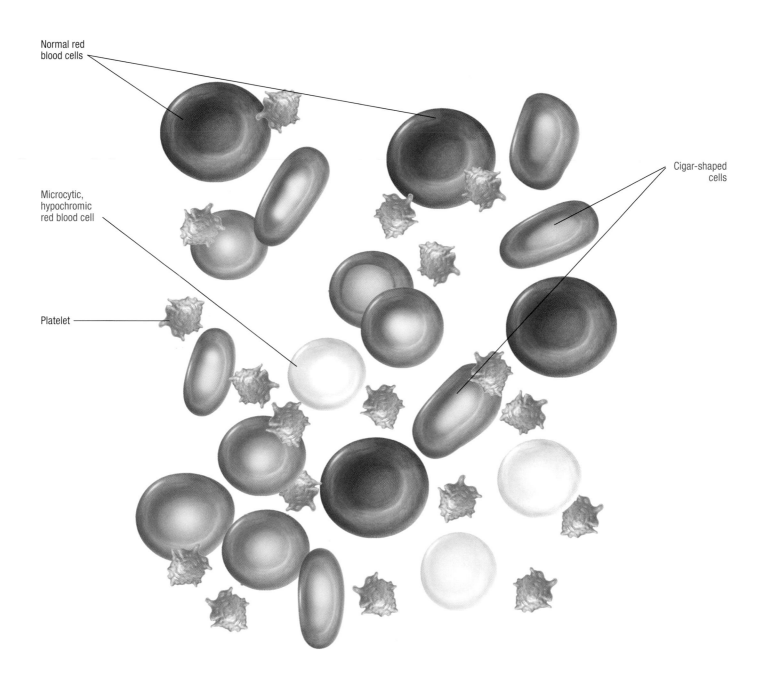

Normal red blood cells

Microcytic, hypochromic red blood cell

Platelet

Cigar-shaped cells

LEUKEMIA

Leukemia is a group of diseases caused by malignant proliferation of white blood cells; each is classified by the dominant cell type. The course of a leukemia may be acute or chronic.
- Acute — large numbers of immature leukocytes; rapid onset and progression
- Chronic — excessive mature leukocytes in the periphery and bone marrow; slower onset and progression.

 AGE ALERT
The most common malignancies in children are the leukemias. Each specific type has its own prognosis, but generally, the prognosis in children is better than in adults.

Causes
No definitive cause identified.
Possible risk factors:
- Genetic predisposition
- Immunologic factors
- Environmental exposure to chemicals, radiation
- Predisposing disease.

Chronic myeloid leukemia (CML):
- In almost 90% of patients, Philadelphia, or Ph[1] chromosome; translocated long arm of chromosome 22, usually to chromosome 9.

Pathophysiology
Acute leukemia is characterized by malignant proliferation of white blood cell precursors (blasts) in bone marrow or lymph tissue and their accumulation in peripheral blood, bone marrow, and body tissues. Leukemic cells inhibit normal bone marrow production of erythrocytes, platelets, and immune function. Its most common forms and the characteristic cells are the following:
- acute lymphoblastic (or lymphocytic) leukemia (ALL) — lymphocyte precursors (lymphoblasts)
- acute myeloid leukemias, known collectively as acute non-lymphocytic leukemia (ANLL):
- acute myeloblastic (or myelogenous) leukemia — myeloid precursors (myeloblasts)
- acute monoblastic (monocytic) leukemia — monocyte precursors (monoblasts)
- other types of ANLL — acute myelomonocytic leukemia, acute erythroleukemia.

Chronic myeloid leukemia (CML) proceeds in two distinct phases:
- insidious chronic phase — anemia and bleeding disorders

- blastic crisis or acute phase — rapid proliferation of myeloblasts, the most primitive granulocyte precursors.
Chronic lymphocytic leukemia (CLL) — abnormal small lymphocytes in lymphoid tissue, blood, and bone marrow.

Signs and symptoms
Acute leukemias:
- Sudden high fever, thrombocytopenia, abnormal bleeding
- Nonspecific signs and symptoms, including weakness, pallor, chills
- Also, for ALL, AML, and acute monoblastic leukemia: possible dyspnea, anemia, fatgue, malaise, tachycardia, palpitations, systolic ejection murmur, abdominal and bone pain.
CLL:
- Early stages: fatigue, malaise, fever, nodular enlargement
- Late stages: severe fatigue, weight loss, liver or spleen enlargement, bone tenderness
- With disease progression and bone marrow involvement: anemia; pallor; weakness; dyspnea; tachycardia; palpitations; bleeding; opportunistic fungal, viral, and bacterial infections
CML:
- Anemia, thrombocytopenia
- Hepatosplenomegaly
- Sternal and rib tenderness
- Low-grade fever
- Anorexia, weight loss
- Renal calculi or gouty arthritis
- Prolonged infection
- Ankle edema

Diagnostic tests
- Complete blood count with differential
- Bone marrow aspirate, bone marrow biopsy
- Lumbar puncture
- Special pathology stains, immunophenotyping, cytogenetic analysis
- Chromosome analysis of peripheral blood or bone marrow.

Treatment
- Antibiotic, antifungal, antiviral drugs
- Systemic chemotherapy
- Granulocyte injections
- Transfusion of blood and blood products
- Bone marrow transplantation.

HISTOLOGIC DIAGNOSIS OF LEUKEMIAS

Acute lymphocytic leukemia

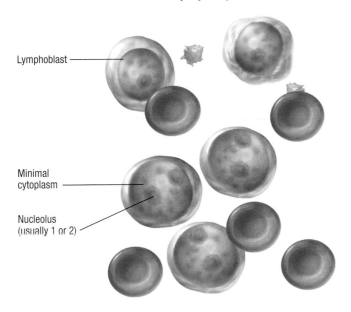

Lymphoblast

Minimal cytoplasm

Nucleolus (usually 1 or 2)

Acute myelogenous leukemia

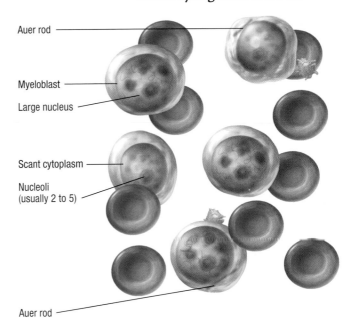

Auer rod

Myeloblast

Large nucleus

Scant cytoplasm

Nucleoli (usually 2 to 5)

Auer rod

Chronic lymphocytic leukemia

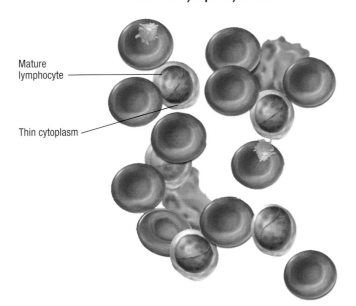

Mature lymphocyte

Thin cytoplasm

Chronic myeloid leukemia

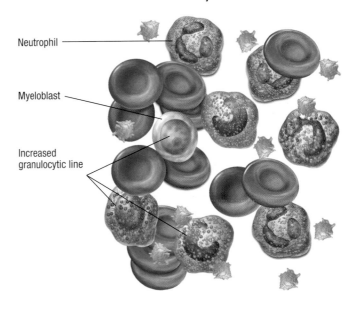

Neutrophil

Myeloblast

Increased granulocytic line

MALIGNANT LYMPHOMAS

Malignant lymphomas (also known as non-Hodgkin's lymphomas and lymphosarcomas) are a heterogeneous group of malignant diseases originating in lymph nodes and other lymphoid tissue. Malignant lymphomas are two to three times more common in males than in females. Since the early 1970s, their incidence has increased by more than 80%, to about 55,000 new cases annually in the United States. The reason for the increase is unknown, although acquired immunodeficiency syndrome (AIDS) is partly attributable. Nodular lymphomas have a better prognosis than the diffuse form of the disease, but in both, the prognosis is worse than in Hodgkin's disease.

Causes

- Direct cause unknown
- Possible viral etiology
- Exposure to toxins — benzene, gasoline, pesticides, herbicides.

 AGE ALERT
Malignant lymphomas occur in all age-groups, but incidence rises with age (median age is 50).

Pathophysiology

Malignant lymphoma is pathophysiologically similar to Hodgkin's disease, but Reed-Sternberg cells are not present, and the specific mechanism of lymph node destruction is different. The abnormal lymphoid tissue is identified by its tissue architecture and patterns of infiltration. These lymphomas are defined as *follicular, interfollicular, mantle,* or *medullary,* depending on the distribution of malignant cells in specific regions of the lymph node. The tissue is then described by the pattern of infiltration as *diffuse* or *nodular.*

Signs and symptoms

- Enlarged tonsils and adenoids
- Painless, rubbery enlargement of lymphatic tissue (lymphadenopathy), usually cervical or supraclavicular nodes.
    In children:
- Cervical nodes usually affected first
- Dyspnea and coughing.
    In advancing disease:
- Symptoms specific to involved structure
- Systemic complaints — fatigue, malaise, weight loss, fever, night sweats.

Diagnostic tests

- Biopsy of tissue removed during exploratory laparotomy — differentiates malignant lymphoma from Hodgkin's disease
- Histologic evaluation and immunophenotyping of biopsied lymphatic tissue
- Radiologic studies — bone and chest X-rays, lymphangiography, liver and spleen scans, computed tomography scan of the abdomen, excretory urography.

Treatment

- Radiation therapy — mainly in the early, localized stage of disease.
- Total nodal irradiation
- Chemotherapy with combinations of antineoplastic agents
- Autologous or allogeneic blood stem cell transplantation after relapse.

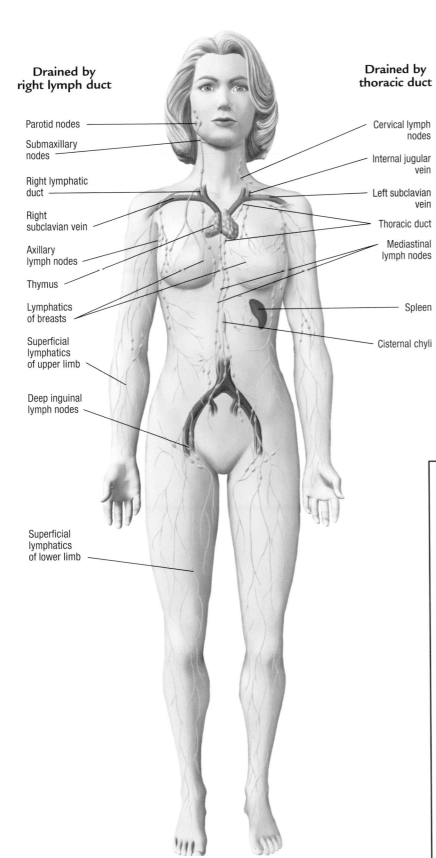

Drained by right lymph duct

Parotid nodes

Submaxillary nodes

Right lymphatic duct

Right subclavian vein

Axillary lymph nodes

Thymus

Lymphatics of breasts

Superficial lymphatics of upper limb

Deep inguinal lymph nodes

Superficial lymphatics of lower limb

Drained by thoracic duct

Cervical lymph nodes

Internal jugular vein

Left subclavian vein

Thoracic duct

Mediastinal lymph nodes

Spleen

Cisternal chyli

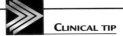

>>> **CLINICAL TIP**

CERVICAL LYMPHADENOPATHY

This person has characteristic lymphadenopathy (of the cervical lymph nodes) due to lymphoma.

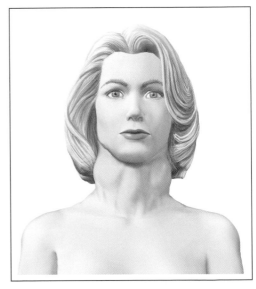

MULTIPLE MYELOMA

Multiple myeloma, also known as malignant plasmacytoma or plasma cell myeloma, is a disseminated malignant neoplasia of marrow plasma cells that infiltrates bone to produce osteolytic lesions throughout the skeleton (flat bones, vertebrae, skull, pelvis, ribs). Multiple myeloma annually strikes about 14,000 people in the United States — mostly men over age 40.

Prognosis is usually poor because diagnosis is commonly made after the disease has already infiltrated the vertebrae, pelvis, skull, ribs, clavicles, and sternum. By then, skeletal destruction is widespread and vertebral collapse is imminent. Without treatment, about half of all patients die within 6 months of diagnosis. Early diagnosis and treatment prolong the lives of many patients by 3 to 5 years. Death usually follows complications, such as infection, renal failure, hematologic imbalance, fractures, hypercalcemia, hyperuricemia, or dehydration.

Causes

Primary cause unknown.
   Possible links:
- Translocations involving chromosome 14
- Autoimmune diseases or allergies
- Environmental toxins
- Chemicals in agricultural products or added during food processing.

Pathophysiology

Plasma cells are normal leukocytes that secrete immunoglobulins. When plasma cells become malignant, they reproduce uncontrollably and create many abnormal immunoglobulins. During this process, they invade the bone marrow, then the bone matrix, causing osteolytic lesions of the bone. Myeloma cells then proliferate outside of the bone marrow in all lymphatic tissues where plasma cells normally are present. Since plasma cells are in virtually all body organs, all body systems may be affected by this proliferation and abnormal immunoglobulin production. The severity of renal failure correlates with the amount of immunoglobulin protein found in the urine. Infiltration and precipitation of immunoglobulin light chains (Bence-Jones protein) in the distal tubules causes myeloma nephrosis.

Signs and symptoms

- Severe, constant back and rib pain that increases with exercise and may be worse at night
- Arthritic symptoms — achy pain; swollen, tender joints
- Fever, malaise
- Evidence of peripheral neuropathy (such as paresthesia)
- Evidence of diffuse osteoporosis and pathologic fractures.
   In advanced disease:
- Acute symptoms of vertebral compression; loss of body height — 5″ (12.5 cm) or more
- Thoracic deformities (ballooning)
- Anemia, weight loss
- Severe, recurrent infection such as pneumonia may follow damage to nerves associated with respiratory function
- Radiologic evidence of multiple, sharply circumscribed osteolytic (punched out) lesions, particularly on the skull, pelvis, and spine.

Diagnostic tests

- Complete blood count
- Urine studies for Bence Jones protein and hypercalciuria
- Bone marrow aspiration
- Serum electrophoresis
- X-rays of skull, pelvis, spine
- Excretory urography to assess renal involvement.

Treatment

- Chemotherapy to suppress plasma cell growth and control pain
- Autologous hematopoietic blood cell transfusion
- Autologous bone marrow transplantation
- Adjuvant local radiation
- Melphalan–prednisone combination in high intermittent or low continuous daily doses
- Analgesics for pain.

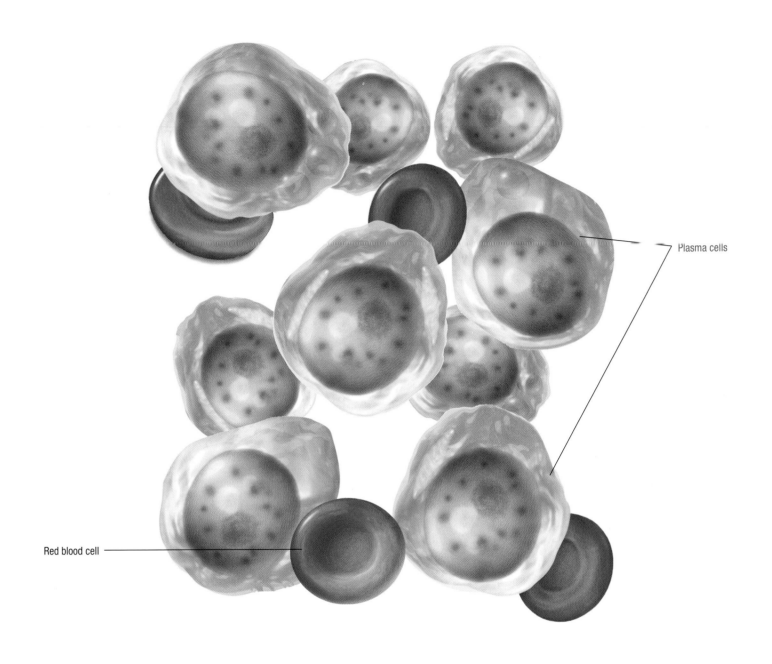

Plasma cells

Red blood cell

PERNICIOUS ANEMIA

Malabsorption of vitamin B_{12} causes pernicious anemia, the most common type of megaloblastic anemia. If not treated, pernicious anemia is fatal. Its manifestations subside with treatment, but some neurologic deficits may be permanent.

 AGE ALERT
Onset typically occurs between ages 50 and 60, and incidence increases with age. It is rare in children. Elderly patients are likely to have a dietary deficiency of B_{12} in addition to or instead of poor absorption.

Causes
- Genetic predisposition (suggested by familial incidence)
- Immunologically related disorder, such as thyroiditis, myxedema, Graves' disease (significantly higher incidence in these patients)
- Iatrogenic — partial or subtotal gastrectomy
- Aging — progressive loss of vitamin B_{12} absorption.

Pathophysiology
Decreased production of hydrochloric acid in the stomach and a deficiency of intrinsic factor, normally secreted by the parietal cells of the gastric mucosa and essential for vitamin B_{12} absorption in the ileum, characterize pernicious anemia. The resulting vitamin B_{12} deficiency inhibits cell growth, particularly of red blood cells (RBCs), leading to production of few, deformed, macrocytic RBCs having poor oxygen-carrying capacity. It also causes neurologic damage by impairing myelin formation.

Signs and symptoms
- Classic triad — weakness, sore tongue, numbness and tingling in extremities.
  Other common manifestations:
- Pale lips and gums
- Faintly jaundiced sclera and pale to bright yellow skin
- Susceptibility to infection, especially of the genitourinary tract.

Gastrointestinal:
- Nausea, vomiting, anorexia, weight loss, flatulence, diarrhea, constipation from disturbed digestion
- Gingival bleeding and tongue inflammation (may hinder eating and intensify anorexia).
  Neurologic:
- Neuritis; weakness in extremities
- Peripheral numbness and paresthesia
- Disturbed position sense
- Lack of coordination; ataxia; impaired fine finger movement
- Positive Babinski and Romberg signs
- Light-headedness
- Altered vision (diplopia, blurred vision), taste, and hearing (tinnitus); optic muscle atrophy
- Loss of bowel and bladder control; and, in males, impotence
- Irritability, poor memory, headache, depression, and delirium; may be temporary, but irreversible central nervous system changes may have occurred before treatment.
  Cardiovascular:
- Palpitations, wide pulse pressure, dyspnea, orthopnea, tachycardia, premature beats, and, eventually, heart failure.

Diagnostic tests
- Hemoglobin and mean corpuscular volume
- Serum vitamin B_{12}
- Bone marrow aspiration
- Gastric analysis for free hydrochloric acid
- Schilling test for excretion of radiolabeled vitamin B_{12} (definitive test for pernicious anemia).

Treatment
- Early parenteral vitamin B_{12} replacement — can reverse pernicious anemia, minimize complications, and possibly prevent permanent neurologic damage
- Concomitant iron and folic acid replacement
- After initial response — lifelong monthly self-administered maintenance dose of vitamin B_{12}
- Blood transfusions.

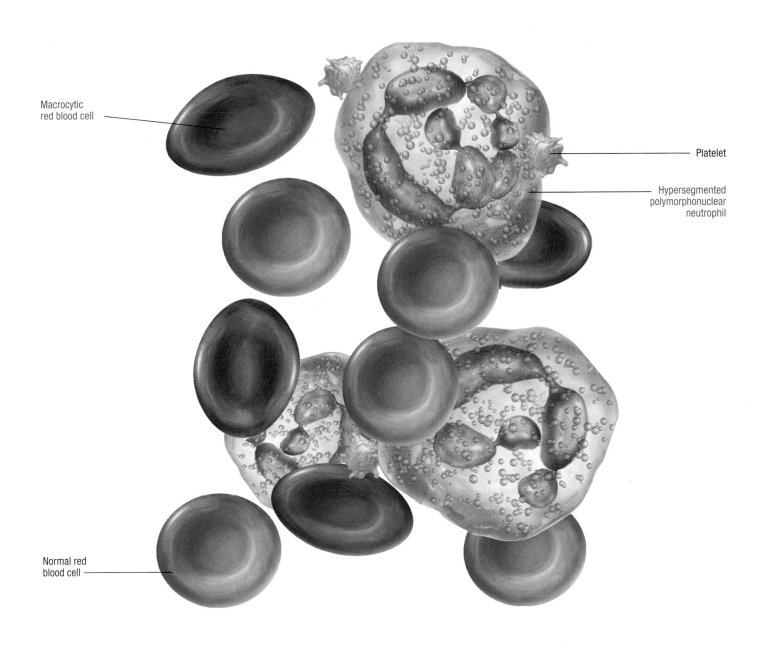

Macrocytic
red blood cell

Platelet

Hypersegmented
polymorphonuclear
neutrophil

Normal red
blood cell

POLYCYTHEMIA VERA

Polycythemia vera is a chronic disorder characterized by increased red blood cell (RBC) mass, erythrocytosis, leukocytosis, thrombocytosis; elevated hemoglobin level; and low or normal plasma volume. This disease is also known as primary polycythemia, erythremia, or polycythemia rubra vera. It occurs most commonly among Jewish males of European descent.

AGE ALERT
Polycythemia vera usually occurs between ages 40 and 60; it seldom affects children.

Prognosis depends on age at diagnosis, treatment, and complications. In untreated polycythemia, mortality is high and associated with thrombosis, hyperviscosity, or expanded blood volume. Additionally, myeloid metaplasia (ectopic hematopoiesis in the liver and spleen) with myelofibrosis (fibrous tissue in bone marrow) and acute leukemia may develop.

Causes

Unknown, but probably related to a clonal stem cell defect.

Pathophysiology

In polycythemia vera, uncontrolled and rapid cellular reproduction and maturation cause proliferation or hyperplasia of all bone marrow cells (panmyelosis). Increased RBC mass makes the blood abnormally viscous and inhibits blood flow through the microcirculation. Diminished blood flow and thrombocytosis set the stage for intravascular thrombosis.

CLINICAL TIP

Secondary polycythemia is excessive production of circulating RBCs due to hypoxia, tumor, or disease. It occurs in approximately 2 of every 100,000 people living at or near sea level; the incidence increases among those living at high altitudes.

Spurious polycythemia is characterized by an increased hematocrit but decreased plasma volume. It usually affects middle-aged people and is more common in men than in women. Causes include dehydration, hypertension, thromboembolic disease, or elevated serum cholesterol or uric acid.

Signs and symptoms

- Feeling of fullness in the head, dizziness, headache
- Ruddy cyanosis (plethora) of nose
- Clubbing of digits
- Painful pruritus
- Splenomegaly.

Diagnostic tests

- Complete blood count, hematocrit, platelet count
- Arterial oxygen saturation
- Endogenous erythroid colony-forming assay; serum erythropoietin
- Serum iron
- Vitamin B_{12} assay
- Bone marrow biopsy.

Treatment

- Phlebotomy to reduce RBC mass
- Myelosuppressive therapy with hydroxyurea
- Interferon-alfa.

Densely packed red blood cells

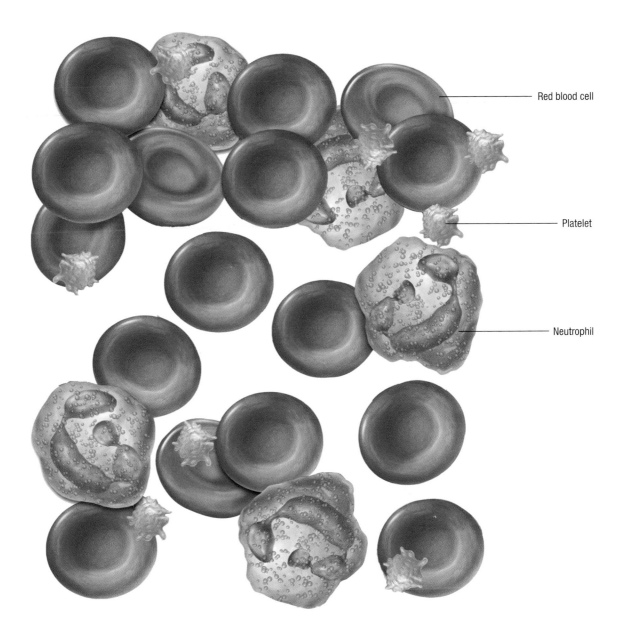

Red blood cell

Platelet

Neutrophil

SICKLE CELL ANEMIA

A congenital hemolytic anemia that occurs primarily but not exclusively in African-Americans, sickle cell anemia results from a defective hemoglobin (Hb) molecule (Hb S) that causes red blood cells (RBCs) to become sickle-shaped. Such cells clog capillaries and impair circulation, resulting in chronic ill health (fatigue, dyspnea on exertion, swollen joints), periodic crises, long-term complications, and early death.

If both parents are carriers of sickle cell trait (or another hemoglobinopathy), each child has a 25% chance of developing sickle cell anemia. Overall, 1 in every 400 to 600 black children has sickle cell anemia. The defective Hb S–producing gene may have persisted because, in areas where malaria is endemic, the heterozygous sickle cell trait provides resistance to malaria and is actually beneficial.

 AGE ALERT
Half of patients with sickle cell anemia once died by their early twenties; few lived to middle age. Earlier diagnosis and more effective treatment have improved the prognosis of sickle cell anemia. Most patients now survive into adulthood.

Causes
- Homozygous inheritance of the gene that produces Hb S
- Heterozygous inheritance of this gene results in sickle cell trait, which is usually asymptomatic.

Pathophysiology
Hemoglobin S becomes insoluble whenever hypoxia occurs. As a result, these RBCs become rigid and elongated, forming a crescent or sickle shape. Such sickling can produce hemolysis (cell destruction). In addition, these altered cells make blood more viscous and tend to accumulate in smaller blood vessels and capillaries and smaller blood vessels. The result is loss of normal circulation, swelling, tissue infarctions, and pain. Furthermore, the blockage causes anoxic changes that lead to further sickling and obstruction. Aplastic (megaloblastic) crisis results from bone marrow depression associated with infection, usually viral. Autosplenectomy, in which splenic damage and scarring is so extensive that the spleen shrinks and becomes impalpable, occurs in patients with long-term disease. It increases susceptibility to *Streptococcus pneumoniae* sepsis, which can be fatal without prompt treatment.

Signs and symptoms
- Cardiomegaly, systolic and diastolic murmurs
- Pulmonary infarctions (which may result in cor pulmonale)
- Stroke
- Chronic fatigue, unexplained dyspnea or dyspnea on exertion
- Ischemic leg ulcers (especially around the ankles)
- Increased susceptibility to infection.
  Occlusive or infarctive crises:
- Severe abdominal, thoracic, muscular, or bone pain
- Worsening jaundice, dark urine.
  Aplastic crisis:
- Pallor
- Lethargy, sleepiness, coma
- Dyspnea
- Markedly decreased bone marrow activity, RBC hemolysis.

Diagnostic tests
Electrophoresis for Hb S. (This should be done on umbilical cord blood samples at birth or heel puncture to screen newborns at risk.)

 CLINICAL TIP
During early childhood, palpation may reveal splenomegaly, but, as the child grows older, the spleen shrinks.

Treatment
- Prophylactic penicillin before age 4 months
- Oral hydroxyurea to reduce the number of painful crises
- Hospitalization and transfusion of packed RBCs if hemoglobin drops suddenly or condition deteriorates rapidly.
  Sequestration crisis:
- Sedation
- Analgesics
- Blood transfusion
- Oxygen
- Large amounts of oral or I.V. fluids.

PERIPHERAL BLOOD SMEAR IN SICKLE CELL ANEMIA

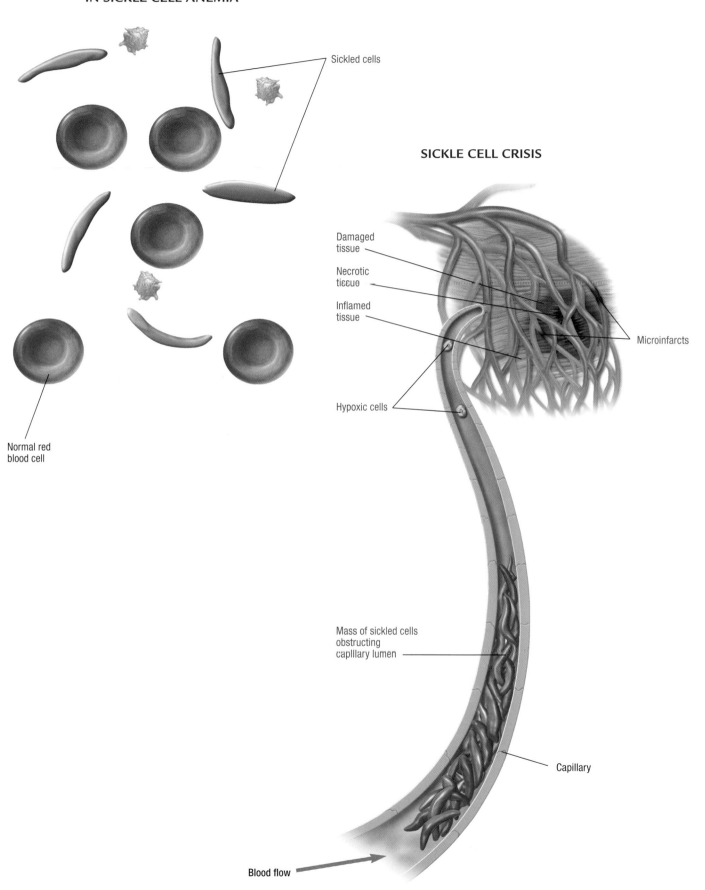

Sickled cells

Normal red blood cell

SICKLE CELL CRISIS

Damaged tissue

Necrotic tissue

Inflamed tissue

Microinfarcts

Hypoxic cells

Mass of sickled cells obstructing capillary lumen

Capillary

Blood flow

THALASSEMIA

Thalassemia, a group of hereditary hemolytic anemias, is characterized by defective synthesis in the polypeptide chains of the protein component of hemoglobin. Red blood cell (RBC) synthesis is also impaired.

Thalassemias are most common in people of Mediterranean ancestry (especially Italian and Greek, who develop the form called β-thalassemia). People whose ancestors originated in Africa, southern China, southeast Asia, and India develop the form called α-thalassemia, which reflects deletion of one or more of four hemoglobin genes. Prognosis varies with the number of deleted genes.

In β-thalassemia, the most common form of this disorder, synthesis of the beta-polypeptide chain is defective. It occurs in three clinical forms: *major, intermedia,* and *minor.* The severity of the resulting anemia depends on whether the patient is homozygous or heterozygous for the thalassemic trait. The prognosis varies:
- thalassemia major — patients seldom survive to adulthood
- thalassemia intermedia — children develop normally into adulthood; puberty usually delayed
- thalassemia minor — normal life span.

Causes
β-thalassemia:
- Thalassemia major or intermedia — homozygous inheritance of a partially dominant autosomal gene
- Thalassemia minor — heterozygous inheritance of the same gene.

α-thalassemia:
- Deletion of one or more of four genes.

Pathophysiology
In β-thalassemia, total or partial deficiency of beta-polypeptide chain production impairs hemoglobin synthesis and results in continual production of fetal hemoglobin beyond the neonatal period. Normally, immunoglobulin synthesis switches from gamma- to beta-polypeptides at the time of birth. This conversion doesn't happen in thalassemic infants. Their red cells are hypochromic and microcytic. In α-thalassemia, a much reduced quantity of alpha-globin chains is produced.

Signs and symptoms
Thalassemia major (also known as Cooley's anemia, Mediterranean disease, and erythroblastic anemia):
- At birth — no symptoms
- Infants ages 3 to 6 months — pallor; yellow skin and sclera
- Infants ages 6 to 12 months — severe anemia, bone abnormalities, failure to thrive, and life-threatening complications

- Splenomegaly or hepatomegaly, with abdominal enlargement; frequent infections; bleeding tendencies (especially nose bleeds); anorexia
- Small body, large head (characteristic features); possible mental retardation
- Facial features similar to Down syndrome in infants, due to thickened bone at the base of the nose from bone marrow hyperactivity.

Thalassemia intermedia:
- Some degree of anemia, jaundice, and splenomegaly
- Signs of hemosiderosis, such as hemoptysis, iron deficiency anemia, or paroxysmal nocturnal hemoglobinemia — due to increased intestinal absorption of iron.

Thalassemia minor:
- Usually produces no symptoms
- Mild anemia, often overlooked.

α-thalassemia syndromes — silent carrier, α-thalassemia trait, hemoglobin H disease, hydrops fetalis:
- Reflect the number of gene deletions present
- Range from asymptomatic to incompatible with life.

Diagnostic tests
- Complete blood count, red cell morphology, reticulocyte count, hemoglobin, hematocrit
- Quantitative hemoglobin electrophoresis
- Bilirubin; urinary and fecal urobilinogen levels
- Serum folate
- Skull and long bone X-rays.

Treatment
- Iron supplements contraindicated in all forms of thalassemia.

β-thalassemia major —essentially supportive:
- Prompt treatment with appropriate antibiotics for infections
- Folic acid supplements
- Transfusions of packed RBCs to increase hemoglobin levels (used judiciously to minimize iron overload)
- Splenectomy and bone marrow transplantation (effectiveness has not been confirmed).

β-thalassemia intermedia and thalassemia minor:
- No treatment.

α-thalassemia:
- Blood transfusions
- In utero transfusion for hydrops fetalis.

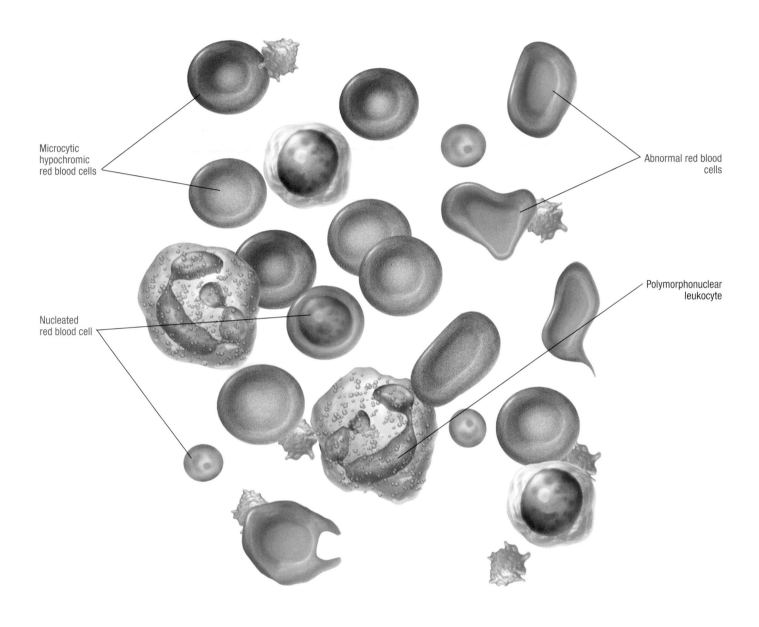

Microcytic
hypochromic
red blood cells

Abnormal red blood
cells

Nucleated
red blood cell

Polymorphonuclear
leukocyte

ACQUIRED IMMUNODEFICIENCY SYNDROME

Human immunodeficiency virus (HIV) infection may cause acquired immunodeficiency syndrome (AIDS). Although characterized by gradual destruction of cell-mediated (T cell) immunity, AIDS also affects humoral immunity and even autoimmunity through the central role of the CD4+ (helper) T lymphocyte in all immune reactions. The resulting immunodeficiency makes the patient susceptible to opportunistic infections, cancers, and other abnormalities that define AIDS.

 AGE ALERT
HIV is predominantly an infection of young people, with most cases involving persons between ages 17 and 55. However, it has also been reported in elderly men and women.

The incidence is increasing faster among women than men, and heterosexual transmission of HIV now predominates. Most women with heterosexually transmitted HIV infection report having had sexual contact with an I.V. drug user. An increase in the incidence of AIDS among women of childbearing age-group is expected to cause an increase in the number of children with HIV infection.

Causes
- HIV-I retrovirus transmitted by contact with infected blood or body fluids.
  High risk populations:
- Homosexual or bisexual men
- I.V. drug users
- Neonates of infected women
- Recipients of contaminated blood or blood products
- Heterosexual partners of persons in high-risk groups.

Pathophysiology
The natural history of AIDS begins with infection by the HIV retrovirus, which is detectable only by laboratory tests, and ends with death. Twenty years of data strongly suggest that HIV isn't transmitted by casual household or social contact. The HIV virus may enter the body by any of several routes involving the transmission of blood or body fluids; for example:
- direct inoculation during intimate sexual contact
- transfusion of contaminated blood or blood products
- use of contaminated needles
- transplacental or postpartum transmission.
  HIV strikes helper T cells bearing the CD4+ antigen. Normally a receptor for major histocompatibility complex (MHC) molecules, the antigen serves as a receptor for the retrovirus and allows it to enter the cell. Viral binding also requires the presence of a coreceptor on the cell surface. The virus also may infect CD4+ antigen-bearing cells of the GI tract, uterine cervix, and neuroglia.

Like other retroviruses, HIV copies its genetic material in a reverse manner compared with other viruses and cells. Through the action of reverse transcriptase, HIV produces DNA from its viral RNA. Transcription is often poor, leading to mutations, some of which make HIV resistant to antiviral drugs. The viral DNA enters the nucleus of the cell and is incorporated into the host cell's DNA, where it is transcribed into more viral RNA. If the host cell reproduces, it duplicates the HIV DNA along with its own and passes it on to the daughter cells. Thus, the host cell carries this information and, if activated, replicates the virus. Viral enzymes, proteases, arrange the structural components and RNA into viral particles that move to the periphery of the host cell, where the virus buds and emerges from the host cell — free to infect other cells.

HIV replication may lead to cell death or the virus may become latent. HIV infection leads to profound pathology, either directly through destruction of CD4+ cells, other immune cells, and neuroglial cells, or indirectly through the secondary effects of CD4+ T-cell dysfunction and resulting immunosuppression.

Signs and symptoms
Latency:
- Mononucleosis-like syndrome, which may be attributed to flu or another virus; may remain asymptomatic for years.
  Symptomatic phase:
- Persistent generalized lymphadenopathy
- Nonspecific symptoms, including weight loss, fatigue, night sweats
- Fevers related to altered function of CD4+ cells, immunodeficiency, and infection of other CD4+ antigen-bearing cells
- Neurologic symptoms
- Opportunistic infection, cancer.

Diagnostic tests
- Immunoassay for HIV infection
- CD4+ T-cell count.

Treatment
Antiretroviral agents:
- Protease inhibitors
- Nucleoside reverse-transcriptase inhibitors
- Nonnucleoside reverse-transcriptase inhibitors.
  Additional treatment:
- Immunomodulatory agents
- Human granulocyte colony-stimulating growth factor
- Anti-infective and antineoplastic agents
- Supportive therapy, including nutritional support, fluid and electrolyte replacement therapy, pain relief, and psychological support.

MANIFESTATIONS OF HIV INFECTION AND AIDS

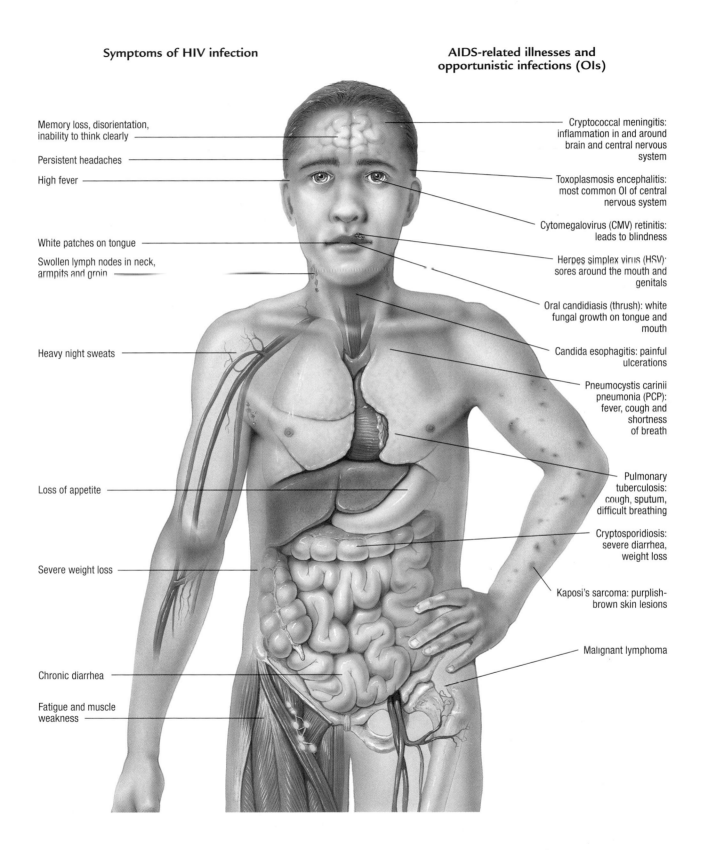

Symptoms of HIV infection

Memory loss, disorientation, inability to think clearly

Persistent headaches

High fever

White patches on tongue

Swollen lymph nodes in neck, armpits and groin

Heavy night sweats

Loss of appetite

Severe weight loss

Chronic diarrhea

Fatigue and muscle weakness

AIDS-related illnesses and opportunistic infections (OIs)

Cryptococcal meningitis: inflammation in and around brain and central nervous system

Toxoplasmosis encephalitis: most common OI of central nervous system

Cytomegalovirus (CMV) retinitis: leads to blindness

Herpes simplex virus (HSV): sores around the mouth and genitals

Oral candidiasis (thrush): white fungal growth on tongue and mouth

Candida esophagitis: painful ulcerations

Pneumocystis carinii pneumonia (PCP): fever, cough and shortness of breath

Pulmonary tuberculosis: cough, sputum, difficult breathing

Cryptosporidiosis: severe diarrhea, weight loss

Kaposi's sarcoma: purplish-brown skin lesions

Malignant lymphoma

ALLERGIC RHINITIS

Allergic rhinitis is a reaction to airborne (inhaled) allergens. Depending on the allergen, the resulting rhinitis and conjunctivitis may occur seasonally (hay fever) or year-round (perennial allergic rhinitis). Allergic rhinitis is the most common atopic allergic reaction, affecting over 20 million Americans.

AGE ALERT
Allergic rhinitis is most prevalent in young children and adolescents, but occurs in all age-groups.

Causes
- Immunoglobulin E (IgE)-mediated type I hypersensitivity response to an environmental antigen (allergen) in a genetically susceptible person
  Common triggers:
- Wind-borne pollens:
- spring: oak, elm, maple, alder, birch, cottonwood
- summer: grasses, sheep sorrel, English plantain
- autumn: ragweed, other weeds
- Perennial allergens and irritants:
- dust mite excreta, fungal spores, molds
- feather pillows
- cigarette smoke
- animal dander.

Pathophysiology
During primary exposure to an allergen, T cells recognize the foreign allergens and release chemicals that instruct B cells to produce specific antibodies called immunoglobulin E (IgE). IgE antibodies attach themselves to mast cells. Mast cells with attached IgE can remain in the body for years, ready to react when they next encounter the same allergen.

The second time the allergen enters the body, it comes into direct contact with the IgE antibodies attached to the mast cells. This stimulates the mast cells to release chemicals, such as histamine, which initiate a response that causes tightening of the smooth muscles in the airways; dilation of small blood vessels; increased mucus secretion in the nasal cavity and airways; and itching.

Signs and symptoms
Seasonal allergic rhinitis:
- Paroxysmal sneezing
- Profuse watery rhinorrhea; nasal obstruction or congestion
- Pruritus of nose and eyes
- Pale, cyanotic, edematous nasal mucosa
- Red, edematous eyelids and conjunctivae.
  Perennial allergic rhinitis:
- Chronic nasal obstruction, commonly extending to eustachian tube
- Conjunctivitis and other extranasal effects are rare.

Diagnostic tests
- Microscopic examination of sputum and nasal secretions
- Immunoassay for IgE
- Skin testing paired with tested responses to environmental stimuli.

Treatment
- Antihistamines
- Inhaled intranasal steroids
- Desensitization with injections of extracted allergens.

Primary exposure

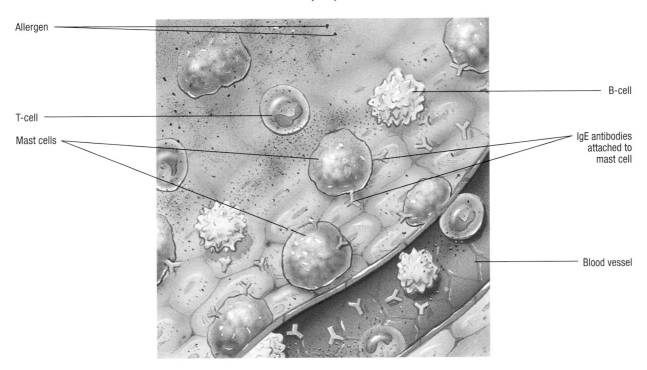

Allergen

T-cell

Mast cells

B-cell

IgE antibodies attached to mast cell

Blood vessel

Reexposure

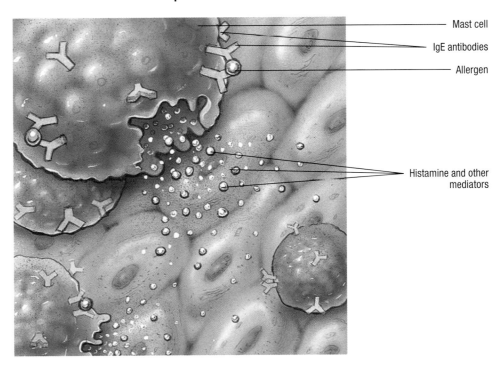

Mast cell

IgE antibodies

Allergen

Histamine and other mediators

ANAPHYLAXIS

Anaphylaxis is an acute, potentially life-threatening type I (immediate) hypersensitivity reaction marked by sudden onset of rapidly progressive urticaria (vascular swelling in skin, accompanied by itching) and respiratory distress. With prompt recognition and treatment, prognosis is good. A severe reaction may precipitate vascular collapse, leading to systemic shock and, sometimes, death. Typically occuring within minutes, the reaction can occur up to 1 hour after reexposure to an antigen.

Causes

Ingestion of or other systemic exposure to sensitizing drugs or other substances, such as:
- serums (usually horse serum), vaccines, allergen extracts
- diagnostic chemicals, such as sulfobromophthalein, sodium dehydrocholate, radiographic contrast media
- enzymes such L-asparginase in chemotherapeutic regimens
- hormones, such as insulin
- penicillin or other antibiotics, sulfonamides
- salicylates
- food proteins, as in legumes, nuts, berries, seafood, egg albumin
- sulfite food additives, common in dried fruits and vegetables, salad bars
- insect venom.

CLINICAL TIP

Latex allergy is a hypersensitivity reaction to products that contain natural latex derived from the sap of a rubber tree, not synthetic latex. Natural latex is increasingly present in products at home and at work. Hypersensitivity reactions can range from local dermatitis to life-threatening anaphylactic reaction.

Pathophysiology

Anaphylaxis requires previous sensitization or exposure to the specific antigen, resulting in immunoglobulin E (IgE) production by plasma cells in the lymph nodes and enhancement by helper T cells. IgE antibodies then bind to membrane receptors on mast cells in connective tissue and basophils in the blood.

On reexposure, immunoglobulins M and G (IgM and IgG) recognize the antigen as foreign and bind to it. Destruction of the antigen by the complement cascade begins. Continued antigen presence activates IgE on basophils, which promotes the release of mediators, including histamine, serotonin, and slow-reacting substance of anaphylaxis (SRS-A). The sudden release of histamine causes vasodilation and increases capillary permeability.

Activated IgE also stimulates mast cells in connective tissue along the venule walls to release more histamine and eosinophil chemotactic factor of anaphylaxis (ECF-A). These substances produce disruptive lesions that weaken the venules.

In the lungs, histamine causes endothelial cells to burst and endothelial tissue to tear away from surrounding tissue. Fluids leak into the alveoli, and SRS-A prevents the alveoli from expanding, thus reducing pulmonary compliance.

At the same time, basophils and mast cells begin to release prostaglandins and bradykinin along with histamine and serotonin. These chemical mediators spread through the body in the circulation, triggering systemic responses: vasodilation, smooth muscle contraction, and increased mucus production. The mediators also induce vascular collapse by increasing vascular permeability, which leads to decreased peripheral resistance and plasma leakage from the vessels to the extravascular tissues. Consequent reduction of blood volume causes hypotension, hypovolemic shock, and cardiac dysfunction.

Signs and symptoms

- Sudden physical distress within seconds or minutes after exposure to an allergen
- Delayed or persistent reaction may occur up to 24 hours later. The severity of the reaction relates inversely to the interval between exposure to the allergen and the onset of symptoms.

Usual initial symptoms:
- Feeling of impending doom or fright
- Sweating
- Sneezing, shortness of breath, nasal pruritus, urticaria, angioedema.

Systemic manifestations:
- Hypotension, shock, cardiac arrhythmias
- Edema of the upper respiratory tract, resulting in hypopharyngeal and laryngeal obstruction
- Hoarseness, stridor, wheezing, and accessory muscle use
- Severe stomach cramps, nausea, diarrhea, and urinary urgency and incontinence.

Diagnostic tests

No single diagnostic test can identify anaphylaxis.

Treatment

- Immediate administration of epinephrine to reverse bronchoconstriction and cause vasoconstriction
- Tracheostomy or endotracheal intubation and mechanical ventilation
- Oxygen therapy
- I.V. vasopressors
- Longer-acting epinephrine, corticosteroids, antihistamines, histamine-2 blocker
- Albuterol mini-nebulizer treatment
- Volume expanders.

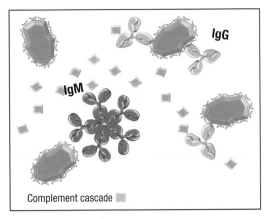

1. Response to antigen
Immunoglobulins M and G (IgM and IgG) recognize and bind the antigen.

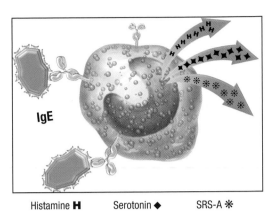

2. Release of chemical mediators
Activated IgE on basophils promotes the release of mediators: histamine, serotonin, and slow-reacting substance of anaphylaxis.

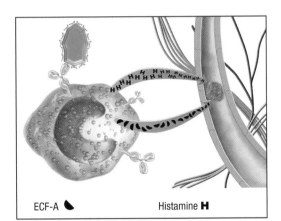

3. Intensified response
Mast cells release more histamine and eosinophil chemotactic factor of anaphylaxis (ECF-A), which create venule-weakening lesions.

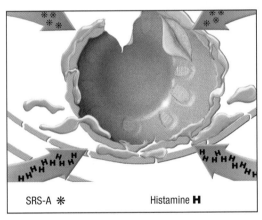

4. Respiratory distress
In the lungs, histamine causes endothelial cell destruction and fluid leak into alveoli.

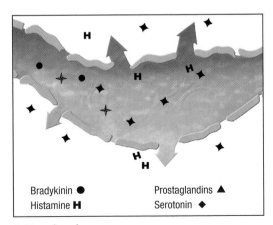

5. Deterioration
Meanwhile, mediators increase vascular permeability, causing fluid leak from the vessels.

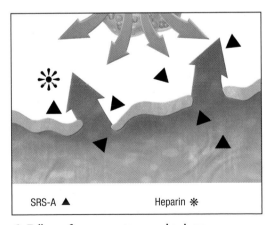

6. Failure of compensatory mechanisms
Endothelial cell damage causes basophils and mast cells to release heparin and mediator-neutralizing substances. However, anaphylaxis is now irreversible.

ANKYLOSING SPONDYLITIS

A chronic, usually progressive inflammatory bone disease, ankylosing spondylitis primarily affects the sacroiliac, apophyseal, and costovertebral joints, along with adjacent soft tissue. The disease (also known as rheumatoid spondylitis and Marie-Strümpell disease) usually begins in the sacroiliac joints and gradually progresses to the lumbar, thoracic, and cervical regions of the spine. Deterioration of bone and cartilage can lead to formation of fibrous tissue and eventual fusion of the spine or peripheral joints.

Ankylosing spondylitis may be equally prevalent in both sexes. Progressive disease is well recognized in men, but the diagnosis is commonly overlooked or missed in women, who tend to have more peripheral joint involvement.

Causes
- Direct cause unknown
- Familial tendency; more than 90% of patients are positive for human leukocyte antigen (HLA)-B27
- Presence of circulating immune complexes suggests immunologic activity.

Pathophysiology
Spondylitis involves inflammation of one or more vertebrae. Ankylosing spondylitis is a chronic inflammatory disease that predominantly affects the joints between the vertebrae of the spine, and the joints between the spine and the pelvis. Involvement of the peripheral joints or soft tissues is a rare occurrence. It eventually causes the affected vertebrae to fuse or grow together. The disease waxes and wanes, it can go into remission, exacerbation, or arrest at any stage.

Signs and symptoms
- Intermittent low back pain that is usually most severe in the morning or after a period of inactivity
- Stiffness and limited motion of the lumbar spine
- Pain and limited expansion of the chest
- Peripheral arthritis involving shoulders, hips, and knees
- Hip deformity and associated limited range of motion
- Upper lobe pulmonary fibrosis (mimics tuberculosis).

Diagnostic tests
- HLA-B27 assay
- X-ray
- Erythrocyte sedimentation rate
- Alkaline phosphatase
- Serum immunoglobulin A
- Rheumatoid factor.

Treatment
- No treatment that reliably halts progression
- Physical therapy to delay further deformity — good posture, stretching and deep-breathing exercises and, in some patients, braces and lightweight supports
- Anti-inflammatory nonsteroidal analgesics, such as aspirin, indomethacin, sulfasalazine
- Surgery for severe hip or spinal involvement; spinal surgery carries high risk of spinal cord damage and requires long convalescence.

Lateral view

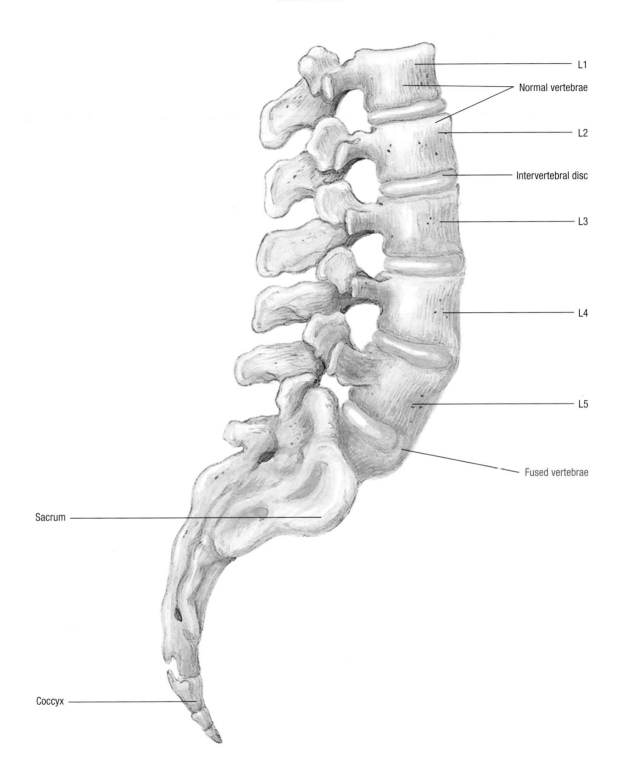

L1

Normal vertebrae

L2

Intervertebral disc

L3

L4

L5

Fused vertebrae

Sacrum

Coccyx

LUPUS ERYTHEMATOSUS

Lupus erythematosus is a chronic inflammatory disorder of the connective tissues that appears in two forms: *discoid* lupus erythematosus, which affects only the skin, and *systemic* lupus erythematosus (SLE), which affects multiple organ systems as well as the skin and can be fatal. The remainder of the section addresses only SLE.

SLE is characterized by recurring remissions and exacerbations, which are especially common during the spring and summer. SLE strikes women 8 times as often as men, increasing to 15 times as often during childbearing years. The prognosis improves with early detection and treatment but remains poor for patients who develop cardiovascular, renal, or neurologic complications, or severe bacterial infections.

Causes
Direct cause unknown.

Interrelated immunologic, environmental, hormonal, and genetic factors:
- Physical or mental stress
- Streptococcal or viral infections
- Exposure to sunlight or ultraviolet light
- Immunization
- Pregnancy
- Abnormal estrogen metabolism
- Drugs, including procainamide, hydralazine, anticonvulsants; less frequently, penicillins, sulfa drugs, oral contraceptives.

Pathophysiology
Autoimmunity is believed to be the prime mechanism in SLE. The body produces antibodies against components of its own cells, such as the antinuclear antibody (ANA), and immune complex disease follows. Patients with SLE may produce antibodies against many different tissue components, such as red blood cells, neutrophils, platelets, lymphocytes, or almost any organ or tissue in the body.

Signs and symptoms
- Onset either acute or insidious
- No characteristic clinical pattern
- May involve any organ system; all symptoms reflect tissue injury and subsequent inflammation and necrosis resulting from the invasion by immune complexes.

Diagnostic tests
- Complete blood count with differential; platelet count
- Erythrocyte sedimentation rate
- Serum electrophoresis
- ANA and lupus erythematosus cell tests
- Anti–double-stranded deoxyribonucleic acid antibody test
- Additional autoantibody testing, such as extractable nuclear antigen antibody tests Smith antigen (highly specific for SLE)
- Lupus anticoagulant and anticardiolipin tests.

Treatment
- Nonsteroidal anti-inflammatory compounds
- Topical corticosteroid creams
- Intralesional corticosteroids or antimalarials
- Systemic corticosteroids
- High-dose steroids and cytotoxic therapy.

ORGANS AFFECTED BY SYSTEMIC LUPUS ERYTHEMATOSUS

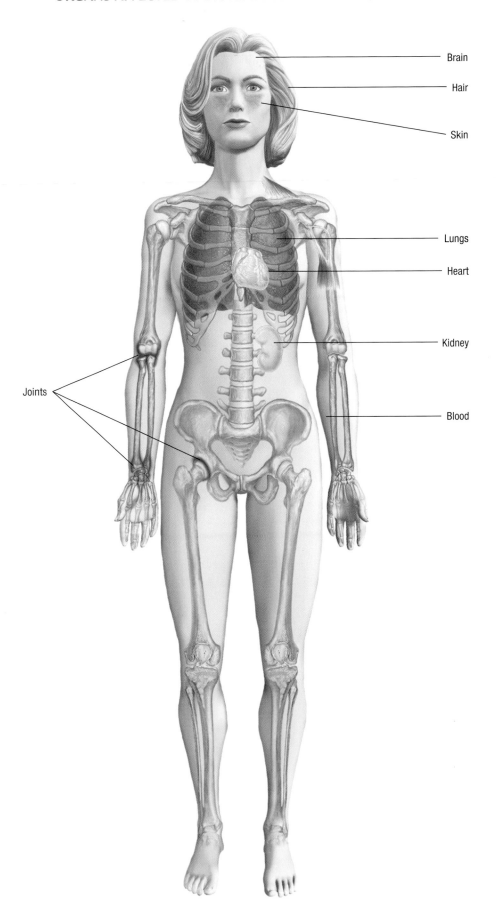

Brain

Hair

Skin

Lungs

Heart

Kidney

Joints

Blood

Rheumatoid arthritis

Rheumatoid arthritis (RA) is a chronic, systemic inflammatory disease that primarily attacks peripheral joints and the surrounding muscles, tendons, ligaments, and blood vessels. Partial remissions and unpredictable exacerbations mark the course of this potentially crippling disease. Rheumatoid arthritis strikes women three times more often than men.

AGE ALERT
RA can occur at any age, but 80% of the patients develop rheumatoid arthritis between ages 35 and 50.

Causes
Direct cause unknown.
Proposed mechanisms:
• Abnormal immune activation (in a genetically susceptible person) leading to inflammation, complement activation, and cell proliferation in joints and tendon sheaths
• Infection (viral or bacterial), hormone action, or lifestyle factors.

Pathophysiology
The body develops IgM antibody against the body's own IgG (also called rheumatoid factor [RF]). RF aggregates into complexes, generates inflammation, causing eventual cartilage damage and triggering other autoimmune responses.

If not arrested, the inflammatory process in the joints occurs in four stages:
• Congestion and edema of the synovial membrane and joint capsule cause synovitis. Infiltration by lymphocytes, macrophages, and neutrophils continues the local inflammatory response. These cells, as well as fibroblast-like synovial cells, produce enzymes that help to degrade bone and cartilage.
• Pannus — thickened layers of granulation tissue — covers and invades cartilage and eventually destroys the joint capsule and bone.
• Fibrous ankylosis — fibrous invasion of the pannus and scar formation — occludes the joint space. Bone atrophy and misalignment cause visible deformities and disrupt the articulation of opposing bones, causing muscle atrophy and imbalance and, possibly, partial dislocations (subluxations).
• Fibrous tissue calcifies, resulting in bony ankylosis and total immobility.

Signs and symptoms
• Nonspecific symptoms, most likely related to the initial inflammatory reactions, precede inflammation of the synovium.

As the disease progresses:
• Specific localized, bilateral, and symmetric articular symptoms, frequently in the fingers at the proximal interphalangeal, metacarpophalangeal, and metatarsophalangeal joints, possibly extending to the wrists, knees, elbows, and ankles from inflammation of the synovium
• Stiffening of affected joints after inactivity, especially on arising in the morning
• Joint pain and tenderness, at first only with movement but eventually even at rest
• Flexion deformities or hyperextension of metacarpophalangeal joints, subluxation of the wrist, and stretching of tendons pulling the fingers to the ulnar side (ulnar drift), or characteristic "swan's neck" appearance or "boutonnière" deformity.

Extra-articular findings:
• Gradual appearance of rheumatoid nodules — subcutaneous, round or oval, nontender masses (20% of RF-positive patients), usually on elbows, hands, or Achilles' tendon
• Vasculitis possibly leading to skin lesions, leg ulcers, and multiple systemic complications
• Pericarditis, pulmonary nodules or fibrosis, pleuritis, or inflammation of the sclera and overlying tissues of the eye
• Peripheral neuropathy with numbness or tingling in the feet or weakness and loss of sensation in the fingers.

Diagnostic tests
• X-ray
• RF titer
• Synovial fluid analysis
• Serum protein electrophoresis
• Erythrocyte sedimentation rate, C-reactive protein levels.

Treatment
• Salicylates, particularly aspirin; nonsteroidal anti-inflammatory agents
• Antimalarials
• Corticosteroids
• Methotrexate, cyclosporine, azathioprine in early disease
• Supportive measures, including rest, splinting to rest inflamed joints, range-of-motion exercises, physical therapy, heat applications for chronic disease and ice application for acute episodes
• Synovectomy, osteotomy, tendon transfers
• Joint reconstruction or total joint replacement
• Arthrodesis (joint fusion).

JOINTS TYPICALLY AFFECTED BY RHEUMATOID ARTHRITIS

Knee

Hand and wrist

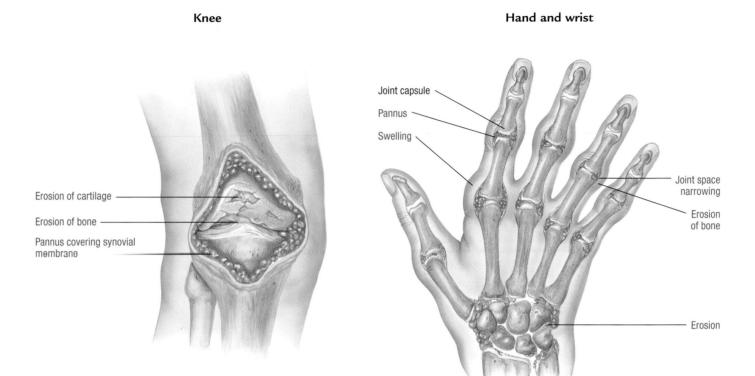

Erosion of cartilage

Erosion of bone

Pannus covering synovial membrane

Joint capsule

Pannus

Swelling

Joint space narrowing

Erosion of bone

Erosion

Hip

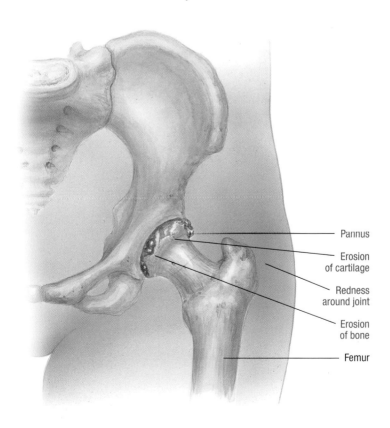

Pannus

Erosion of cartilage

Redness around joint

Erosion of bone

Femur

SCLERODERMA

Scleroderma (also known as systemic sclerosis) is an uncommon disease of diffuse connective tissue. Degenerative and fibrotic changes in the skin, blood vessels, synovial membranes, skeletal muscles, and internal organs (especially the esophagus, intestinal tract, thyroid, heart, lungs, and kidneys) follow the initial inflammation. The seven forms of scleroderma are diffuse systemic sclerosis, localized, linear, chemically induced localized, eosinophilia myalgia syndrome, toxic oil syndrome, and graft-versus-host disease.

Scleroderma affects women three to four times more often than men, especially between ages 30 and 50. The peak incidence is in people ages 50 to 60.

Causes

Direct cause unknown.
Possible causes include:
- Systemic exposure to silica dust or polyvinyl chloride
- Anticancer agents such as bleomycin; nonnarcotic analgesics such as pentazocine hydrochloride
- Abnormal immune response
- Underlying vascular cause, tissue changes initiated by persistent perfusion defect.

Pathophysiology

Scleroderma usually begins in the fingers and extends proximally to the upper arms, shoulders, neck, and face. The skin atrophies, edema and infiltrates containing CD4+ T cells surround the blood vessels, and inflamed collagen fibers become edematous and degenerative, losing strength and elasticity. The dermis becomes tightly bound to the underlying structures, resulting in atrophy of the affected appendages and destruction of the distal phalanges by osteoporosis. As the disease progresses, the fibrosis and atrophy can affect other areas, including muscles and joints.

Signs and symptoms

- Early symptoms — Raynaud's phenomenon (blanching, cyanosis, and erythema of the fingers and toes); progressive phalangeal resorption may shorten the fingers
- Localized scleroderma — patchy skin changes with a teardrop-like appearance known as *morphea*
- Linear scleroderma — band of thickened skin on the face or extremities that severely damages underlying tissues, causing atrophy and deformity
- Limited systemic sclerosis — skin thickening, commonly limited to distal extremities and face, but can involve internal organs
- CREST syndrome: **C**alcinosis, **R**aynaud's phenomenon, **E**sophageal dysfunction, **S**clerodactyly, **T**elangiectasia — a benign subtype of limited systemic sclerosis
- Diffuse systemic sclerosis — generalized skin thickening and involvement of internal organs.

Diagnostic tests

- Erythrocyte sedimentation rate, rheumatoid factor, antinuclear antibody test results
- X-rays — hand, chest, GI
- Skin biopsy.

Treatment

No cure.
To preserve normal body functions and minimize complications:
- Immunosuppressants, vasodilators, antihypertensives
- Digital sympathectomy, cervical sympathetic blockade
- Possible surgical debridement
- Antacids, soft, bland diet
- Angiotensin-converting enzyme inhibitor
- Physical therapy, heat therapy.

Thin, shiny skin on fingers

Flexed, stiff fingers

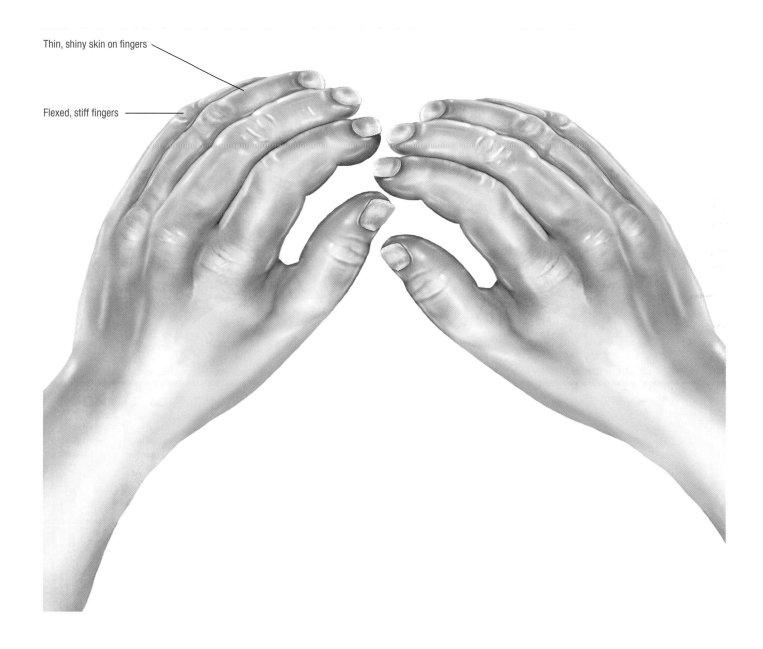

ADRENAL HYPOFUNCTION

Adrenal hypofunction is classified as primary or secondary. *Primary* adrenal hypofunction or insufficiency (*Addison's disease*) originates within the adrenal gland and is characterized by the decreased secretion of mineralocorticoids, glucocorticoids, and androgens. It's defined as destruction of more than 90% of both adrenal glands and is usually caused by an autoimmune process. Addison's disease is relatively uncommon and can occur at any age and in both sexes. *Secondary* adrenal hypofunction is due to impaired pituitary secretion of adrenocorticotropin (ACTH) and is characterized by decreased glucocorticoid secretion.

With early diagnosis and adequate replacement therapy, the prognosis for adrenal hypofunction is good.

CLINICAL TIP

Adrenal crisis (Addisonian crisis) is a critical deficiency of mineralocorticoids and glucocorticoids in patients with chronic adrenal insufficiency. It generally follows sepsis, trauma, surgery, omission of steroid therapy, or other acute physiologic stress. This medical emergency mandates immediate, vigorous treatment.

Causes
Primary hypofunction (Addison's disease):
- Bilateral adrenalectomy
- Hemorrhage into adrenal gland
- Neoplasms
- Tuberculosis, histoplasmosis, cytomegalovirus
- Family history of autoimmune disease.
    Secondary hypofunction (glucocorticoid deficiency):
- Hypopituitarism (causing decreased ACTH secretion)
- Abrupt withdrawal of long-term corticosteroid therapy
- Removal of an ACTH-secreting tumor
- Pituitary injury by tumor or infiltrative or autoimmune process.

Pathophysiology
Addison's disease is a chronic condition that results from partial or complete adrenal destruction. In most cases, cellular atrophy is limited to the cortex, although medullary involvement may occur, resulting in catecholamine deficiency.

ACTH acts primarily to regulate the adrenal release of glucocorticoids (primarily cortisol); mineralocorticoids, including aldosterone; and sex steroids that supplement those produced by the gonads. ACTH secretion is controlled by corticotropin-releasing hormone from the hypothalamus and by negative feedback control by the glucocorticoids.

Cortisol deficiency causes decreased liver gluconeogenesis. Glucose levels of patients on insulin may be dangerously low.

Aldosterone deficiency causes increased renal sodium loss and enhances potassium reabsorption. Sodium excretion causes a reduction in water volume that leads to hypotension.

Androgen deficiency may result in decreased hair growth in axillary and pubic areas, loss of erectile function, or decreased libido.

Signs and symptoms
Primary hypofunction:
- Weakness, fatigue
- Nausea, vomiting, anorexia, weight loss
- Conspicuous bronze color of the skin, especially on hands, elbows, and knees; darkening of scars
- Cardiovascular abnormalities, including orthostatic hypotension, decreased cardiac size and output, and weak, irregular pulse
- Decreased tolerance for even minor stress
- Fasting hypoglycemia
- Craving for salty food.
    Secondary hypofunction:
- Similar to primary hypofunction; differences include:
– hyperpigmentation absent because ACTH and melanocyte-stimulating hormone levels are low
– possibly normal blood pressure and electrolyte balance because aldosterone secretion is near normal
– usually normal androgen secretion.
    Addisonian crisis:
- Profound weakness and fatigue
- Nausea, vomiting, dehydration
- Hypotension
- Confusion.

Diagnostic tests
Adrenal hypofunction:
- Plasma cortisol levels
- Metyrapone test
- Rapid ACTH stimulation test.
    Acute adrenal insufficiency with typical Addisonian symptoms:
- Plasma cortisol levels
- Serum sodium and potassium levels
- Fasting blood glucose levels
- Blood urea nitrogen levels
- Hematocrit; lymphocyte and eosinophil counts
- X-ray.

Treatment
Primary or secondary adrenal hypofunction:
- Lifelong corticosteroid replacement, usually with cortisone or hydrocortisone, which have a mineralocorticoid effect
- I.V. hydrocortisone.
    Primary adrenal hypofunction:
- Oral fludrocortisone, a synthetic mineralocorticoid, to prevent dangerous dehydration, hypotension, hyponatremia, and hyperkalemia.

Adrenal hormones

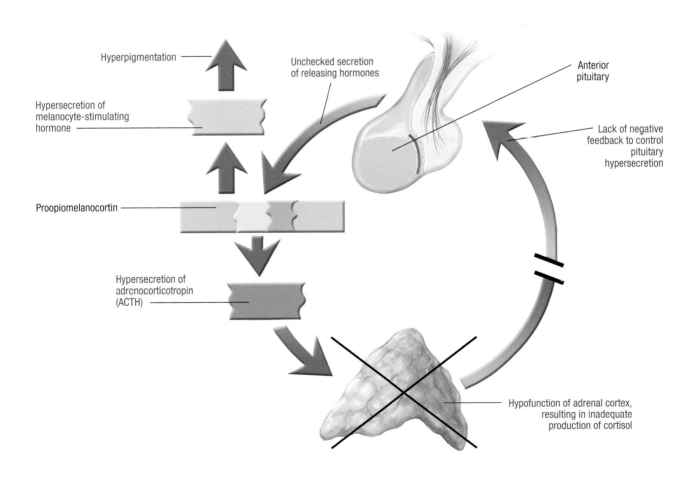

Adrenal gland

Adrenal gland cross section

Cortex
- Mineralocorticoids
- Glucocorticoids
- Androgens
- Estrogens

Medulla
- Norepinephrine
- Epinephrine

Blocked secretion of cortisol in primary adrenal hypofunction

Hyperpigmentation

Unchecked secretion of releasing hormones

Anterior pituitary

Hypersecretion of melanocyte-stimulating hormone

Lack of negative feedback to control pituitary hypersecretion

Proopiomelanocortin

Hypersecretion of adrenocorticotropin (ACTH)

Hypofunction of adrenal cortex, resulting in inadequate production of cortisol

CUSHING'S SYNDROME

Cushing's syndrome is a cluster of clinical abnormalities caused by excessive adrenocortical hormones (particularly cortisol) or related corticosteroids and, to a lesser extent, androgens and aldosterone. Cushing's disease (adrenocorticotropin [ACTH] excess) accounts for about 70% of the cases of Cushing's syndrome.

AGE ALERT
Cushing's syndrome caused by ectopic corticotropin secretion is more common in adult men, with the peak incidence between ages 40 and 60. In 30% of patients, Cushing's syndrome results from a cortisol-secreting tumor. Adrenal tumors, rather than pituitary tumors, are more common in children, especially girls.

The annual incidence of endogenous cortisol excess in the United States is 2 to 4 cases per 1 million people per year. The incidence of Cushing's syndrome resulting from exogenous administration of cortisol is uncertain, but it's known to be much greater than that of endogenous types. The prognosis for endogenous Cushing's syndrome is guardedly favorable with surgery, but morbidity and mortality are high without treatment. About 50% of the individuals with untreated Cushing's syndrome die within 5 years of onset as a result of overwhelming infection, suicide, complications from generalized arteriosclerosis (coronary artery disease), and severe hypertensive disease.

Causes
- Pituitary hypersecretion of ACTH
- Autonomous, ectopic ACTH secretion by a tumor outside the pituitary (usually malignant, frequently a pancreatic tumor or oat cell carcinoma of the lung)
- Administration of synthetic glucocorticoids or steroids.

Pathophysiology
Cortisol excess results in anti-inflammatory effects and excessive catabolism of protein and peripheral fat to support hepatic glucose production. The mechanism may be ACTH-dependent, in which elevated plasma ACTH levels stimulate the adrenal cortex to produce excess cortisol, or ACTH-independent, in which excess cortisol is produced by the adrenal cortex or exogenously administered. This suppresses the hypothalamic-pituitary-adrenal axis, also present in ectopic ACTH-secreting tumors.

Complications associated with Cushing's syndrome are due to the effects of cortisol, the principal glucocorticoid. The complications may include:
- hypertension due to sodium and water retention (common), leading to ischemic heart disease and heart failure
- lipidosis (common)
- peptic ulcer due to increased gastric secretions, pepsin production, and decreased gastric mucus
- impaired glucose tolerance due to increased hepatic gluconeogenesis and insulin resistance.
- frequent infections or slow wound healing due to increased lymphocyte production and suppressed antibody formation
- suppressed inflammatory response
- osteoporosis and pathologic fractures due to increased calcium resorption from bone

Signs and symptoms
- Fat pads above the clavicles, over the upper back (buffalo hump), on the face (moon facies), and throughout the trunk (truncal obesity); slender arms and legs
- Increased susceptibility to infection; decreased resistance to stress
- Hypertension; left ventricular hypertrophy; bleeding and ecchymosis; dyslipidemia
- Increased androgen production — clitoral hypertrophy, mild virilism, hirsutism, and amenorrhea or oligomenorrhea in women; sexual dysfunction
- Sodium and secondary fluid retention, increased potassium excretion, ureteral calculi
- Irritability and emotional lability
- Little or no scar formation; poor wound healing
- Purple striae; facial plethora; acne
- Muscle weakness
- Pathologic fractures; skeletal growth retardation in children.

Diagnostic tests
- Blood and urine glucose levels
- Serum sodium and potassium levels
- Arterial blood gas analysis (metabolic alkalosis)
- Urinary free cortisol levels
- Dexamethasone suppression test
- Blood levels of corticotropin-releasing hormone, ACTH, and various glucocorticoids.

Treatment
- Specific for cause of hypercortisolism-pituitary, adrenal, ectopic
- Surgery for tumors of adrenal or pituitary glands or other tissue, such as lung
- Radiation therapy for tumor
- For inoperable tumor, drugs, such as mitotane or aminoglutethimide to block steroid synthesis.

CLINICAL TIP
Most patients with Cushing's syndrome are treated with transphenoidal surgery, which has a high cure rate (80%). Pharmacotherapy is usually used as adjunctive rather than primary therapy.

MANIFESTATIONS OF CUSHING'S SYNDROME

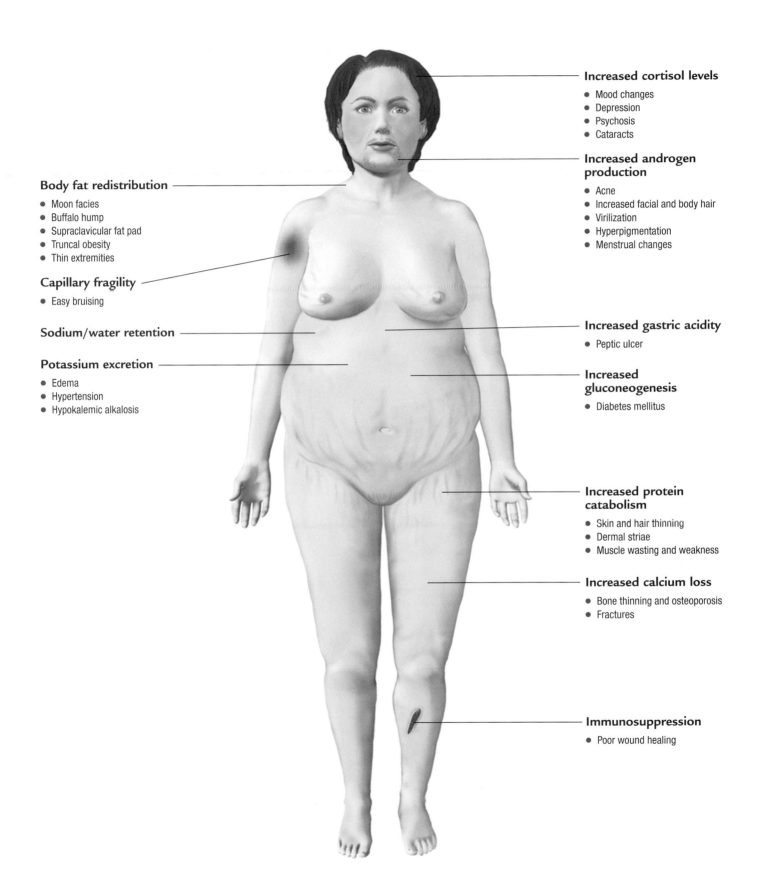

Increased cortisol levels
- Mood changes
- Depression
- Psychosis
- Cataracts

Increased androgen production
- Acne
- Increased facial and body hair
- Virilization
- Hyperpigmentation
- Menstrual changes

Body fat redistribution
- Moon facies
- Buffalo hump
- Supraclavicular fat pad
- Truncal obesity
- Thin extremities

Capillary fragility
- Easy bruising

Sodium/water retention

Potassium excretion
- Edema
- Hypertension
- Hypokalemic alkalosis

Increased gastric acidity
- Peptic ulcer

Increased gluconeogenesis
- Diabetes mellitus

Increased protein catabolism
- Skin and hair thinning
- Dermal striae
- Muscle wasting and weakness

Increased calcium loss
- Bone thinning and osteoporosis
- Fractures

Immunosuppression
- Poor wound healing

Cushing's syndrome   **267**

DIABETES INSIPIDUS

A disorder of water metabolism, diabetes insipidus results from a deficiency of circulating vasopressin (also called antidiuretic hormone, or ADH) or from renal resistance to this hormone. The three forms of diabetes insipidus are neurogenic, nephrogenic, and psychogenic. Neurogenic diabetes insipidus is caused by a deficiency of ADH; nephrogenic diabetes insipidus, by the resistance of renal tubules to ADH. Diabetes insipidus is characterized by excessive fluid intake and hypotonic polyuria. A decrease in ADH levels leads to altered intracellular and extracellular fluid control, causing renal excretion of a large amount of urine.

AGE ALERT
The disorder may start at any age and is slightly more common in men than in women. The incidence is slightly greater today than in the past.

In uncomplicated diabetes insipidus, the prognosis is good with adequate water replacement, and patients usually lead normal lives.

Causes
- Neurogenic: stroke, hypothalamic or pituitary tumor, cranial trauma or surgery, hypophysectomy, aneurysm, thrombosis, infection, immunologic disorders
- Nephrogenic: pyelonephritis, amyloidosis, destructive uropathies, polycystic disease, intrinsic renal disease, end-stage renal failure (less common)
- Psychogenic: primary polydipsia or sarcoidosis
- Transient diabetes insipidus — alcohol, exposure to cold.

Pathophysiology
Diabetes insipidus is related to an insufficiency of ADH, leading to polydipsia and polyuria.

Neurogenic, or *central,* diabetes insipidus is an inadequate ADH response to changes in plasma osmolarity. A lesion of the hypothalamus, infundibular stem, or posterior pituitary partially or completely blocks ADH synthesis, transport, or release.

Neurogenic diabetes insipidus has an acute onset. A three-phase syndrome can occur, which involves:
- progressive loss of nerve tissue and increased diuresis
- normal diuresis
- polyuria and polydipsia, reflecting permanent loss of the ability to secrete adequate ADH.

Nephrogenic diabetes insipidus is caused by an inadequate renal response to ADH. The collecting duct's permeability to water does not increase in response to ADH. Nephrogenic diabetes insipidus is generally related to disorders and drugs that damage the renal tubules or inhibit the generation of cyclic adenosine monophosphate in the tubules. Drugs include lithium carbonate, general anesthetics such as methoxyflurane, and demeclocycline. In addition, hypokalemia or hypercalcemia impairs the renal response to ADH. A rare genetic form of nephrogenic diabetes insipidus is an X-linked recessive trait.

Psychogenic diabetes insipidus is caused by an extremely large fluid intake. This primary polydipsia may be idiopathic or reflect psychosis or sarcoidosis. The polydipsia and resultant polyuria wash out ADH more quickly than it can be replaced. Chronic polyuria may overwhelm the renal medullary concentration gradient, rendering the kidneys partially or totally unable to concentrate urine.

Regardless of the cause, insufficient ADH causes the immediate excretion of large volumes of dilute urine and consequent plasma hyperosmolality. In conscious individuals, the thirst mechanism is stimulated, usually for cold liquids. If diabetes insipidus ensues, severe dehydration, shock, and renal failure can result.

Signs and symptoms
- Polydipsia and polyuria up to 20 L/day (cardinal symptoms)
- Sleep disturbance and fatigue
- Headache and visual disturbance
- Abdominal fullness, anorexia, and weight loss.

Diagnostic tests
- Urine osmolality and specific gravity
- Water deprivation test to identify vasopressin deficiency
- Serum sodium.

Treatment
- Vasopressin to control fluid balance and prevent dehydration until the cause of diabetes insipidus can be identified and eliminated.

CLINICAL TIP
In contrast to DI, the syndrome of inappropriate antidiuretic hormone secretion (SIADH) results when excessive ADH secretion is triggered by stimuli other than increased extracellular fluid osmolarity and decreased extracellular fluid volume, reflected by hypotension. SIADH is a relatively common complication of surgery or critical illness. The prognosis varies with the degree of disease and the speed at which it develops. SIADH usually resolves within 3 days of effective treatment.

MECHANISM OF ADH DEFICIENCY

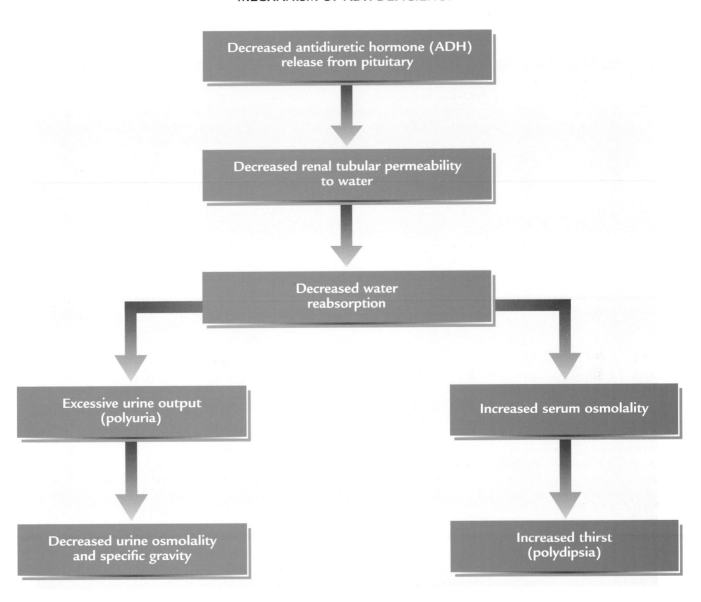

> **CLINICAL TIP**

LABORATORY VALUES FOR PATIENTS WITH DIABETES INSIPIDUS

Value	Normal	Diabetes insipidus (DI)
Serum ADH	1 to 5 pg/ml	Decreased in central DI, may be normal with nephrogenic or psychogenic DI
Serum osmolality	285 to 300 mOsm/kg	>300 mOsm/kg
Serum sodium	135 to 145 mEq/L	>145 mEq/L
Urine osmolality	300 to 1400 mOsm/kg	<300 mOsm/kg
Urine specific gravity	1.005 to 1.030	<1.005
Urine output	1 to 1.5 L/24 hr	30 - 40 L/24 hours
Fluid intake	1 to 1.5L/24 hr	>50 L/24 hours

Diabetes mellitus

Diabetes mellitus is a metabolic disorder characterized by hyperglycemia resulting from lack of insulin, lack of insulin effect, or both. Three general classifications are recognized:
- Type 1 — absolute insulin insufficiency
- Type 2 — insulin resistance with varying degrees of insulin secretory defects
- Gestational diabetes — manifested during pregnancy.

 AGE ALERT
Although possible at any age, Type 1 usually manifests before age 30. It requires exogenous insulin and dietary management.
   Type 2 usually occurs in obese adults after age 40. It's treated with diet and exercise combined with various antidiabetic drugs; treatment may include insulin therapy.

Causes
- Heredity
- Environment (infection, toxins)
- Stress, diet, lack of exercise in genetically susceptible persons.

Pathophysiology
Type 1 and Type 2 diabetes mellitus are two separate and distinct pathophysiological entities. In persons genetically susceptible to *Type 1* diabetes, a triggering event, possibly a viral infection, causes production of autoantibodies which kill the beta cells of the pancreas. This leads to a decline in and ultimate lack of insulin secretion. Insulin deficiency, when more than 90% of the beta cells have been destroyed, leads to hyperglycemia, enhanced lipolysis, and protein catabolism.

Type 2 diabetes mellitus is a chronic disease caused by one or more of the following factors: impaired insulin production, inappropriate hepatic glucose production, or peripheral insulin receptor insensitivity. Genetic factors are significant, and onset is accelerated by obesity and a sedentary lifestyle. Added stress can be a pivotal factor.

Gestational diabetes mellitus is glucose intolerance during pregnancy in a woman not previously diagnosed with diabetes. This may occur if placental hormones counteract insulin, causing insulin resistance. It's a significant risk factor for future Type 2 diabetes mellitus.

Signs and symptoms
- Polyuria and polydipsia
- Nausea; anorexia (common) or polyphagia (occasional)
- Weight loss (usually 10% to 30%; persons with Type 1 diabetes often have almost no body fat at diagnosis)
- Headaches, fatigue, lethargy, reduced energy levels, impaired school or work performance
- Muscle cramps, irritability, emotional lability
- Vision changes, such as blurring
- Numbness and tingling
- Abdominal discomfort and pain; diarrhea or constipation.

Diagnostic tests
In men and nonpregnant women:
- Two of the following criteria obtained more than 24 hours apart, using the same test twice or any combination:
- fasting plasma glucose level of 126 mg/dl or more on at least two occasions
- typical symptoms of uncontrolled diabetes and random blood glucose level of 200 mg/dl or more
- blood glucose level of 200 mg/dl or more 2 hours after ingesting 75 g of oral dextrose
- Other criteria:
- diabetic retinopathy on ophthalmologic examination
- other diagnostic and monitoring tests, including urinalysis for acetone and glycosylated hemoglobin (reflects glycemic control over the past 2 to 3 months).

In pregnant women:
- Positive glucose tolerance test — high peak blood sugar levels after ingestion of glucose (1g/kg body weight) and delayed return to fasting levels.

Treatment
Type 1 diabetes mellitus:
- Insulin replacement, meal planning, and exercise (current forms of insulin replacement include mixed-dose, split mixed-dose, and multiple daily injection regimens and continuous subcutaneous insulin infusions)
- Pancreas transplantation (currently requires chronic immunosuppression).

Type 2 diabetes mellitus:
- Oral antidiabetic drugs to stimulate endogenous insulin production, increase insulin sensitivity at the cellular level, suppress hepatic gluconeogenesis, and delay GI absorption of carbohydrates (drug combinations may be used)
- Exogenous insulin, alone or with oral antidiabetic drugs, to optimize glycemic control.

Type 1 and Type 2 diabetes mellitus:
- Individualized meal plan designed to meet nutritional needs, control blood glucose and lipid levels, and reach and maintain appropriate body weight
- Weight reduction (obese patient with Type 2 diabetes mellitus) or high calorie allotment, depending on growth stage and activity level (Type 1 diabetes mellitus).

Gestational diabetes:
- Medical nutrition therapy and exercise
- Alpha glucosidase inhibitors, injected insulin, or both (if euglycemia not achieved)
- Counseling on the high risk for gestational diabetes in subsequent pregnancies and Type 2 diabetes later in life
- Exercise and weight control to help avert Type 2 diabetes.

 CLINICAL TIP
Although patients with Type 2 diabetes are able to suppress development of ketones under basal conditions, they may develop diabetic ketoacidosis in the presence of precipitating factors such as sepsis.

POTENTIAL LONG-TERM COMPLICATIONS OF DIABETES MELLITUS

Loss of vision

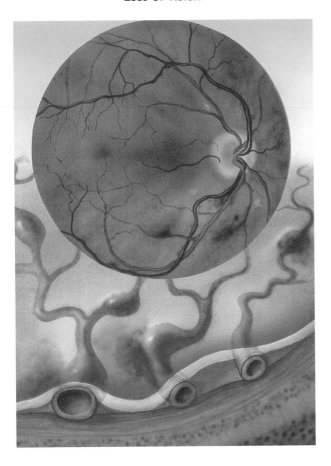

Nerve damage

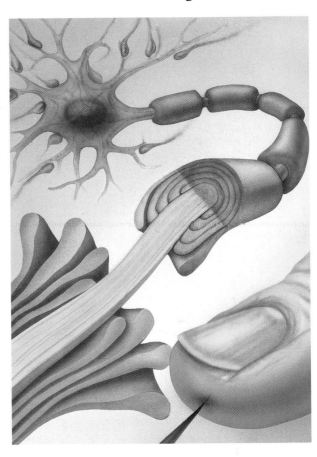

Poor circulation

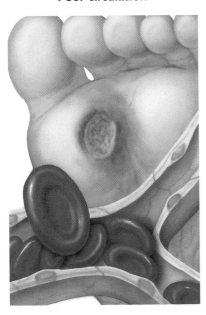

Heart disease

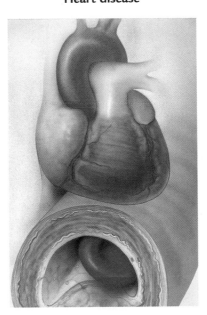

Kidney failure

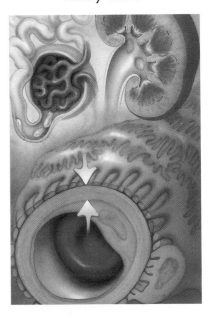

GROWTH HORMONE EXCESS

Growth hormone (GH) excess that begins in adulthood (after epiphyseal closure) is called *acromegaly*. GH excess that is present before closure of the epiphyseal growth plates of the long bones causes *pituitary gigantism*. In both cases, the result is increased growth of bone, cartilage, and other tissues, as well as increased carbohydrate catabolism and protein synthesis. In gigantism, a proportional overgrowth of all body tissues before epiphyseal closure causes remarkable height increases — as much as 6 inches (15 cm) a year. Acromegaly is rare; its prevalence is about 70 people per million in the United States, affecting men and women equally. GH excess is a slow but progressive disease that shortens life if untreated. Morbidity and mortality tend to be related to coronary artery disease and hypertension secondary to prolonged exposure to excessive growth hormone.

AGE ALERT
Most cases of acromegaly are diagnosed in the fourth and fifth decades, but the disease is usually present for years before diagnosis. Gigantism affects infants and children, causing them to reach as much as three times the normal height for their age. Affected adults may reach a height of more than 7.5 feet (203 cm).

Causes
GH excess is caused by eosinophilic or mixed-cell adenomas of the anterior pituitary gland.

Pathophysiology
A GH-secreting tumor creates an unpredictable GH secretion pattern, which replaces the usual peaks at 1 to 4 hours after the onset of sleep. Elevated GH and somatomedin levels stimulate growth of all tissues. In pituitary gigantism, the epiphyseal plates aren't closed, and so the excess GH stimulates linear growth. It also increases the bulk of bones and joints and causes enlargement of internal organs and metabolic abnormalities. In acromegaly, the excess GH increases bone density and width, and the proliferation of connective and soft tissues.

Signs and symptoms
Acromegaly:
- Soft-tissue thickening that causes enlargement of hands, feet, nose, mandible, supraorbital ridge, and ears
- Severe headache, central nervous system impairment, bitemporal hemianopia (defective vision), loss of visual acuity, and blindness (if the intrasellar tumor compresses the optic chiasm or nerves)
- Marked prognathism and malocclusion of teeth; may interfere with chewing
- Laryngeal hypertrophy, paranasal sinus enlargement, thickening of the tongue — causing the voice to sound deep and hollow

- Arrowhead appearance of distal phalanges on X-rays, thickened fingers
- Sweating, oily skin, hypertrichosis, new skin tags (typical)
- Irritability, hostility, various psychological disturbances
- Bow legs, barrel chest, arthritis, osteoporosis, kyphosis
- Glucose intolerance, clinical diabetes mellitus
- Hypertension and arteriosclerosis (effects of prolonged excessive GH secretion)
- Hypermetabolism
- Weakness, arthralgia.
  Gigantism:
- Backache, arthralgia, arthritis
- Excessive height
- Headache, vomiting, seizure activity, visual disturbances, papilledema
- Deficiencies of other hormone systems if GH-producing tumor destroys other hormone-secreting cells
- Glucose intolerance and diabetes mellitus.

Diagnostic tests
- Plasma GH level measured by radioimmunoassay
- Somatomedin-C, a metabolite of GH
- Glucose suppression test
- Skull X-ray, computed tomography scan, magnetic resonance imaging
- Blood glucose levels.

Treatment
- Tumor removal by cranial or transsphenoidal hypophysectomy or pituitary radiation therapy
- Mandatory surgery for a tumor causing blindness or other severe neurologic disturbances
- Postoperative replacement of thyroid, cortisone, and gonadal hormones
- Bromocriptine and octreotide to inhibit GH synthesis.

CLINICAL TIP
Growth hormone (somatotropin) *deficiency* results from hypofunction of the anterior pituitary gland with a resulting decreased secretion of GH. GH deficiency includes a group of childhood disorders characterized by subnormal growth velocity, delayed bone age, and a subnormal response to at least two stimuli for release of the hormone. Gonadotropin deficiency may be evident. Fatal convulsions, due to fasting hypoglycemia, may occur — especially during periods of stress. A "distinctive" GH deficiency syndrome presents with abnormal body composition, impaired physical performance, decreased quality of life, and increased mortality. GH deficiency in adults usually has no clinical signs and symptoms.

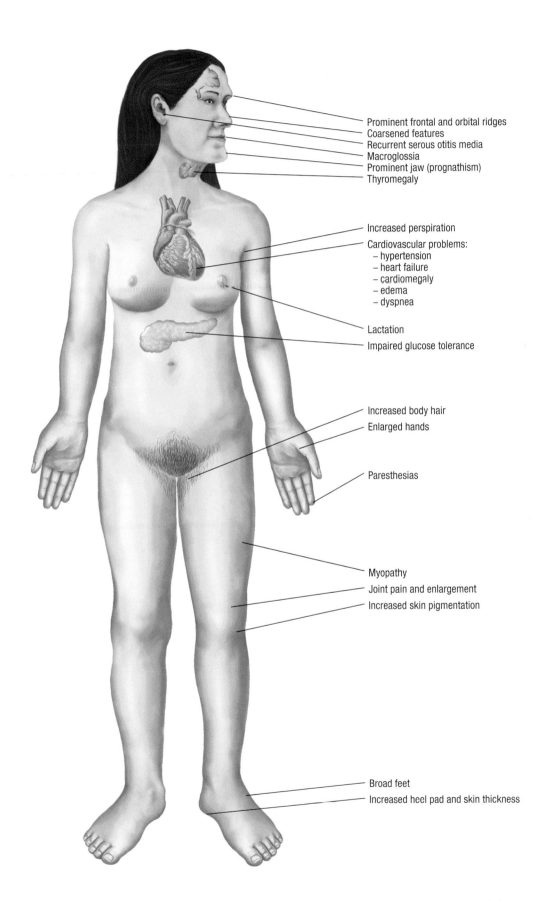

Prominent frontal and orbital ridges
Coarsened features
Recurrent serous otitis media
Macroglossia
Prominent jaw (prognathism)
Thyromegaly

Increased perspiration
Cardiovascular problems:
 – hypertension
 – heart failure
 – cardiomegaly
 – edema
 – dyspnea

Lactation
Impaired glucose tolerance

Increased body hair
Enlarged hands

Paresthesias

Myopathy
Joint pain and enlargement
Increased skin pigmentation

Broad feet
Increased heel pad and skin thickness

HYPERPARATHYROIDISM

Hyperparathyroidism results from excessive secretion of parathyroid hormone (PTH) from one or more of the four parathyroid glands. PTH promotes bone resorption, and hypersecretion leads to hypercalcemia and hypophosphatemia. Renal and GI absorption of calcium increase. Primary hyperparathyroidism is commonly diagnosed when an asymptomatic patient has elevated calcium levels in routine laboratory tests. It affects women two to three times more frequently than men and is seen most frequently in women older than age 40.

CLINICAL TIP

Hypoparathyroidism, which is much rarer than hyperparathyroidism, is caused by disease, injury, or congenital malfunction of the parathyroid glands. Because the parathyroid glands primarily regulate calcium balance, hypoparathyroidism causes hypocalcemia and consequent neuromuscular symptoms ranging from paresthesia to tetany. The clinical effects of hypoparathyroidism are usually correctable with replacement therapy. Some complications of long-term hypocalcemia, such as cataracts and basal ganglion calcifications, are irreversible.

Causes

Primary hyperparathyroidism:
- Most commonly a single adenoma
- Multiple endocrine neoplasia (all four glands usually involved).

Secondary hyperparathyroidism:
- Rickets, vitamin D deficiency, chronic renal failure, and osteomalacia due to phenytoin.

Pathophysiology

Overproduction of PTH by a tumor or hyperplastic tissue increases intestinal calcium absorption, reduces renal calcium clearance, and increases bone calcium release. Response to this excess varies for each patient for unknown reasons.

Hypophosphatemia results when excessive PTH inhibits renal tubular phosphate reabsorption. It aggravates hypercalcemia by increasing the sensitivity of the bone to PTH. Pathologic fractures may be a presenting symptom.

A hypocalcemia-producing abnormality outside the parathyroids can cause excessive compensatory production of PTH, or secondary hyperparathyroidism.

Signs and symptoms

Primary hyperparathyroidism:
- Polyuria, nephrocalcinosis, or recurring nephrolithiasis and consequent renal insufficiency
- Chronic low back pain and easy fracturing
- Bone tenderness, chondrocalcinosis

- Osteopenia and osteoporosis, especially of vertebrae
- Erosions of juxta-articular (adjoining joint) surface
- Subchondral fractures
- Traumatic synovitis
- Pseudogout
- Pancreatitis causing constant, severe epigastric pain that radiates to the back
- Peptic ulcers, causing abdominal pain, anorexia, nausea, and vomiting
- Muscle weakness and atrophy, particularly in the legs
- Psychomotor and personality disturbances, depression, overt psychosis
- Stupor, and possibly coma
- Skin necrosis, cataracts, calcium microthrombi to lungs and pancreas, anemia, and subcutaneous calcification.

Secondary hyperparathyroidism:
- Same features of calcium imbalance as in primary hyperparathyroidism
- Skeletal deformities of the long bones (such as rickets)
- Symptoms of the underlying disease.

Diagnostic tests

Primary disease:
- Serum PTH by radioimmunoassay
- X-ray
- Microscopic bone examination by X-ray spectrophotometry
- Urine and serum calcium, chloride, phosphorus, and alkaline phosphatase levels
- Uric acid and creatinine; basal gastric acid secretion and serum immunoreactive gastrin
- Serum amylase (may indicate acute pancreatitis).

Secondary disease:
- Serum calcium and phosphorus level.

Treatment

Primary hyperparathyroidism:
- Surgery to remove the adenoma or, depending on the extent of hyperplasia, all but half of one gland, to provide normal PTH levels
- Treatments to decrease calcium levels — forcing fluids, limiting dietary intake of calcium, promoting sodium and calcium excretion through forced diuresis
- Oral sodium or potassium phosphate; subcutaneous calcitonin; I.V. mithramycin or biphosphonate
- I.V. magnesium and phosphate; sodium phosphate solution by mouth or retention enema; possibly supplemental calcium, vitamin D, or calcitriol.

Secondary hyperparathyroidism:
- Vitamin D to correct the underlying cause of parathyroid hyperplasia; oral calcium preparation to correct hyperphosphatemia in the patient with kidney disease
- Dialysis in patient with renal failure to decrease phosphorus levels.

PATHOGENESIS OF HYPERPARATHYROIDISM

Tumor or hyperplastic tissue secretes excess PTH

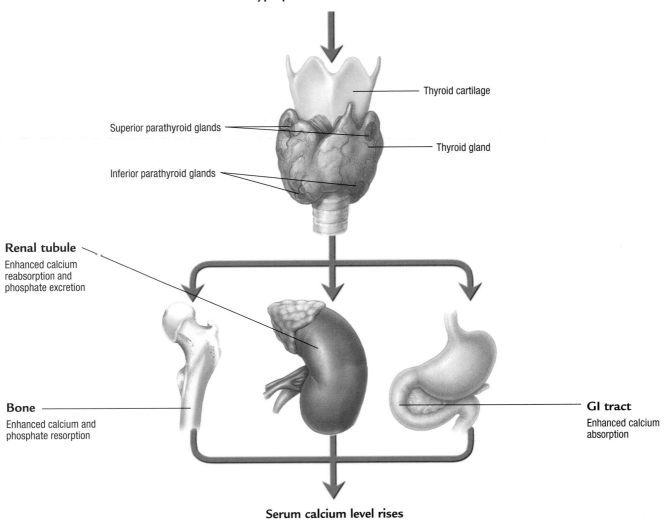

Thyroid cartilage

Superior parathyroid glands

Thyroid gland

Inferior parathyroid glands

Renal tubule

Enhanced calcium reabsorption and phosphate excretion

Bone

Enhanced calcium and phosphate resorption

GI tract

Enhanced calcium absorption

Serum calcium level rises

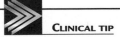

CLINICAL TIP

BONE RESORPTION IN PRIMARY HYPERPARATHYROIDISM

In hyperparathyroidism, body mechanisms sacrifice bone to preserve intracellular calcium levels. X-rays may show diffuse demineralization of bones, bone cysts, outer cortical bone absorption, and subperiosteal erosion of the phalanges and distal clavicles. Microscopic examination of the bone with tests such as X-ray spectrophotometry typically demonstrates increased bone turnover.

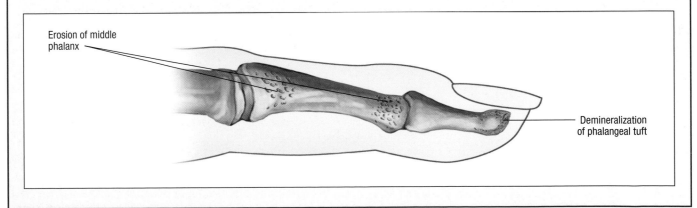

Erosion of middle phalanx

Demineralization of phalangeal tuft

HYPERTHYROIDISM

Hyperthyroidism, or thyrotoxicosis, is a metabolic imbalance that results from the overproduction of thyroid hormone. The most common form is Graves' disease, an autoimmune disorder that increases thyroxine (T_4) production, enlarges the thyroid gland (goiter), and causes multiple system changes.

AGE ALERT
Incidence of Graves' disease is greatest in women between ages 30 and 60, especially those with a family history of thyroid abnormalities; only 5% of patients are younger than age 15.

Causes
- Inherited predisposition, probably autosomal recessive gene
- Other endocrine abnormalities
- Defect in suppressor T-lymphocyte function and consequent production of autoantibodies
- Excessive dietary intake of iodine or possibly stress — can precipitate clinical thyrotoxicosis
- Stress, such as surgery, infection, toxemia of pregnancy, or diabetic ketoacidosis — can precipitate thyroid storm.

Pathophysiology
The thyroid gland secretes the thyroid precursor thyroxine (T_4), the thyroid hormone triiodothyronine (T_3), and thyrocalcitonin. T_4 and T_3 stimulate protein, lipid, and carbohydrate metabolism primarily through catabolic pathways. Thyrocalcitonin removes calcium from the blood and incorporates it into bone. Biosynthesis, storage, and release of thyroid hormones are controlled by the hypothalamic-pituitary axis through a negative-feedback loop.

Thyrotropin-releasing hormone (TRH) from the hypothalamus stimulates the release of thyroid-stimulating-hormone (TSH) by the pituitary. Circulating T_3 levels provide negative feedback through the hypothalamus to decrease TRH levels, and through the pituitary to decrease TSH levels.

Graves' disease is an autoimmune disorder characterized by the production of autoantibodies that attach to and then stimulate TSH receptors on the thyroid gland.

Pituitary tumors with TSH-producing cells are rare, as is hypothalamic disease causing TRH excess.

Signs and symptoms
- Enlarged thyroid (goiter)
- Nervousness, tremor, and palpitations
- Heat intolerance, sweating
- Weight loss despite increased appetite
- Frequent bowel movements
- Exophthalmos (characteristic, but absent in many patients with thyrotoxicosis).

Other signs and symptoms, common because thyrotoxicosis profoundly affects virtually every body system:
- Difficulty concentrating; fine tremor, shaky handwriting, and clumsiness; emotional instability and mood swings ranging from occasional outbursts to overt psychosis

- Moist, smooth, warm, flushed skin; fine, soft hair; premature patchy graying and increased hair loss in both sexes; friable nails and onycholysis; pretibial myxedema, producing thickened skin; accentuated hair follicles; sometimes itchy or painful raised red patches of skin with occasional nodule formation; microscopic examination showing increased mucin deposits
- Systolic hypertension, tachycardia, full bounding pulse, wide pulse pressure, cardiomegaly, increased cardiac output and blood volume, visible point of maximal impulse, paroxysmal supraventricular tachycardia and atrial fibrillation (especially in elderly people), and occasional systolic murmur at the left sternal border
- Increased respiratory rate, dyspnea on exertion and at rest; nausea and vomiting; soft stools or diarrhea; liver enlargement
- Weakness, fatigue, and muscle atrophy; rare coexistence with myasthenia gravis; possibly generalized or localized paralysis associated with hypokalemia; and, rarely, acropachy
- Oligomenorrhea or amenorrhea, decreased fertility, increased incidence of spontaneous abortion (females), gynecomastia (males), diminished libido (both sexes).

Thyroid storm:
- Extreme irritability, hypertension, tachycardia, vomiting, temperature up to 106° F (41.1° C), delirium, and coma.

Diagnostic tests
- Radioimmunoassay for T_4 and T_3
- TSH levels
- Thyroid scan (contraindicated during pregnancy)
- Ultrasonography.

Treatment
- Antithyroid drugs — thyroid hormone antagonists, including propylthiouracil and methimazole, to block thyroid hormone synthesis; propranolol until antithyroid drugs reach their full effect — to manage tachycardia and other peripheral effects of excessive hypersympathetic activity
- Single oral dose of radioactive iodine (^{131}I)
- Surgery and lifelong regular medical supervision — most patients become hypothyroid, sometimes as long as several years after surgery.

CLINICAL TIP
With treatment, most patients can lead normal lives. However, thyroid storm — an acute, severe exacerbation of thyrotoxicosis — is a medical emergency that may have life-threatening cardiac, hepatic, or renal consequences.

THYROID GLAND AND ITS HORMONES

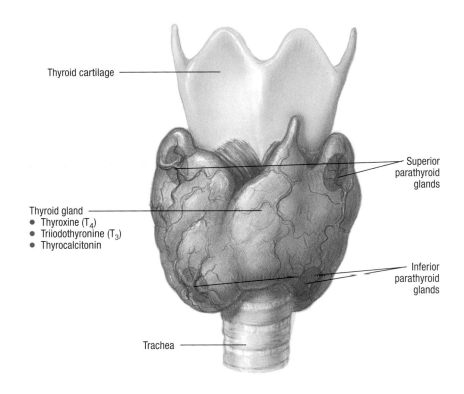

Thyroid cartilage

Superior parathyroid glands

Thyroid gland
- Thyroxine (T$_4$)
- Triiodothyronine (T$_3$)
- Thyrocalcitonin

Inferior parathyroid glands

Trachea

HISTOLOGIC CHANGES IN GRAVES' DISEASE

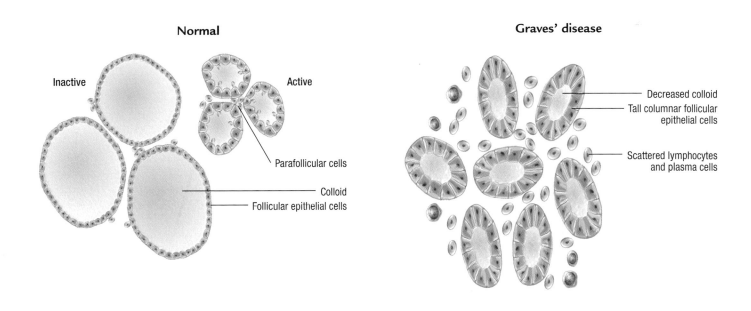

Normal

Inactive

Active

Parafollicular cells

Colloid

Follicular epithelial cells

Graves' disease

Decreased colloid

Tall columnar follicular epithelial cells

Scattered lymphocytes and plasma cells

HYPOPITUITARISM

Hypopituitarism, also known as panhypopituitarism, is a complex syndrome marked by metabolic dysfunction, sexual immaturity, and growth retardation (when it occurs in childhood). The cause is a deficiency of the hormones secreted by the anterior pituitary gland. Panhypopituitarism is a partial or total failure of all six of this gland's vital hormones — adrenocorticotropin (ACTH), thyroid-stimulating hormone (TSH), luteinizing hormone (LH), follicle-stimulating hormone (FSH), growth hormone (GH), and prolactin.

 AGE ALERT
Partial and complete forms of hypopituitarism affect adults and children; in children, these diseases may cause dwarfism and delayed puberty. The prognosis may be good with adequate replacement therapy and correction of the underlying causes.

Primary hypopituitarism usually develops in a predictable pattern. It generally starts with decreased gonadotropin (FSH and LH) levels and consequent hypogonadism, reflected by cessation of menses in women and impotence in men. GH deficiency follows, causing short stature, delayed growth, and delayed puberty in children. Subsequent decreased TSH levels cause hypothyroidism, and, finally, decreased ACTH levels result in adrenal insufficiency, possibly leading to adrenal crisis. When hypopituitarism follows surgical ablation or trauma, the pattern of hormonal events may not necessarily follow that sequence. Damage to the hypothalamus or neurohypophysis may cause diabetes insipidus.

Causes

Primary hypopituitarism:
- Tumor of the pituitary gland
- Congenital defect (hypoplasia or aplasia of the pituitary gland)
- Pituitary infarction (most often from postpartum hemorrhage)
- Partial or total hypophysectomy by surgery, irradiation, or chemical agents
- Granulomatous disease, such as tuberculosis

- Idiopathic or autoimmune origin (occasionally).
  Secondary hypopituitarism:
- Deficiency of releasing hormones produced by the hypothalamus, either idiopathic or resulting from infection, trauma, or a tumor.

Pathophysiology

Hypopituitarism describes the low secretion of an anterior pituitary hormone, and *panhypopituitarism* describes the low secretion of all anterior pituitary hormones. Both can result from malfunction of the pituitary gland or the hypothalamus. The result is a lack of stimulation of target endocrine organs and some degree of deficiency of the target organ hormone; however, this may not be discovered until the body is stressed and the expected increases in secretions from the target organs don't occur.

Signs and symptoms

- ACTH deficiency: weakness, fatigue, weight loss, fasting hypoglycemia, and altered mental function; loss of axillary and pubic hair; orthostatic hypotension and hyponatremia
- TSH deficiency: weight gain, constipation, cold intolerance, fatigue, and coarse hair
- Gonadotropin deficiency: sexual dysfunction, infertility
- Antidiuretic hormone deficiency: diabetes insipidus
- Prolactin deficiency: lactation dysfunction or gynecomastia.

Diagnostic tests

- ACTH, FSH, GH, LH, TSH levels
- Computed tomography or magnetic resonance imaging of pituitary and target glands (adrenal cortex, thyroid, gonads).

Treatment

- Replacement of hormones (cortisol, thyroxine, androgen or cyclic estrogen) secreted by the target glands; prolactin not replaced
- Clomiphene or cyclic gonadotropin-releasing hormone to induce ovulation in female patient of reproductive age.

Anterior pituitary

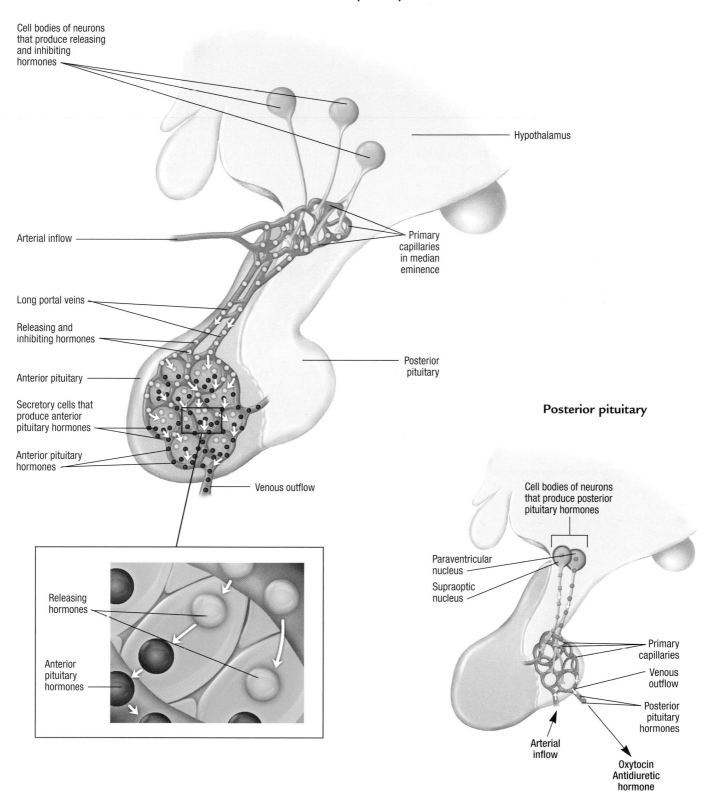

Cell bodies of neurons that produce releasing and inhibiting hormones

Hypothalamus

Arterial inflow

Primary capillaries in median eminence

Long portal veins

Releasing and inhibiting hormones

Anterior pituitary

Posterior pituitary

Secretory cells that produce anterior pituitary hormones

Anterior pituitary hormones

Venous outflow

Posterior pituitary

Releasing hormones

Anterior pituitary hormones

Cell bodies of neurons that produce posterior pituitary hormones

Paraventricular nucleus

Supraoptic nucleus

Primary capillaries

Venous outflow

Posterior pituitary hormones

Arterial inflow

Oxytocin Antidiuretic hormone

HYPOTHYROIDISM

Hypothyroidism results from hypothalamic, pituitary, or thyroid insufficiency or resistance to thyroid hormone. The disorder can progress to life-threatening myxedema coma. Hypothyroidism is more prevalent in women than men; in the United States, the incidence is increasing significantly in people ages 40 to 50.

AGE ALERT
Hypothyroidism occurs primarily after age 40 and is particularly underdiagnosed in elderly persons. After age 65, prevalence increases to as much as 10% in females and 3% in males.

A deficiency of thyroid hormone secretion during fetal development and early infancy results in infantile cretinism (congenital hypothyroidism). Cretinism is three times more common in girls than boys. If untreated, irreversible mental retardation can result.

Subacute thyroiditis, painless thyroiditis, and postpartum thyroiditis are self-limited conditions that usually follow an episode of hyperthyroidism. Untreated subclinical hypothyroidism in adults is likely to become overt at a rate of 5% to 20% per year.

Causes
Primary (disorder of thyroid gland):
• Thyroidectomy or radiation therapy (particularly with iodine 131)
• Inflammation, chronic autoimmune thyroiditis (Hashimoto's thyroiditis), or such conditions as amyloidosis and sarcoidosis (rare)
   Secondary (failure to stimulate normal thyroid function):
• Inadequate production of thyroid hormone
• Use of such antithyroid medications as propylthiouracil
• Pituitary failure to produce thyroid-stimulating hormone (TSH)
• Inborn errors of thyroid hormone synthesis
• Iodine deficiency (usually dietary).
• Hypothalamic failure to produce thyrotropin-releasing hormone (TRH).

Pathophysiology
Hypothyroidism may reflect a malfunction of the hypothalamus, pituitary, or thyroid gland, all of which are part of the same negative-feedback mechanism. However, disorders of the hypothalamus and pituitary rarely cause hypothyroidism. Primary hypothyroidism is most common.

Chronic autoimmune thyroiditis, also called chronic lymphocytic thyroiditis, occurs when autoantibodies destroy thyroid gland tissue. Chronic autoimmune thyroiditis associated with goiter is called Hashimoto's thyroiditis. The cause of this autoimmune process is unknown, although heredity has a role,

and specific human leukocyte antigen subtypes are associated with greater risk.

Outside the thyroid, antibodies can reduce the effect of thyroid hormone in two ways. First, antibodies can block the TSH receptor and prevent the production of TSH. Second, cytotoxic antithyroid antibodies may attack thyroid cells.

Signs and symptoms
• Typical, vague, early clinical features — weakness, fatigue, forgetfulness, sensitivity to cold, unexplained weight gain, constipation
• Myxedema — decreasing mental stability; coarse, dry, flaky, inelastic skin; puffy face, hands, and feet; hoarseness; periorbital edema; upper eyelid droop; dry, sparse hair; thick, brittle nails (as disorder progresses)
• Cardiovascular involvement — decreased cardiac output, slow pulse rate, signs of poor peripheral circulation, congestive heart failure, cardiomegaly (occasionally).
   Other common effects:
• Anorexia, abdominal distention, menorrhagia, decreased libido, infertility, ataxia, and nystagmus; reflexes with delayed relaxation time (especially Achilles' tendon)
• Progression to myxedema coma — usually gradual but may develop abruptly when stress aggravates severe or prolonged hypothyroidism —progressive stupor, hypoventilation, hypoglycemia, hyponatremia, hypotension, hypothermia.

Diagnostic tests
• Radioimmunoassay for thyroid hormones triiodothyronine (T_3) and thyroxine (T_4)
• TSH level
• Thyroid panel to differentiate primary hypothyroidism, secondary hypothyroidism, and euthyroid sick syndrome (impaired peripheral conversion of thyroid hormone due to a suprathyroidal illness, such as severe infection)
• Serum cholesterol, alkaline phosphatase, and triglyceride levels
• Complete blood count and peripheral smear.
   Myxedema coma:
• Serum sodium, blood pH, and partial pressure of carbon dioxide.

Treatment
• Gradual lifelong thyroid hormone replacement with T_4 and, occasionally, T_3
• Surgical excision, chemotherapy, or radiation for tumors.

AGE ALERT
Elderly patients should be started on a very low dose of T_4, such as 25 mcg every morning, to avoid cardiac problems. TSH levels guide gradual increases in dosage.

Normal

Hashimoto's thyroiditis

Inactive   Active

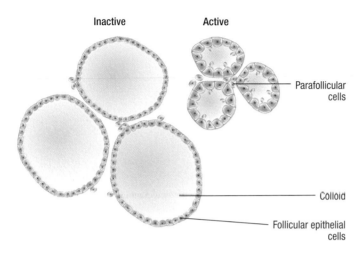

Parafollicular cells

Colloid

Follicular epithelial cells

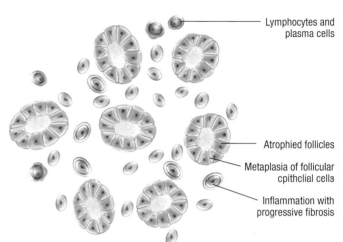

Lymphocytes and plasma cells

Atrophied follicles

Metaplasia of follicular cpithclial cells

Inflammation with progressive fibrosis

CLINICAL TIP

FACIAL MANIFESTATIONS OF MYXEDEMA

Before the era of rapid laboratory diagnosis and hormone replacement therapy, severe hypothyroidism was diagnosed by typical facial features.

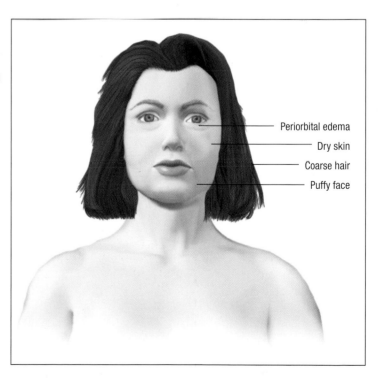

Periorbital edema

Dry skin

Coarse hair

Puffy face

SIMPLE GOITER

Simple (or nontoxic) goiter is a thyroid gland enlargement that isn't caused by inflammation or a neoplasm, and is commonly classified as endemic or sporadic. Inherited defects may be responsible for insufficient thyroxine (T_4) synthesis or impaired iodine metabolism. Because families tend to congregate in a single geographic area, this familial factor may contribute to the incidence of both endemic and sporadic goiters.

Causes
Endemic goiter:
- Inadequate dietary iodine.
  Sporadic goiter:
- Large amounts of foods containing agents that inhibit T_4 production, such as rutabagas, cabbage, soybeans, peanuts, peaches, peas, strawberries, spinach, radishes
- Drugs such as propylthiouracil, iodides, phenylbutazone, para-aminosalicylic acid, cobalt, lithium; may cross placenta and affect fetus.

Pathophysiology
Goiters can occur in the presence of hypothyroidism, hyperthyroidism, or normal levels of thyroid hormone. In the presence of a severe underlying disorder, compensatory responses may cause both thyroid enlargement (goiter) and hypothyroidism. Simple goiter occurs when the thyroid gland can't secrete enough thyroid hormone to meet metabolic requirements. As a result, the thyroid gland enlarges to compensate for inadequate hormone synthesis, a compensation that usually overcomes mild to moderate hormonal impairment.

Endemic goiter usually results from inadequate secretion of thyroid hormone secondary to inadequate dietary intake of iodine associated with such factors as iodine-depleted soil or malnutrition. Since the introduction of iodized salt in the United States, cases of endemic goiter have virtually disappeared.

Sporadic goiter is triggered by certain drugs or foods that inhibit or block production of thyroid hormones.

Signs and symptoms
- Enlarged thyroid — ranging from mild enlargement to massive, multinodular goiter
- Respiratory distress
- Dysphagia
- Venous engorgement; development of collateral venous circulation in the chest
- Dizziness or syncope (Pemberton's sign) when the patient raises her arms above her head.

Diagnostic tests
- Thyroid-stimulating hormone (TSH) level
- Serum T_4 concentrations
- Radioactive iodine (^{131}I) uptake test.

Treatment
- Exogenous thyroid hormone replacement with levothyroxine (treatment of choice) — inhibits TSH secretion and allows gland to rest
- Small doses of iodide (Lugol's iodine or potassium iodide solution) — commonly relieves goiter due to iodine deficiency
- Avoidance of known goitrogenic drugs and foods
- For large goiter that's unresponsive to treatment — subtotal thyroidectomy.

RECOGNIZING TYPES OF GOITERS

Toxic goiter (Graves' disease)

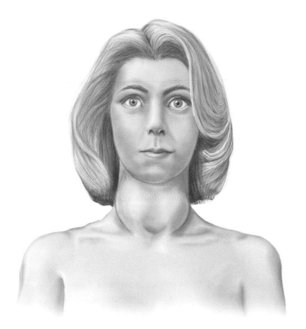

Simple (nontoxic) goiter

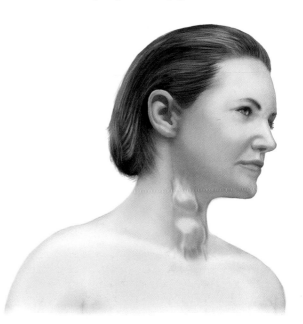

Nodular goiter

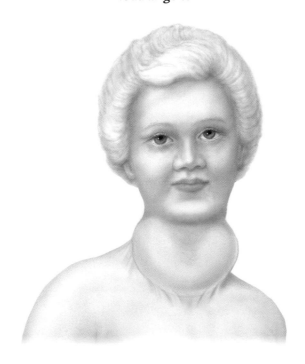

THYROID CANCER

Thyroid carcinoma is the most common endocrine malignancy. It occurs in all age groups, especially in people who have had radiation treatment of the neck area.

Causes

Direct cause unknown.

Predisposing factors:

● Prolonged thyroid-stimulating hormone (TSH) stimulation due to radiation exposure or heredity
● Familial predisposition
● Chronic goiter.

Pathophysiology

Papillary carcinoma accounts for half of all thyroid cancers in adults. Most common in young adult females, it is the least virulent form of thyroid cancer and metastasizes slowly. *Follicular carcinoma* is less common but more likely to recur and metastasize to the regional nodes and through blood vessels into the bones, liver, and lungs. *Medullary carcinoma* originates in the parafollicular cells derived from the last branchial pouch and contains amyloid and calcium deposits. It can produce thyrocalcitonin, histaminase, adrenocorticotropin (producing Cushing's syndrome), and prostaglandin E_2 and F_3 (producing diarrhea). This rare form of thyroid cancer is familial, associated with pheochromocytoma, and completely curable when detected before it causes symptoms. Untreated, it progresses rapidly. Seldom curable by resection, anaplastic tumors resist radiation and metastasize rapidly.

Signs and symptoms

● Painless nodule; hard nodule in an enlarged thyroid gland; or palpable lymph nodes and thyroid enlargement
● Hoarseness, dysphagia, dyspnea, pain on palpation

● Hypothyroidism (low metabolism, mental apathy, and sensitivity to cold) or hyperthyroidism (hyperactivity, restlessness, and sensitivity to heat)
● Diarrhea, anorexia, irritability, vocal cord paralysis
● Symptoms of distant metastasis.

Diagnostic tests

● Thyroid scan
● Needle biopsy
● Computed tomography scan; ultrasonography; chest X-ray
● Serum alkaline phosphatase; serum calcitonin assay.

Treatment

● Papillary or follicular cancer — total or subtotal thyroidectomy; modified node dissection (bilateral or unilateral) on the side of the primary cancer

CLINICAL TIP

Before surgery, tell the patient to expect temporary voice loss or hoarseness lasting several days after surgery.

● Medullary, giant, or spindle cell cancer — total thyroidectomy and radical neck excision
● Inoperable cancer or postoperatively in lieu of radical neck excision — radiation (^{131}I) with external radiation
● To increase tolerance to surgery and radiation — adjunctive thyroid suppression with exogenous thyroid hormones and simultaneous administration of an adrenergic blocking agent such as propranolol
● Metastasis — radiation (^{131}I); chemotherapy for symptomatic, widespread metastasis is limited.

CLINICAL TIP

Hypocalcemia may develop if parathyroid glands are removed.

Anterior view

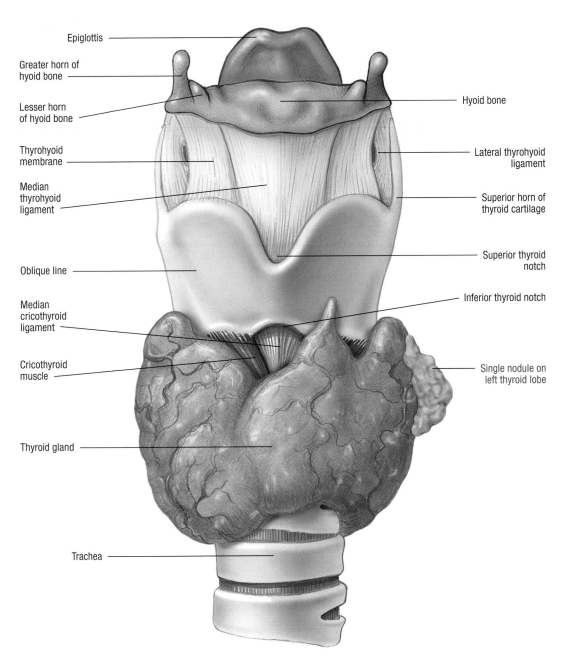

Epiglottis

Greater horn of
hyoid bone

Lesser horn
of hyoid bone

Thyrohyoid
membrane

Median
thyrohyoid
ligament

Oblique line

Median
cricothyroid
ligament

Cricothyroid
muscle

Thyroid gland

Trachea

Hyoid bone

Lateral thyrohyoid
ligament

Superior horn of
thyroid cartilage

Superior thyroid
notch

Inferior thyroid notch

Single nodule on
left thyroid lobe

ABNORMAL UTERINE BLEEDING

Abnormal uterine bleeding refers to endometrial bleeding without recognizable organic lesions. It is the indication for almost 25% of gynecologic surgical procedures. The prognosis varies with the cause. Correction of hormonal imbalance or structural abnormality yields a good prognosis.

Causes
- Polycystic ovarian syndrome
- Obesity — enzymes in peripheral adipose tissue convert the androgen androstenedione to estrogens
- Immaturity of the hypothalamic-pituitary-ovarian mechanism (postpubertal teenagers)
- Anovulation (women in their late thirties or early forties)
- Hormone-producing ovarian tumor.

Pathophysiology
Irregular bleeding is associated with hormonal imbalance and absence of ovulation (anovulation). When progesterone secretion is absent but estrogen secretion continues, the endometrium proliferates and become hypervascular. When ovulation does not occur, the endometrium randomly breaks down, and exposed vascular channels cause prolonged and excessive bleeding. In most cases of abnormal uterine bleeding, the endometrium shows no pathologic changes. However, in chronic unopposed estrogen stimulation (as from a hormone-producing ovarian tumor), the endometrium may show hyperplastic or malignant changes.

Signs and symptoms
- Metrorrhagia — episodes of vaginal bleeding between menses
- Hypermenorrhea (also termed menorrhagia) — heavy or prolonged menses, longer than 8 days
- Chronic polymenorrhea (menstrual cycle less than 18 days) or oligomenorrhea (infrequent menses)
- Fatigue due to anemia
- Infertility due to anovulation.

Diagnostic tests
- Progesterone trial
- Ovulatory cycle body temperature monitoring
- Serum progesterone
- Studies ruling out other causes of excessive vaginal bleeding, such as cancer, polyps, pregnancy, infection
- Dilatation and curettage or office endometrial biopsy
- Hemoglobin and hematocrit.

Treatment
- High-dose estrogen-progestogen combination therapy (oral contraceptives) to control endometrial growth and reestablish a normal cyclic pattern of menstruation (usually given four times daily for 5 to 7 days even though bleeding usually stops in 12 to 24 hours; drug choice and dosage determined by patient's age and cause of bleeding); maintenance therapy with lower dose combination oral contraceptives
- Progestogen therapy — alternative in many women, especially those susceptible to adverse effects of estrogen such as thrombophlebitis
- I.V. estrogen followed by progesterone or combination oral contraceptives if the patient is young (more likely to be anovulatory) and severely anemic (if oral drug therapy is ineffective)
- Iron replacement or transfusions of packed cells or whole blood, as indicated, due to anemia caused by recurrent bleeding.

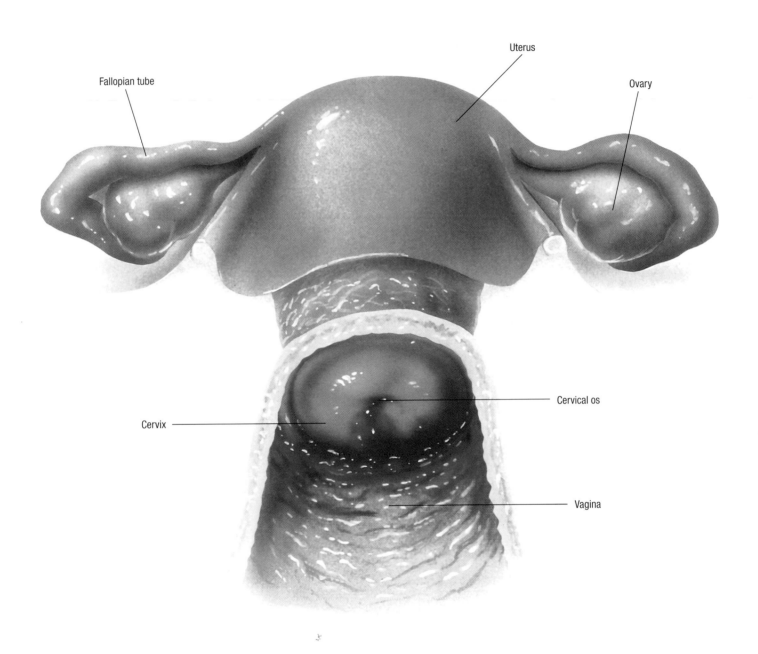

Fallopian tube

Uterus

Ovary

Cervical os

Cervix

Vagina

Amenorrhea

Amenorrhea is the *abnormal* absence of menstruation. Absence of menstruation is normal before puberty, after menopause, or during pregnancy and lactation; it's pathologic at any other time. Primary amenorrhea is the absence of menarche in an adolescent (after age 16 years). Secondary amenorrhea is the absence of menstruation for at least 3 months after the normal onset of menarche. Primary amenorrhea occurs in 0.3% of women; secondary amenorrhea, in 1% to 3% of women. Prognosis is variable, depending on the specific cause. Surgical correction of outflow tract obstruction is usually curative.

Causes

- Anovulation due to deficient secretion of:
- estrogen
- gonadotropins
- luteinizing hormone
- follicle-stimulating hormone (FSH)
- Lack of ovarian response to gonadotropins
- Constant presence of progesterone or other endocrine abnormalities
- Endometrial adhesions (Asherman syndrome)
- Ovarian, adrenal, or pituitary tumor
- Emotional disorders — common in patients with depression or anorexia nervosa:
- mild emotional disturbances tend to distort the ovulatory cycle
- severe psychic trauma may abruptly change the bleeding pattern or completely suppress one or more full ovulatory cycles
- Malnutrition or intense exercise — suppresses hormonal changes initiated by the hypothalamus.

Pathophysiology

The mechanism varies depending on the cause and whether the defect is structural, hormonal, or both. Women who have adequate estrogen levels but a progesterone deficiency don't ovulate and are thus infertile. In primary amenorrhea, the hypothalamic-pituitary-ovarian axis is dysfunctional. Because of anatomic defects of the central nervous system, the ovary doesn't receive the hormonal signals that normally initiate the development of secondary sex characteristics and the beginning of menstruation.

Secondary amenorrhea can result from any of several mechanisms, including:

- central — hypogonadotropic hypoestrogenic anovulation
- uterine — such as Asherman syndrome, in which severe scarring has replaced functional endometrium
- premature ovarian failure.

Signs and symptoms

- Absence of menstruation
- Vasomotor flushes
- Vaginal atrophy
- Hirsutism
- Acne (secondary amenorrhea).

Diagnostic tests

- X-ray to determine bone age (confirms primary amenorrhea)
- Sensitive pregnancy test
- Pituitary gonadotropin levels
- Thyroid panel
- Appropriate X-rays, laparoscopy, biopsy to identify ovarian, adrenal, or pituitary tumor.
    Tests to identify dominant or missing hormones:
- Microscopic examination of cervical mucus to detect "ferning" (an estrogen effect)
- Vaginal cytologic examination
- Endometrial biopsy
- Serum progesterone level
- Serum androgen levels
- Urinary 17-ketosteroid levels
- Plasma FSH level.

Treatment

- Appropriate hormone replacement to reestablish menstruation
- Treatment of the cause of amenorrhea not related to hormone deficiency — for example, surgery for amenorrhea due to a tumor
- Inducing ovulation — for example, with clomiphene citrate in women with intact pituitary gland and amenorrhea secondary to gonadotropin deficiency, polycystic ovarian disease, or excessive weight loss or gain
- FSH and human menopausal gonadotropins for women with pituitary disease
- Reassurance and emotional support (psychiatric counseling if amenorrhea results from emotional disturbances)
- Teaching the patient how to keep an accurate record of her menstrual cycles.

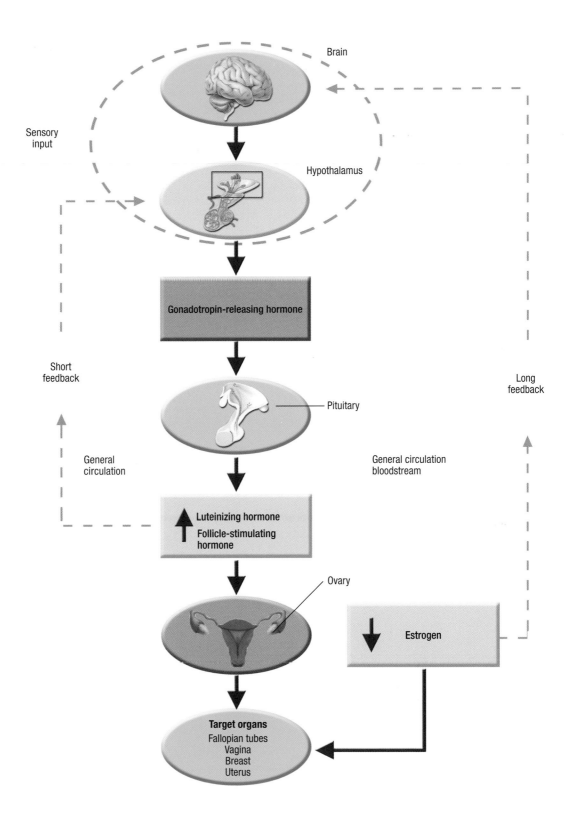

BENIGN BREAST CONDITIONS

Also incorrectly known as fibrocystic disease of the breast, this disorder of benign changes in breast tissue is usually bilateral.

 AGE ALERT
Fibrocystic change is the most common benign breast disorder, affecting an estimated 10% of women ages 21 and younger, 25% of women ages 22 and older, and 50% of postmenopausal women.

Although most lesions are benign, some may proliferate and show atypical cellular growth. Fibrocystic change by itself is not a precursor to breast cancer, but if atypical cells are present, the risk for breast carcinoma increases.

Causes
Exact cause unknown.
Proposed causes:
● Estrogen excess and progesterone deficiency during luteal phase of menstrual cycle
● Environmental toxins that inhibit cyclic guanosine monophosphate enzymes:
– methylxanthines — caffeine (coffee), theophylline (tea), theobromine (chocolate)
– tyramine — in cheese, wine, nuts
– tobacco.

Pathophysiology
Breast tissue appears to respond to hormonal stimulation, although the exact mechanism is unknown. Cysts may form with lobular or subareolar areas. Cysts are classified as microcysts (smaller than 1 mm) and macrocysts (3 mm or larger). In *ductal epithelial proliferation* (hyperplasia), the ducts below the areola and the nipple dilate, and the ductal epithelium may undergo metaplastic changes. Fibrotic areas may form as a result of inflammation caused by either the cysts or ductal hyperplasia.

Signs and symptoms
● Breast pain due to inflammation and nerve root stimulation (most common symptom), beginning 4 to 7 days into the luteal phase of the menstrual cycle and continuing until the onset of menstruation
● Pain in the upper outer quadrant of both breasts (common site)
● Palpable lumps that increase in size premenstrually and are freely moveable (about 50% of all menstruating women)
● Granular feeling of breasts on palpation
● Occasional greenish-brown to black nipple discharge that contains fat, proteins, ductal cells, and erythrocytes (ductal hyperplasia).

Diagnostic tests
● Ultrasonography to distinguish cystic (fluid-filled) from solid masses
● Tissue biopsy to distinguish benign from malignant changes
● Cytologic analysis of bloody aspirate to rule out malignancy.

Treatment
● Symptomatic to relieve pain, including:
– diet low in caffeine and fat and high in fruits and vegetables
– support bra
● Draining of painful cysts under local anesthesia
● Synthetic androgens (danazol) for severe pain (occasionally).

BENIGN BREAST CONDITIONS

Fibrocystic changes

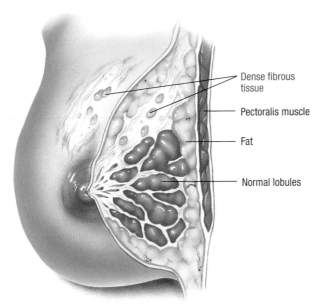

- Dense fibrous tissue
- Pectoralis muscle
- Fat
- Normal lobules

Breast cyst

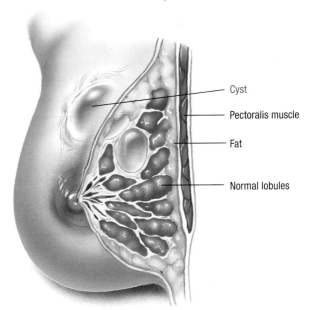

- Cyst
- Pectoralis muscle
- Fat
- Normal lobules

BENIGN BREAST TUMORS

Intraductal papilloma

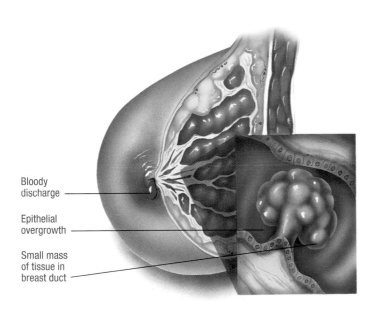

- Bloody discharge
- Epithelial overgrowth
- Small mass of tissue in breast duct

Fibroadenoma

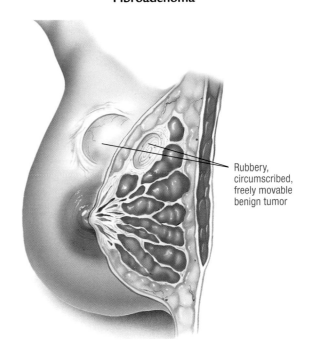

- Rubbery, circumscribed, freely movable benign tumor

BENIGN PROSTATIC HYPERPLASIA

In benign prostatic hyperplasia (BPH), also known as benign prostatic hypertrophy, the prostate gland enlarges enough to compress the urethra and cause overt urinary obstruction. Depending on the size of the enlarged prostate, the age and health of the patient, and the extent of obstruction, BPH is treated symptomatically or surgically.

 AGE ALERT
BPH is common, affecting up to 50% of men over age 50 and 75% of men over age 80.

Causes
- Age-associated changes in hormone activity
- Arteriosclerosis
- Inflammation
- Metabolic or nutritional disturbances.

Pathophysiology
Androgenic hormone production decreases with age, causing imbalance in androgen and estrogen levels and high levels of dihydrotestosterone, the main prostatic intracellular androgen. The shift in hormone balance induces the early, nonmalignant changes of BPH in periurethral glandular tissue. The growth of the fibroadenomatous nodules (masses of fibrous glandular tissue) progresses to compress the remaining normal gland (nodular hyperplasia). The hyperplastic tissue is mostly glandular, with some fibrous stroma and smooth muscle. As the prostate enlarges, it may extend into the bladder and obstruct urinary outflow by compressing or distorting the prostatic urethra. Progressive bladder distention may lead to formation of a pouch that retains urine when the rest of the bladder empties. This retained urine may lead to calculus formation or cystitis.

Signs and symptoms
Presenting signs and symptoms:
- Reduced urinary stream caliber and force
- Urinary hesitancy
- Feeling of incomplete voiding, interrupted stream.

As obstruction increases:
- Frequent urination with nocturia
- Sense of urgency
- Retention, dribbling, incontinence
- Possible hematuria.

Diagnostic tests
- Excretory urography
- Cystoscopy
- Blood urea nitrogen and serum creatinine levels
- Prostate-specific antigen (PSA)
- Urinalysis and urine cultures
- Cystourethroscopy if symptoms are severe — definitive diagnosis.

Treatment
Conservative therapy includes:
- prostate massages
- sitz baths
- fluid restriction for bladder distention
- antimicrobials for infection
- regular ejaculation
- alpha-adrenergic blockers (terazosin, prazosin)
- medical management to reduce risk of urinary retention (finasteride)
- continuous drainage with a urinary catheter to alleviate urine retention (high-risk patients).

To relieve intolerable symptoms, surgical procedures may include:
- suprapubic (transvesical) resection
- transurethral resection
- retropubic (extravesical) resection allowing direct visualization; usually maintains potency and continence
- suprapubic cystostomy under local anesthetic if indwelling urinary catheter can't be passed transurethrally
- laser excision to relieve prostatic enlargement
- nerve-sparing surgery to reduce common complications
- indwelling urinary catheter for urine retention
- balloon dilation of urethra and prostatic stents to maintain urethral patency.

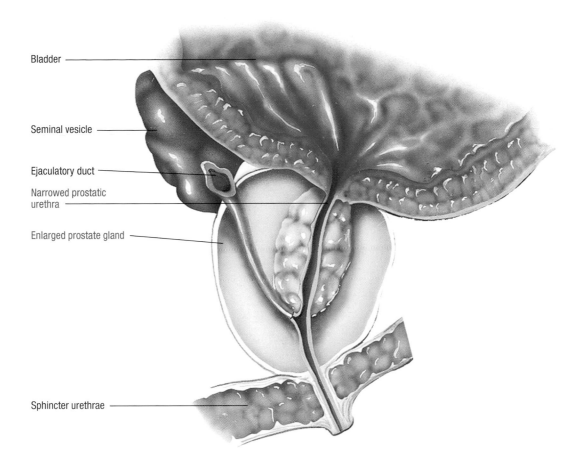

Bladder

Seminal vesicle

Ejaculatory duct

Narrowed prostatic urethra

Enlarged prostate gland

Sphincter urethrae

CLINICAL TIP

PALPATING THE PROSTATE GLAND

This useful tool in detecting early signs of prostatic enlargement includes the following steps:

- Have patient stand and lean over the exam table; if he can't do this, have him lie on his left side with his right knee and hip flexed or with both knees drawn to his chest
- Inspect the skin of the perineal, anal, and posterior scrotal walls
- Insert lubricated gloved finger into the rectum
- Palpate the prostate through the anterior rectal wall
- The gland should feel smooth and rubbery, about the size of a walnut.

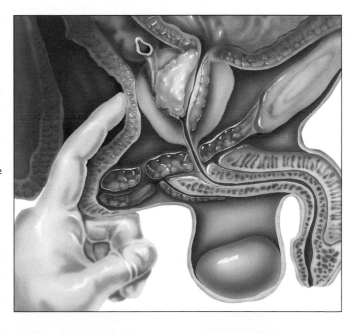

BREAST CANCER

Breast cancer is the most common cancer affecting women and is the number two killer (after lung cancer) of women ages 35 to 54. It rarely occurs in men. The 5-year survival rate for localized breast cancer has improved from 72% in the 1940s to 97% today because of earlier diagnosis and the variety of treatments now available. Lymph node involvement is the most valuable prognostic predictor. With adjuvant therapy, 70% to 75% of women with negative nodes will survive 10 years or more, compared with 20% to 25% of women with positive nodes.

AGE ALERT
Breast cancer may develop any time after puberty but is most common after age 50 (about 20% of cases occur in women under age 30 and about 70% in women over age 50).

Causes

High-risk factors:
- Family history of breast cancer, particularly first-degree relatives (mother, sister, and/or maternal aunt)
- Positive tests for genetic mutations (BRCA 1 and BRCA 2)
- Long menstrual cycles
- Early menarche, late menopause
- Nulliparous or first pregnancy after age 30
- History of unilateral breast cancer or ovarian cancer
- Exposure to low-level radiation.
  Lower risk factors:
- Pregnancy before age 20, history of multiple pregnancies
- Native American or Asian ancestry.

Pathophysiology

Breast cancer occurs more commonly in the left breast than the right and more commonly in the outer upper quadrant. Slow-growing breast cancer may take up to 8 years to become palpable at 3/8" (1 cm) in size. It spreads by way of the lymphatic system and the bloodstream, through the right side of the heart to the lungs, and eventually to the other breast, the chest wall, liver, bone, and brain.

The estimated growth rate of breast cancer is referred to as "doubling time," or the time it takes the malignant cells to double in number. Survival time for breast cancer is based on tumor size and spread; the number of involved nodes is the single most important factor in predicting survival time.

Breast cancer is classified by histologic appearance and location of the lesion, as follows:
- adenocarcinoma — arising from the epithelium
- intraductal — within the ducts (includes Paget's disease)
- infiltrating — in parenchymal tissue of the breast
- inflammatory (rare) — overlying skin becomes edematous, inflamed, and indurated; reflects rapid tumor growth
- lobular carcinoma in situ — involves glandular lobes
- medullary or circumscribed — large tumor, rapid growth rate.

The descriptive terms should be coupled with a staging or nodal status classification system. The most commonly used staging system is the TNM (tumor size, nodal involvement, metastatic progress).

Signs and symptoms
- Lump or mass in the breast, breast pain
- Change in symmetry or size of the breast
- Change in skin — thickening, scaly skin around the nipple, dimpling, edema (peau d'orange), or ulceration
- Change in skin temperature (a warm, hot, or pink area)
- Unusual drainage or discharge
- Change in nipple (itching, burning, erosion, or retraction)
- Pathologic bone fractures, hypercalcemia
- Edema of the arm.

CLINICAL TIP
A spontaneous discharge of any kind in a non-breastfeeding, nonlactating woman warrants investigation; suspect any greenish-black, white, creamy, serous, or bloody discharge.

Diagnostic tests
- Mammography
- Needle biopsy, surgical biopsy
- Ultrasonography to distinguish a fluid-filled cyst from a tumor; can be used instead of an invasive surgical biopsy
- Bone scan, computed tomography scan, alkaline phosphatase levels, liver function studies, liver biopsy to detect distant metastases
- Estrogen and progesterone receptor assay of tumor tissue.

Treatment

Surgical:
- Lumpectomy — may be done as outpatient procedure if tumor is small with no evidence of axillary node involvement; in many cases, radiation therapy is combined with this surgery
- Lumpectomy and dissection of axillary lymph nodes — leaves breast intact
- Simple mastectomy — removes breast but not lymph nodes or pectoral muscles
- Modified radical mastectomy — removes breast and axillary lymph nodes
- Radical mastectomy (now seldom used) — removes breast, axillary lymph nodes, and pectoralis major and minor muscles.
  Other treatments:
- Reconstructive surgery if no advanced disease
- Chemotherapy — adjuvant or primary therapy:
- cyclophosphamide, fluorouracil, methotrexate, doxorubicin, vincristine, paclitaxel, prednisone
- Tamoxifen (estrogen antagonist) — adjuvant treatment of choice for postmenopausal patients with positive estrogen receptor status; has also been found to reduce risk of breast cancer in women at high risk
- Peripheral stem cell therapy for advanced disease
- Primary radiation therapy before or after tumor removal:
- effective for small tumors in early stages with no evidence of distant metastasis
- helps make inflammatory breast tumors more surgically manageable
- also used to prevent or treat local recurrence
- Estrogen, progesterone, androgen, or antiandrogen aminoglutethimide therapy.

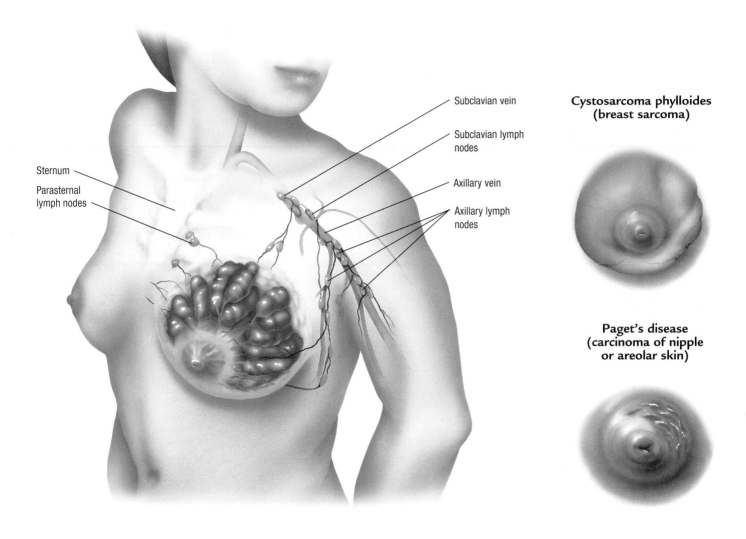

Sternum

Parasternal lymph nodes

Subclavian vein

Subclavian lymph nodes

Axillary vein

Axillary lymph nodes

Cystosarcoma phylloides (breast sarcoma)

Paget's disease (carcinoma of nipple or areolar skin)

Cellular progression to breast cancer

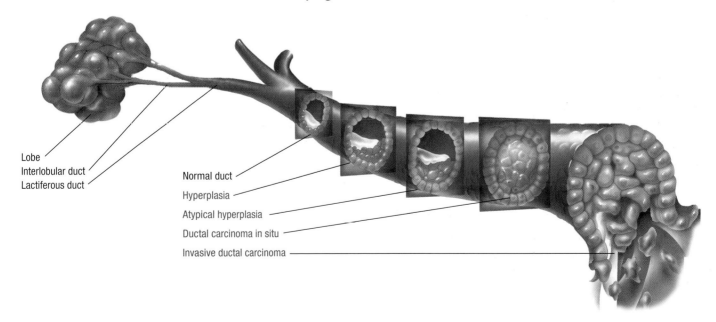

Lobe

Interlobular duct

Lactiferous duct

Normal duct

Hyperplasia

Atypical hyperplasia

Ductal carcinoma in situ

Invasive ductal carcinoma

CERVICAL CANCER

The third most common cancer of the female reproductive system, cervical cancer is classified as either microinvasive or invasive.

Causes

Cause unknown.
Predisposing factors include:
• frequent intercourse at a young age (under age 16)
• multiple sexual partners
• multiple pregnancies
• sexually transmitted diseases (particularly genital human papilloma virus)
• smoking.

Pathophysiology

Preinvasive disease ranges from mild cervical dysplasia, in which the lower third of the epithelium contains abnormal cells, to carcinoma in situ, in which the full thickness of epithelium contains abnormally proliferating cells. Other names for carcinoma in situ include cervical intraepithelial neoplasia and squamous intraepithelial lesion. Preinvasive disease detected early and properly treated is curable in 75% to 90% of cases. If preinvasive disease remains untreated (and depending on the form in which it appears), it may progress to invasive cervical cancer.

In invasive carcinoma, cancer cells penetrate the basement membrane and can spread directly to contiguous pelvic structures or disseminate to distant sites by lymphatic routes.

In almost all cases of cervical cancer (95%), the histologic type is squamous cell carcinoma, which varies from well-differentiated cells to highly anaplastic spindle cells. Only 5% are adenocarcinomas.

 AGE ALERT
Usually, invasive carcinoma occurs in women between ages 30 and 50; rarely, in those under age 20.

Signs and symptoms

Preinvasive disease:
• Often produces no symptoms or other clinically apparent changes.
  Early invasive cervical cancer:
• Abnormal vaginal bleeding
• Persistent vaginal discharge
• Postcoital pain and bleeding.
  Advanced disease:
• Pelvic pain
• Vaginal leakage of urine and feces from a fistula
• Anorexia, weight loss, and anemia.

Diagnostic tests

• Cytologic examination (Papanicolaou smear)
• Colposcopy
• Staining with Lugol's or Schiller's solution (iodine solutions) to identify areas for biopsy when the smear shows abnormal cells but there's no obvious lesion
• Lymphangiography, cystography, scans to detect metastasis.

Treatment

Preinvasive lesions:
• Loop electrosurgical excision procedure (LEEP)
• Cryosurgery
• Laser destruction
• Conization (and frequent Pap smear follow-up)
• Hysterectomy.
  Invasive carcinoma:
• Radical hysterectomy
• Radiation therapy (internal, external, or both)
• Combination of the above two procedures.

Carcinoma in situ   **Squamous cell carcinoma**

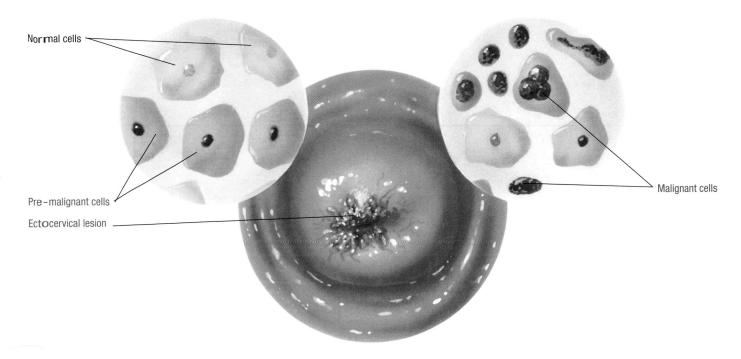

Normal cells

Pre-malignant cells

Ectocervical lesion

Malignant cells

CLINICAL TIP

DIAGNOSIS BY PAP SMEAR

Normal
- Large, surface type squamous cells
- Small, pyknotic nuclei

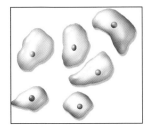

Invasive carcinoma
- Marked pleomorphism
- Irregular nuclei
- Clumped chromatin
- Prominent nucleoli

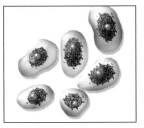

Mild dysplasia
- Mild increase in nuclear:cytoplasmic ratio
- Hyperchromasia
- Abnormal chromatin pattern

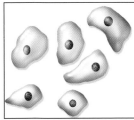

Severe dysplasia, carcinoma in situ
- Basal type cells
- Very high nuclear:cytoplasmic ratio
- Marked hyperchromasia
- Abnormal chromatin

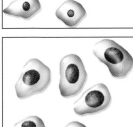

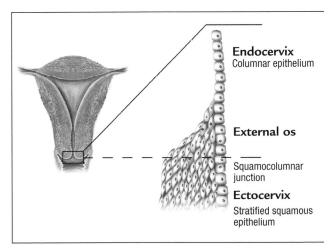

Endocervix
Columnar epithelium

External os

Squamocolumnar junction

Ectocervix
Stratified squamous epithelium

CRYPTORCHIDISM

Cryptorchidism is a congenital disorder in which one or both testes fail to descend into the scrotum, remaining in the abdomen or inguinal canal or at the external ring. Although this condition may be bilateral, it more commonly affects the right testis. True undescended testes remain along the path of normal descent; ectopic testis deviate from that path.

AGE ALERT
Cryptorchidism occurs in 30% of premature male newborns but in only 3% of those born at term. In about 80% of affected infants, the testes descend spontaneously during the first year; in the rest, the testes may descend later. If indicated, surgical therapy is successful in up to 95% of the cases if the infant is treated early enough.

Causes
Primary cause unknown.
Possible causes of cryptorchidism include:
- testosterone deficiency resulting in a defect in the hypothalamic-pituitary-gonadal axis, causing failure of gonadal differentiation and gonadal descent
- structural factors impeding gonadal descent, such as ectopic testis or short spermatic cord
- genetic predisposition in a small number of cases; greater incidence of cryptorchidism in infants with neural tube defects
- in premature newborns — early gestational age; normal descent of testes into the scrotum is in seventh month of gestation.

Pathophysiology
A prevalent but still unsubstantiated theory links undescended testes to the development of the gubernaculum, a fibromuscular band that connects the testes to the scrotal floor and probably helps pull the testes into the scrotum by shortening as the fetus grows. Normally in the male fetus, testosterone stimulates the formation of the gubernaculum. Thus, cryptorchidism may result from inadequate testosterone levels or a defect in the testes or the gubernaculum. Because the undescended testis is maintained at a higher temperature, spermatogenesis is impaired, leading to reduced fertility.

Signs and symptoms
Unilateral cryptorchidism:
- Testis on affected side not palpable in scrotum; scrotum underdeveloped
- Enlarged scrotum on unaffected side due to compensatory hypertrophy (occasionally).
  Uncorrected bilateral cryptorchidism:
- Infertility after puberty despite normal testosterone levels.

Diagnostic tests
- Karyotype to establish genetic sex
- Serum gonadotropin – presence of circulating hormone confirms presence of testes.

Treatment

AGE ALERT
If the testes don't descend spontaneously by age 1, surgical correction is generally indicated. Surgery should be performed before age 2; by this time about 40% of undescended testes can no longer produce viable sperm.

- Orchiopexy to secure the testes in the scrotum and prevent sterility, excessive trauma from abnormal positioning, and harmful psychological effects (usually before age 4 years; optimum age, 1 to 2 years)
- Human chorionic gonadotropin I.M. to stimulate descent (rarely); ineffective for testes located in the abdomen.

VARIETIES OF CRYPTORCHIDISM

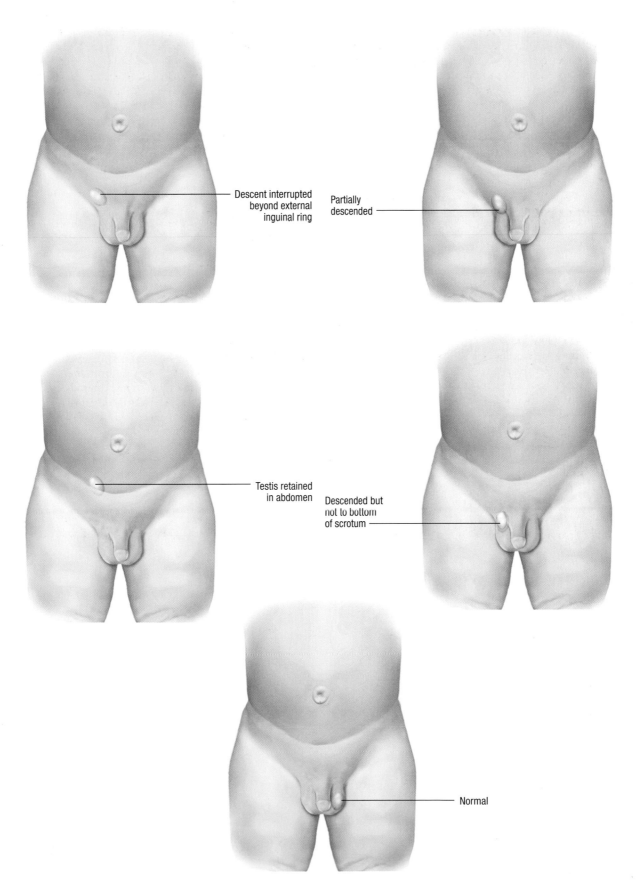

Descent interrupted beyond external inguinal ring

Partially descended

Testis retained in abdomen

Descended but not to bottom of scrotum

Normal

ENDOMETRIAL CANCER

Uterine cancer (cancer of the endometrium) is the most common gynecologic cancer.

 AGE ALERT
Uterine cancer usually affects postmenopausal women between ages 50 and 60; it's uncommon between ages 30 and 40 and extremely rare before age 30. Most premenopausal women who develop uterine cancer have a history of anovulatory menstrual cycles or other hormonal imbalance.

Causes

Primary cause unknown.
Predisposing factors:
- Anovulation, abnormal uterine bleeding
- History of atypical endometrial hyperplasia
- Unopposed estrogen stimulation
- Nulliparity
- Polycystic ovarian syndrome
- Familial tendency
- Obesity, hypertension, diabetes.

Pathophysiology

In most cases, uterine cancer is an adenocarcinoma that metastasizes late, usually from the endometrium to the cervix, ovaries, fallopian tubes, and other peritoneal structures. It may spread to distant organs, such as the lungs and the brain, through the blood or the lymphatic system. Lymph node involvement can also occur. Less common are adenoacanthoma, endometrial stromal sarcoma, lymphosarcoma, mixed mesodermal tumors (including carcinosarcoma), and leiomyosarcoma.

Signs and symptoms

- Uterine enlargement
- Persistent and unusual premenopausal bleeding
- Any postmenopausal bleeding
- Other signs or symptoms, such as pain and weight loss, don't appear until the cancer is well advanced.

Diagnostic tests

- Endometrial, cervical, and endocervical biopsies.
  Positive diagnosis requires baseline data and staging:
- Chest X-ray or computed tomography scan
- Complete blood studies
- Surgical staging — biopsy of organs removed at surgical treatment, selected lymph node sampling, peritoneal washings.

Treatment

- Surgery — generally total abdominal hysterectomy, bilateral salpingo-oophorectomy, or possibly omentectomy with or without pelvic or para-aortic lymphadenectomy
- Radiation therapy — intracavitary or external (or both):
- if tumor is poorly differentiated or histology is unfavorable
- if tumor has deeply invaded uterus or spread to extrauterine sites
- may be curative in some patients
- Hormonal therapy:
- synthetic progesterones, such as medroxyprogesterone or megestrol, for recurrent disease
- tamoxifen as a second-line treatment; 20% to 40% response rate
- Chemotherapy — usually tried when other treatments have failed:
- varying combinations of cisplatin, doxorubicin, etoposide, dactinomycin
- no evidence that they are curative.

PROGRESSION OF ENDOMETRIAL CANCER

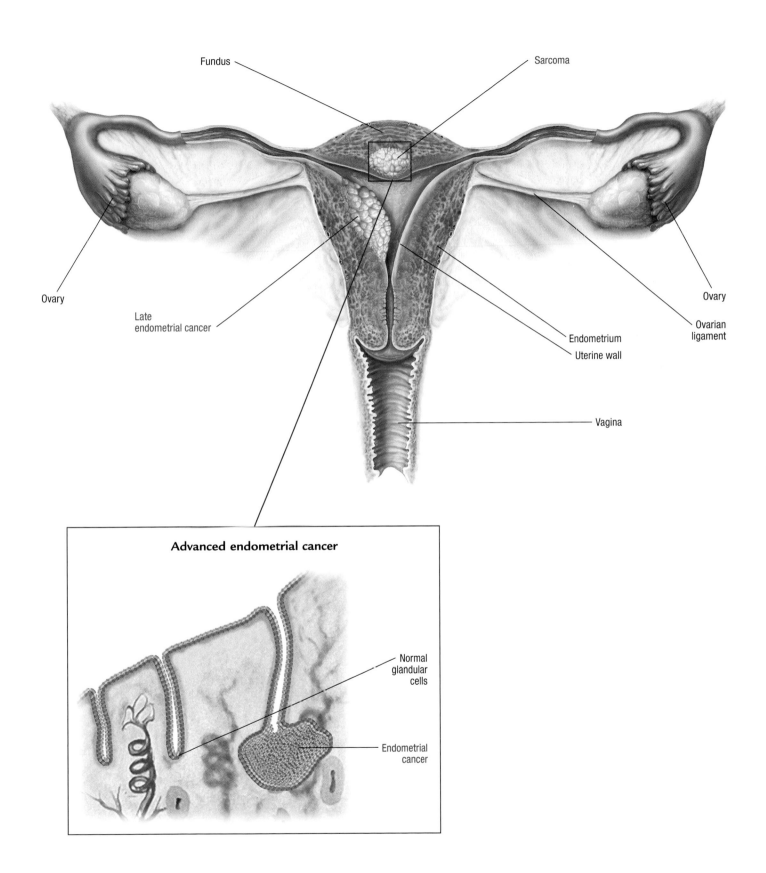

Fundus

Sarcoma

Ovary

Late
endometrial cancer

Ovary

Ovarian
ligament

Endometrium

Uterine wall

Vagina

Advanced endometrial cancer

Normal
glandular
cells

Endometrial
cancer

ENDOMETRIOSIS

Endometriosis is the presence of endometrial tissue outside the lining of the uterine cavity. Ectopic tissue is generally confined to the pelvic area, usually around the ovaries, uterovesical peritoneum, uterosacral ligaments, and cul de sac, but it can appear anywhere in the body.

Active endometriosis may occur at any age, including adolescence. As many as 50% of infertile women may have endometriosis, although the true incidence in both fertile and infertile women remains unknown.

Severe symptoms of endometriosis may have an abrupt onset or may develop over many years. Of women with endometriosis, 30% to 40% become infertile. Endometriosis usually manifests during the menstrual years; after menopause, it tends to subside.

Causes

Primary cause unknown.

Suggested causes (one or more may be true in different women):
- Retrograde menstruation with implantation at ectopic sites; may not be causative alone; occurs in women with no clinical evidence of endometriosis
- Genetic predisposition and depressed immune system
- Coelomic metaplasia (metaplasia of mesothelial cells to the endometrial epithelium caused by repeated inflammation)
- Lymphatic or hematogenous spread to extraperitoneal sites.

Pathophysiology

The ectopic endometrial tissue responds to normal stimulation in the same way as the endometrium, but less predictably. The endometrial cells respond to estrogen and progesterone with proliferation and secretion. During menstruation, the ectopic tissue bleeds, which causes inflammation of the surrounding tissues. This inflammation causes fibrosis, leading to adhesions that produce pain and infertility.

Signs and symptoms

- Classic symptoms — dysmenorrhea, abnormal uterine bleeding, infertility
- Pain — begins 5 to 7 days before menses, peaks, and lasts for 2 to 3 days; severity does not reflect extent of disease

- Depending on site of ectopic tissue:
- ovaries and oviducts: infertility, profuse menses
- ovaries or cul de sac: deep-thrust dyspareunia
- bladder: suprapubic pain, dysuria, hematuria
- large bowel, appendix: abdominal cramps, pain on defecation, constipation; bloody stools
- cervix, vagina, perineum: bleeding from endometrial deposits, painful intercourse.

Diagnostic tests

- Laparoscopy or laparotomy — the only definitive diagnosis.
  Some clinicians recommend:
- empiric trial of gonadotropin-releasing hormone (Gn-RH) agonist therapy to confirm or refute clinical impression before resorting to laparoscopy
- biopsy at the time of laparoscopy; although in some instances, visual inspection confirms diagnosis.

Treatment

Conservative therapy for young women who want to have children:
- Androgens such as danazol
- Progestins and continuous combined oral contraceptives (pseudopregnancy regimen) to relieve symptoms by causing regression of endometrial tissue
- Gn-RH agonists to induce pseudomenopause (medical oophorectomy), causing remission of the disease (commonly used).
  To rule out cancer, when ovarian masses are present:
- Laparoscopic removal of endometrial implants.
  Treatment of last resort for women who don't want to bear children or with extensive disease:
- Total abdominal hysterectomy with or without bilateral salpingo-oophorectomy; success rates vary; unclear whether ovarian conservation is appropriate.

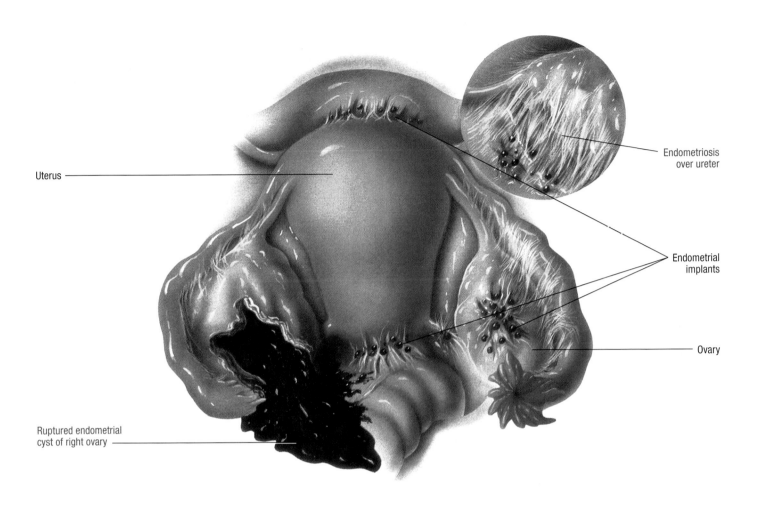

Uterus

Endometriosis over ureter

Endometrial implants

Ovary

Ruptured endometrial cyst of right ovary

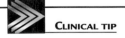

CLINICAL TIP

COMMON SITES OF ENDOMETRIOSIS

Ectopic endometrial tissue can implant almost anywhere in the pelvic peritoneum. It can even invade distant sites, such as the lungs.

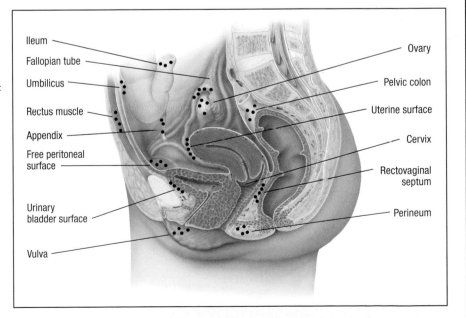

Ileum

Fallopian tube

Umbilicus

Rectus muscle

Appendix

Free peritoneal surface

Urinary bladder surface

Vulva

Ovary

Pelvic colon

Uterine surface

Cervix

Rectovaginal septum

Perineum

FIBROID DISEASE OF UTERUS

Uterine leiomyomas, also known as myomas, fibromyomas, or fibroids, are the most common benign tumors in women. These masses of smooth muscle and fibrous connective tissue are most common in the uterine corpus, although they may appear on the cervix or on the round or broad ligament. Uterine leiomyomas occur in 20% to 25% of women.

The tumors become malignant (leiomyosarcoma) in less than 0.1% of patients, which should serve to comfort women concerned with the possibility of a uterine malignancy in association with a fibroid.

 AGE ALERT
Leiomyomas typically arise after menarche and regress after menopause.

Causes
Primary cause unknown.
Implicated regulators of leiomyoma growth:
- Several growth factors, including epidermal growth factor
- Steroid hormones, including estrogen and progesterone.

Pathophysiology
Leiomyomas are classified according to location: in the uterine wall (intramural), protruding into the endometrial cavity (submucous), or protruding from the serosal surface of the uterus (subserous). Their size varies greatly. They are usually firm and surrounded by a pseudocapsule composed of compressed but otherwise normal uterine myometrium. The uterine cavity may become larger, increasing the endometrial surface area and causing increased uterine bleeding.

Signs and symptoms
- Mostly asymptomatic
- Abnormal bleeding, typically menorrhagia with disrupted submucosal vessels (most common symptom)
- Pain only with:
  - torsion of a pedunculated (stemmed) subserous tumor
  - degenerating leiomyomas (fibroid outgrows its blood supply and shrinks down in size; after myolysis, a laparoscopic procedure to shrink fibroids; after uterine artery embolization)
- Mild hydronephrosis (not believed to be an indication for treatment because renal failure rarely, if ever, results) resulting from pressure on adjacent viscera.

Diagnostic tests
- Complete blood count and differential
- Ultrasonography
- Magnetic resonance imaging.
- Hysterosalpingography, hysteroscopy
- Endometrial biopsy to rule out endometrial cancer in patients over age 35 with abnormal uterine bleeding.

Treatment
Nonsurgical methods:
- Gonadotropin-releasing hormone (Gn-RH) agonists (not a cure, as tumors increase in size after cessation of therapy)
- Nonsteroidal anti-inflammatory drugs.
  Surgical procedures:
- Abdominal, laparoscopic, or hysteroscopic myomectomy (removal of tumors in the uterine muscle)
- Myolysis (a laparoscopic procedure, performed on an outpatient basis); contraindicated in women who desire fertility
- Uterine artery embolization (a promising alternative to surgery, but no existing long-term studies confirm effect on fertility or establish long-term success)
- Hysterectomy; usually isn't the only available option
- Blood transfusions for severe anemia due to excessive bleeding.

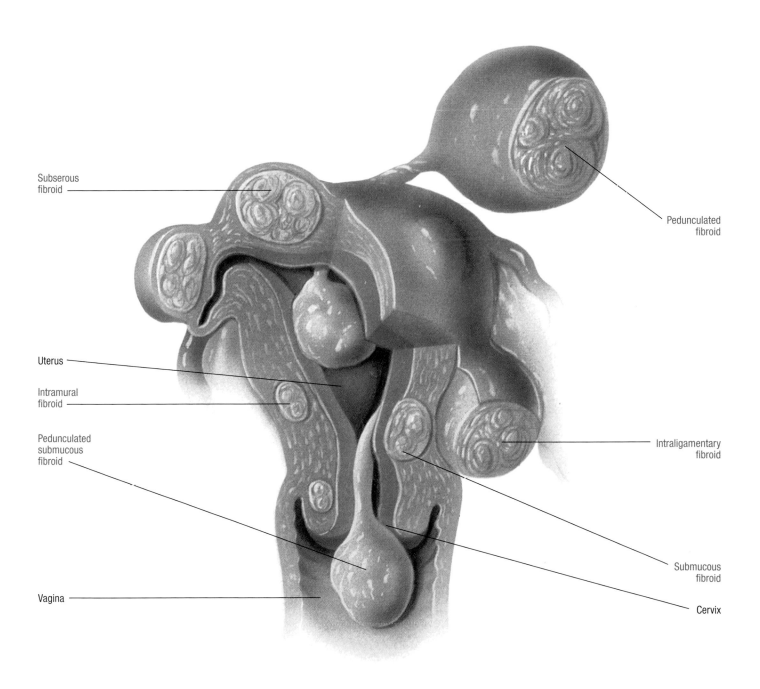

Subserous
fibroid

Pedunculated
fibroid

Uterus

Intramural
fibroid

Pedunculated
submucous
fibroid

Intraligamentary
fibroid

Submucous
fibroid

Vagina

Cervix

HYDROCELE

A hydrocele is a collection of fluid between the visceral and parietal layers of the tunica vaginalis of the testicle or along the spermatic cord. It is the most common cause of scrotal swelling.

Causes
- Congenital malformation (infants)
- Trauma to the testes or epididymis
- Infection of the testes or epididymis
- Testicular tumor.

Pathophysiology
Congenital hydrocele occurs when an opening between the scrotal sac and the peritoneal cavity allows peritoneal fluids to collect in the scrotum. The exact mechanism is unknown.

In adults, the fluid accumulation may be caused by infection, trauma, tumor, an imbalance between the secreting and absorptive capacities of scrotal tissue, or an obstruction of lymphatic or venous drainage in the spermatic cord. Consequent swelling obstructs blood flow to the testes.

Signs and symptoms
- Scrotal swelling and feeling of heaviness
- Inguinal hernia (commonly accompanies congenital hydrocele)
- Fluid collection, presenting as flaccid or tense mass
- Pain with acute epididymal infection or testicular torsion
- Scrotal tenderness due to severe swelling.

Diagnostic tests
- Transillumination to distinguish fluid-filled from solid mass
- Ultrasonography
- Tissue biopsy.

Treatment
- Inguinal hernia with bowel present in the sac: surgical repair
- Tense hydrocele that impedes blood circulation or causes pain: aspiration of fluid and injection of sclerosing drug
- Recurrent hydroceles: excision of tunica vaginalis
- Testicular tumor detected by ultrasound: suprainguinal excision.

 AGE ALERT
Congenital hydrocele commonly resolves spontaneously during the first year of life. Usually, no treatment is indicated.

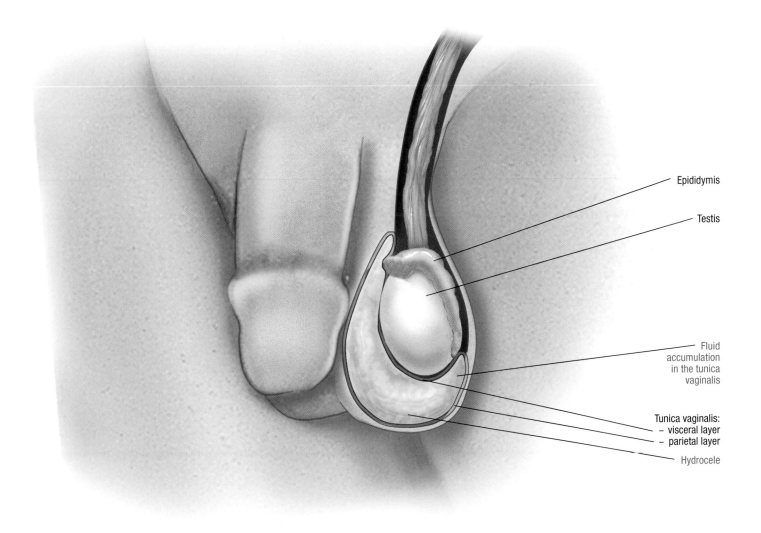

Epididymis

Testis

Fluid
accumulation
in the tunica
vaginalis

Tunica vaginalis:
– visceral layer
– parietal layer

Hydrocele

HYPOSPADIAS AND EPISPADIAS

Among the most common birth defects, congenital anomalies of the ureter, bladder, and urethra occur in about 5% of all births. The abnormality may be obvious at birth or may go unrecognized until symptoms appear.

Hypospadias is a congenital abnormality in which the opening of the urethra is misplaced to the perineal or scrotal region. The defect may be slight to extreme, and it occurs in 1 of 300 live male births. *Epispadias* occurs in 1 in 200,000 infant boys and 1 in 400,000 infant girls. In males, the urethral opening is on the dorsal aspect of the penis; in females, a cleft along the ventral urethral opening extends to the bladder neck.

Causes
- Congenital malformation
- Genetic factors.

Pathophysiology
In *hypospadias*, the urethral opening is on the ventral surface of the penis. A genetic factor is suspected in less severe cases. It is usually associated with a downward bowing of the penis (chordee), making normal urination with the penis elevated impossible. The ventral prepuce may be absent or defective, and the genitalia may be ambiguous. In the rare case of hypospadias in a female, the urethral opening is in the vagina, and vaginal discharge may be present.

Epispadias occurs more commonly in males than females and often accompanies bladder exstrophy, in which a portion of posterior bladder wall protrudes through a defect in the lower abdominal and anterior bladder wall. In mild cases, the orifice is on the dorsum of the glans; in severe cases, on the dorsum of the penis. Affected females have a bifid (cleft into two parts) clitoris and a short, wide urethra. Total urinary incontinence occurs when the urethral opening is proximal to the sphincter.

Signs and symptoms
- Displaced urethral opening
- Altered voiding patterns due to displaced opening of the urethra
- Chordee, or bending of the penis (in hypospadias)
- Ejaculatory dysfunction due to displaced penile opening.

Diagnostic tests
- None, if sexual identification is clear
- If sexual identification unclear, buccal smears or karotyping.

Treatment
- Mild, asymptomatic hypospadias: no treatment
- Severe hypospadias: surgery, preferably before child reaches school age
- Epispadias: multistage surgical repair, almost always necessary.

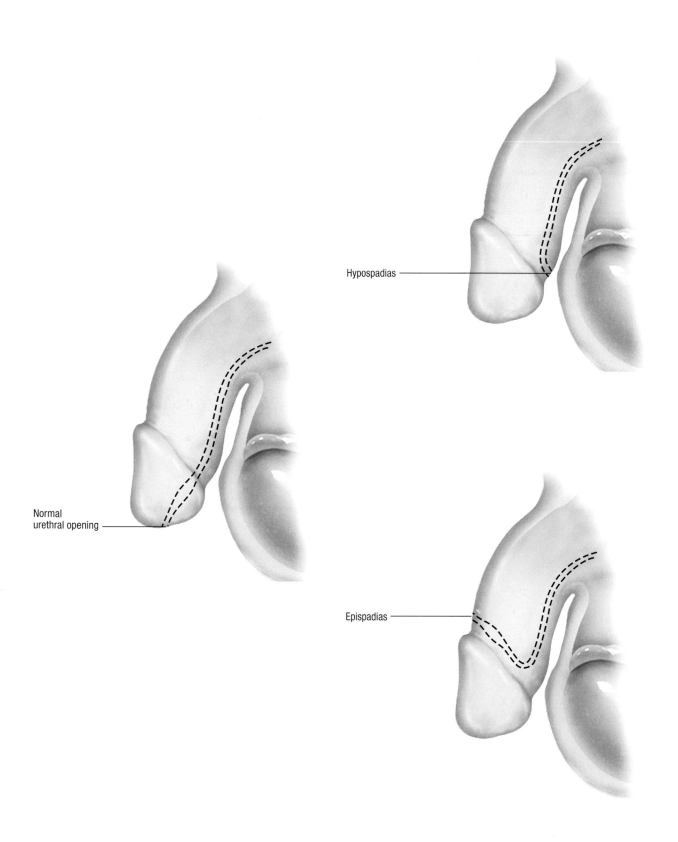

OVARIAN CANCER

Ovarian cancer is the leading gynecologic cause of death in the United States. In women with previously treated breast cancer, metastatic ovarian cancer is more common than cancer at any other site. It may be linked to mutations in the BRCA 1 or BRCA 2 gene.

 AGE ALERT
The greatest number of cases occur in the fifth decade of life. However, ovarian cancer can occur during childhood.

The prognosis varies with the histologic type and stage of the disease. It is generally poor because ovarian tumors produce few early signs and are usually advanced at diagnosis. With early detection and new treatments, about 45% of women with ovarian cancer survive for 5 years; however, the overall survival rate has not improved significantly.

Ovarian cancer occurs in three histologic types: primary epithelial, germ cell, and stromal.
- *Primary epithelial* tumors account for 90% of all ovarian cancers. They include serous cystoadenocarcinoma, mucinous cysto-adenocarcinoma, and endometrioid and mesonephric malignancies. Serous cystoadenocarcinoma is the most common type, accounting for half of all cases.
- *Germ cell* tumors include endodermal sinus malignancies, which secrete alpha-fetoprotein; embryonal carcinoma, a rare ovarian cancer that appears in children; immature teratomas; and dysgerminoma.
- *Stromal* (or sex cord) tumors include granulosa cell tumors, which produce estrogen; granulosa-theca cell tumors; and the rare arrhenoblastomas, which produce androgen and have virilizing effects.

Causes
Exact cause unknown.
Associated factors:
- Infertility, nulliparity
- Familial tendency
- Ovarian dysfunction, irregular menses
- Exposure to asbestos, talc, industrial pollutants.

Pathophysiology
Primary epithelial tumors arise in the Müllerian epithelium; germ cell tumors, in the ovum itself; and sex cord tumors, in the ovarian stroma. Ovarian tumors spread rapidly intraperitoneally by local extension or surface seeding and, occasionally, through the lymphatics and the bloodstream. Generally, extraperitoneal spread is through the diaphragm into the chest cavity, where the tumor may cause pleural effusions. Other metastasis is rare.

Signs and symptoms
- May grow to considerable size before overt symptoms appear
  Occasionally, in the early stages:
- Vague abdominal discomfort, distention
- Mild GI discomfort
- Urinary frequency, pelvic discomfort
- Constipation

- Weight loss.
  Later stages:
- Tumor rupture, torsion, or infection — pain, which, in young patients, may mimic appendicitis
- Granulosa cell tumors — effects of estrogen excess, such as bleeding between periods in premenopausal women
- Arrhenoblastomas (seen rarely) — virilizing effects.
  Advanced ovarian cancer:
- Ascites
- Postmenopausal bleeding and pain (rarely)
- Symptoms of metastatic tumors, most commonly pleural effusion.

Diagnostic tests
- Surgical exploration, including lymph node evaluation and tumor resection, and histologic studies.
  Preoperative evaluation:
- Papanicolaou smear
- Abdominal ultrasonography, computed tomography scan or, preferably, magnetic resonance imaging
- Chest X-ray
- Mammography
- Complete blood count, complete metabolic panel, liver function studies
- Tumor marker studies, such as CA-125 carcinoembryonic antigen and human chorionic gonadotropin.
  In girls or young women with a unilateral encapsulated tumor who wish to maintain fertility:
- Biopsies of the omentum and the uninvolved ovary
- Peritoneal washings for cytologic examination of pelvic fluid.

Treatment
- Varying combinations of surgery, chemotherapy and, in some cases, radiation.
  Conservative treatment for unilateral encapsulated tumor in girl or young woman:
- Resection of the involved ovary
- Careful follow-up, including periodic chest X-rays to rule out lung metastasis.
  More aggressive treatment:
- Total abdominal hysterectomy and bilateral salpingo-oophorectomy with tumor resection, omentectomy, possible appendectomy, lymphadenectomy, tissue biopsies, and peritoneal washings.
  If tumor has matted around other organs or involves organs that can't be resected:
- Surgically debulk tumor implants to less than 2 cm (or smaller) in greatest diameter.
  Chemotherapy:
- May be curative; extends survival time in most patients; largely palliative in advanced disease
- Current standard is combination paclitaxel/platinum-based chemotherapy.
  Radiation therapy:
- Generally not used in the United States because it is largely ineffective and associated with significant morbidity.

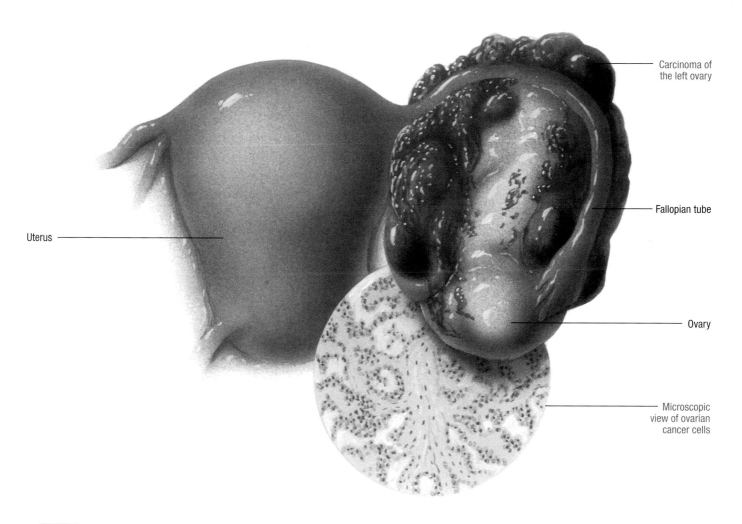

Carcinoma of the left ovary

Fallopian tube

Uterus

Ovary

Microscopic view of ovarian cancer cells

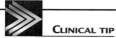

CLINICAL TIP

LIKELY METASTATIC SITES FOR OVARIAN CANCER

Ovarian cancer can metastasize to almost any site. Illustrated are the most common.

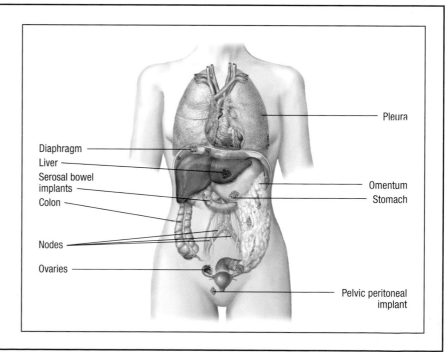

Pleura

Diaphragm

Liver

Serosal bowel implants

Colon

Omentum

Stomach

Nodes

Ovaries

Pelvic peritoneal implant

OVARIAN CYSTS

Ovarian cysts are usually benign sacs that contain fluid or semisolid material. Although these cysts are usually small and produce no symptoms, they may require thorough investigation as possible sites of malignant change. Cysts may be single or multiple (polycystic ovarian disease). Most ovarian cysts are physiologic, or functional; that is, they arise during the normal ovulatory process. Physiologic ovarian cysts include *follicular* cysts, *theca-lutein* cysts, which are commonly bilateral and filled with clear, straw-colored liquid, and *corpus luteum* cysts. *Granulosa-lutein* cysts, which occur within the corpus luteum, manifest as non-neoplastic enlargements of the ovaries. They may appear early and may reach 2 to 2-1/2" [5 to 6 cm] in diameter; however, they usually shrink during the third trimester (rarely needing surgery). Ovarian cysts can develop any time between puberty and menopause, including during pregnancy. The prognosis for benign ovarian cysts is excellent. The presence of a functional ovarian cyst does not increase the risk for malignancy.

Causes
- Granulosa-lutein cysts: excessive accumulation of blood during hemorrhagic phase of menstrual cycle
- Theca-lutein cysts:
- hydatidiform mole, choriocarcinoma
- hormone therapy (human chorionic gonadotropin [HCG] or clomiphene citrate).

Pathophysiology
Follicular cysts are generally very small and arise from follicles that either haven't ruptured or have ruptured and resealed before their fluid is reabsorbed. *Luteal cysts* develop if a mature corpus luteum persists abnormally and continues to secrete progesterone. They consist of blood or fluid that accumulates in the cavity of the corpus luteum and are typically more symptomatic than follicular cysts. When such cysts persist into menopause, they secrete excessive amounts of estrogen in response to the hypersecretion of follicle-stimulating hormone and luteinizing hormone that normally occurs during menopause.

Dermoid cysts are tumors of developmental origin that consist of a fibrous wall lined with stratified epithelium and may contain hair follicles, sweat glands, sebaceous glands, nerve elements, and teeth.

Signs and symptoms
- Large or multiple cysts:
- mild pelvic discomfort, low back pain, dyspareunia
- abnormal uterine bleeding

- Ovarian cysts with torsion: acute abdominal pain similar to that of appendicitis
- Granulosa-lutein cysts:
- in pregnancy: unilateral pelvic discomfort
- in nonpregnant women: delayed menses, followed by prolonged or irregular bleeding.

Diagnostic tests
- Ultrasonography
- Laparoscopy
- Surgery (often during surgery for another condition).

Treatment
- If cyst disappears spontaneously within one to two menstrual cycles — no treatment
- Persisting cyst indicates excision to rule out malignancy
- Functional cysts that appear during pregnancy — analgesics
- Theca-lutein cysts:
- elimination of hydatidiform mole
- destruction of choriocarcinoma
- discontinuation of HCG or clomiphene therapy
- Persistent or suspicious ovarian cyst:
- laparoscopy or exploratory laparotomy with possible ovarian cystectomy or oophorectomy
- if necessary during pregnancy, optimal time is second trimester
- Ruptured corpus luteum cyst:
- culdocentesis to drain intraperitoneal fluid
- surgery for ongoing hemorrhage.

CLINICAL TIP
Polycystic ovarian syndrome is a metabolic disorder characterized by multiple ovarian cysts. About 22% of the women in the United States have the disorder, and about 50% to 80% of these women are obese. Among those who seek treatment for infertility, more than 75% have some degree of polycystic ovarian syndrome, usually manifested by anovulation alone.

A general feature of all anovulation syndromes is a lack of pulsatile release of gonadotropin-releasing hormone. Initial ovarian follicle development is normal. Many small follicles begin to accumulate because there's no selection of a dominant follicle. These follicles may respond abnormally to the hormonal stimulation, causing an abnormal pattern of estrogen secretion during the menstrual cycle.

COMMON OVARIAN CYSTS

Follicular cyst

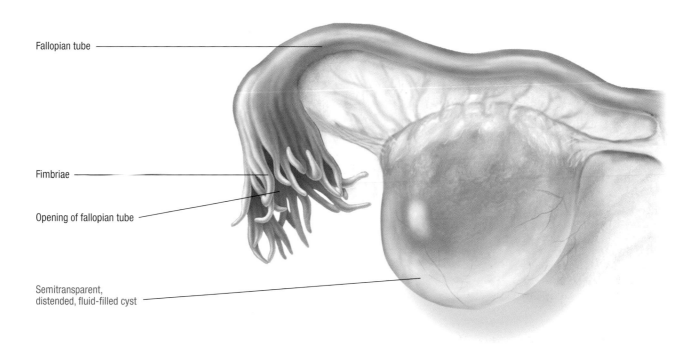

Fallopian tube

Fimbriae

Opening of fallopian tube

Semitransparent,
distended, fluid-filled cyst

Dermoid cyst

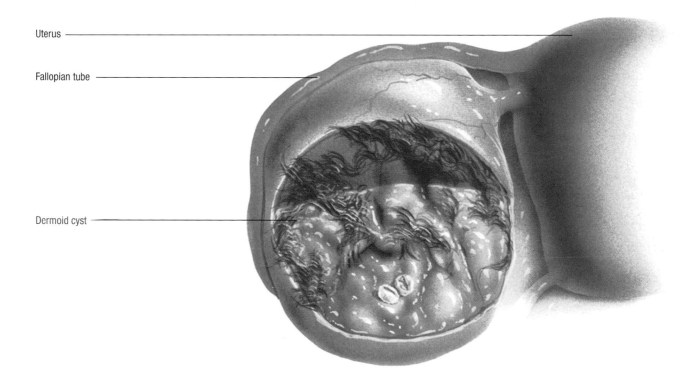

Uterus

Fallopian tube

Dermoid cyst

Pelvic inflammatory disease

Pelvic inflammatory disease (PID) is any acute, subacute, recurrent, or chronic infection of the oviducts and ovaries, with adjacent tissue involvement. It includes inflammation of the fallopian tubes (salpingitis) and ovaries (oophoritis), which can extend to the connective tissue lying between the broad ligaments (parametritis). Early diagnosis and treatment prevent damage to the reproductive system. Untreated PID may cause infertility and may lead to potentially fatal septicemia and shock. PID may also lead to complications that include chronic pelvic pain and formation of scar tissue (adhesions).

Causes

- Infection with aerobic or anaerobic organisms, such as:
- *Neisseria gonorrhoeae* and *Chlamydia trachomatis* (most common)
- staphylococci, streptococci, diphtheroids, *Pseudomonas, Escherichia coli.*
   Predisposing conditions:
- Conization or cauterization of the cervix
- Insertion of an intrauterine device
- Use of a biopsy curette or an irrigation catheter
- Tubal insufflation
- Abortion, pelvic surgery, infection during or after pregnancy.

Pathophysiology

Normally, cervical secretions have a protective and defensive function. Conditions or procedures that alter or destroy cervical mucus impair this bacteriostatic mechanism and allow bacteria present in the cervix or vagina to ascend into the uterine cavity. Uterine infection can also follow the transfer of contaminated cervical mucus into the endometrial cavity by instrumentation. Bacteria may also enter the uterine cavity through the bloodstream or from drainage from a chronically infected fallopian tube, a pelvic abscess, a ruptured appendix, diverticulitis of the sigmoid colon, or other infectious focus.

Uterine infection can result from contamination by one or several common pathogens or may follow the multiplication of normally nonpathogenic bacteria in an altered endometrial environment. Bacterial multiplication is most common during parturition because the endometrium is atrophic, quiescent, and not stimulated by estrogen.

Signs and symptoms

- Profuse, purulent vaginal discharge
- Low-grade fever, malaise
- Lower abdominal pain
- Severe pain on movement of cervix or palpation of adnexa.

Diagnostic tests

- Gram stain and culture of secretions from the endocervix, cul-de-sac, urethra, rectum
- Ultrasonography.

 CLINICAL TIP
According to the Centers for Disease Control and Prevention, the three minimum criteria for clinical diagnosis of PID are:
- **lower abdominal tenderness**
- **bilateral adnexal tenderness**
- **cervical motion tenderness.**

Treatment

- Antibiotic therapy beginning immediately after culture specimens are obtained and reevaluated as soon as laboratory results are available (usually after 24 to 48 hours). Infection may become chronic if treated inadequately. PID therapy regimens should provide broad-spectrum coverage of likely etiologic pathogens: *C. trachomatis, N. gonorrhoeae,* anaerobes, gram-negative rods, and streptococci
- Adequate drainage if pelvic abscess forms
- Ruptured abscess (life-threatening complication):
- total abdominal hysterectomy with bilateral salpingo-oophorectomy
- laparoscopic drainage with preservation of the ovaries and uterus appears to hold promise.

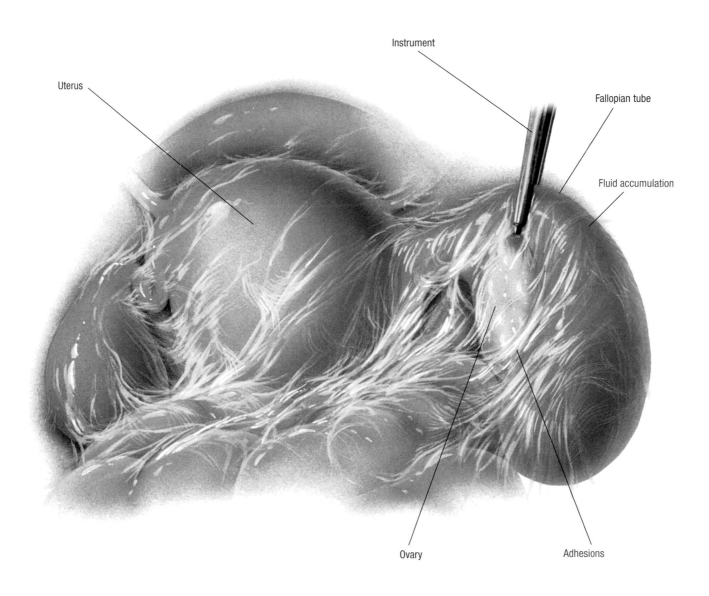

Instrument

Uterus

Fallopian tube

Fluid accumulation

Ovary

Adhesions

PROSTATE CANCER

Prostate cancer is the most common cancer in men over age 50. Adenocarcinoma is its most common form; sarcoma occurs only rarely. Most prostatic carcinomas originate in the posterior prostate gland; the rest originate near the urethra. Malignant prostatic tumors seldom result from the benign hyperplastic enlargement that commonly develops around the prostatic urethra in elderly men. Prostatic cancer seldom produces symptoms until it is advanced.

Causes

Exact cause unknown.
> *Implicated contributing factors:*
- Familial or ethnic predisposition
- Exposure to environmental toxins (radiation, air pollution: arsenic, benzene, hydrocarbons, polyvinyl chlorides)
- Sexually transmitted diseases
- Endogenous hormonal influence
- Diet containing fat from animal products.

Pathophysiology

Although androgens regulate prostate growth and function and may also speed tumor growth, no definite link between increased androgen levels and prostatic cancer has been found.

Incidence of prostate cancer among African-Americans is the highest in the world. Incidence is lowest in Asians.

 AGE ALERT
Incidence of prostate cancer increases with age more rapidly than that of any other cancer.

Signs and symptoms

- None in early stages.
> *Advanced disease:*
- Difficulty initiating a urine stream
- Dribbling, urine retention
- Unexplained cystitis
- Hematuria.

Diagnostic tests

- Prostate-specific antigen (PSA) in men over age 50
- Serum acid phosphatase
- Ultrasound if PSA test positive
- Magnetic resonance imaging, computed tomography scan, excretory urography
- Bone scan
- Biopsy confirms the diagnosis.

Treatment

Therapy aims to return the serum acid phosphatase level to normal; a subsequent rise points to recurrence. Treatment must be chosen carefully, because prostatic cancer usually affects older men, who commonly have coexisting disorders, such as hypertension, diabetes, or cardiac disease. Therapy varies with each stage of the disease and generally includes:
- radiation
- prostatectomy
- orchiectomy
- hormone therapy with synthetic estrogen (diethylstilbestrol) and antiandrogens, such as cyproterone, megestrol, and flutamide; gonadotropin-releasing hormone agonists such as leuprolide
- radical prostatectomy for locally invasive lesions.
> *Metastatic disease:*
- To relieve pain from metastatic bone involvement:
- radiation therapy
- single injection of strontium-89
- Chemotherapy (combinations of cyclophosphamide, doxorubicin, fluorouracil, cisplatin, etoposide, vindesine) offers limited benefit; combining several treatment methods may be most effective.

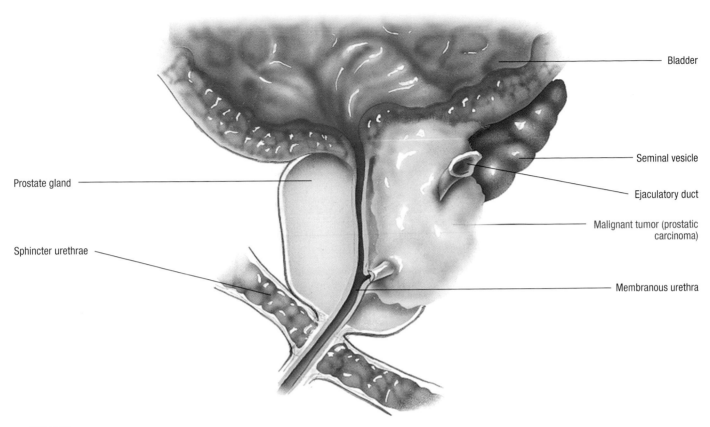

Bladder

Seminal vesicle

Ejaculatory duct

Malignant tumor (prostatic carcinoma)

Prostate gland

Sphincter urethrae

Membranous urethra

CLINICAL TIP

PATHWAY FOR METASTASIS OF PROSTATE CANCER

When primary prostatic lesions metastasize, they typically invade the prostatic capsule, spreading along the ejaculatory ducts in the space between the seminal vesicles or perivesicular fascia.

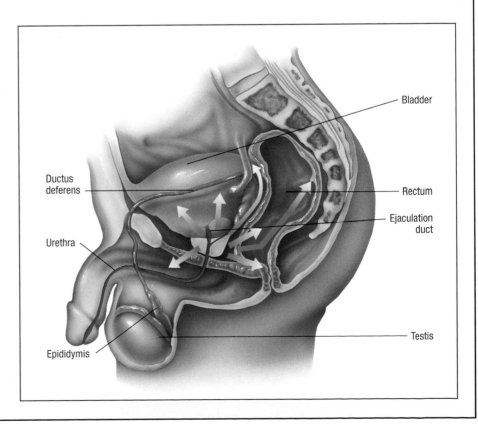

Bladder

Ductus deferens

Rectum

Ejaculation duct

Urethra

Testis

Epididymis

PROSTATITIS

Prostatitis, or inflammation of the prostate gland, may be acute or chronic. It's usually nonbacterial and idiopathic in origin (95% of cases). The nonbacterial form of the disorder is also known as prostatodynia. Acute prostatitis most often results from infection with gram-negative bacteria and is easy to recognize and treat. However, chronic prostatitis, the most common cause of recurrent urinary tract infections (UTIs) in men, is less easy to recognize.

 AGE ALERT
As many as 35% of men over age 50 have chronic prostatitis.

Causes
- Nonbacterial prostatitis — unknown.
- Bacterial prostatitis — *Escherichia coli* (80% of cases); *Klebsiella, Enterobacter, Proteus, Pseudomonas,* streptococci, staphylococci.
  Probable routes of entry:
- Through the blood stream
- Invasion of rectal bacteria through lymphatics
- Reflux of infected bladder urine into prostate ducts
- Infrequent or excessive sexual intercourse
- Procedures such as cystoscopy or catheterization (less commonly)
- From the urethra (chronic prostatitis).

 AGE ALERT
Acute prostatitis is associated with benign prostatic hypertrophy in older men.

Pathophysiology
Spasms in the genitourinary tract or tension in the pelvic floor muscles may cause inflammation and nonbacterial prostatitis.

Bacterial prostatic infections can be the result of a previous or concurrent infection, which stimulates an inflammatory response in the prostate. Inflammation is usually limited to a few of the gland's excretory ducts.

Signs and symptoms
Early acute prostatitis:
- Low back pain, especially when standing
- Perineal fullness, suprapubic tenderness
- Frequent and urgent urination
- Dysuria, nocturia, urinary obstruction
- Cloudy urine.
  Chronic bacterial prostatitis:
- Same urinary symptoms as in acute form but to a lesser degree
- Recurrent symptomatic cystitis.
  Other possible signs:
- Evidence of UTI, such as urinary frequency, burning, cloudy urine
- Painful ejaculation

- Bloody semen
- Persistent urethral discharge
- Erectile dysfunction.

Diagnostic tests
- Pelvic X-ray
- Urine culture
- Comparison of urine cultures of specimens obtained by the Meares and Stamey technique.

 CLINICAL TIP
The Meares and Stamey technique offers a firm diagnosis of prostatitis. The test requires four specimens, as follows:
- when the patient starts voiding
- midstream
- after patient stops voiding and doctor massages the prostate to produce secretions
- final voided specimen.

Treatment
Supportive therapy:
- Bed rest, adequate hydration, analgesics, antipyretics, sitz baths, stool softeners as necessary.
  Acute prostatitis:
- Systemic antibiotic therapy is treatment of choice; may include:
- oral antibiotic indicated by culture and sensitivity testing
- for sepsis: I.V. co-trimoxazole or I.V. gentamicin plus ampicillin until sensitivity test results are known; parenteral therapy for 48 hours to 1 week; then oral agent for 30 more days (with favorable test results and clinical response).
  Chronic prostatitis due to E. coli:
- Co-trimoxazole for at least 6 weeks
- If drug therapy is unsuccessful:
- transurethral resection removing all infected tissue
- total prostatectomy.
  Symptomatic treatment of chronic prostatitis:
- Instruct patient to drink at least 8 glasses of water daily
- Regular careful massage of the prostate to relieve discomfort (vigorous massage may cause secondary epididymitis or septicemia)
- Regular ejaculation to help promote drainage of prostatic secretions
- Anticholingerics and analgesics to help relieve nonbacterial prostatitis symptoms
- Alpha-adrenergic blockers and muscle relaxants to relieve pain
- Continuous low-dose anabolic steroid therapy (effective in some men).

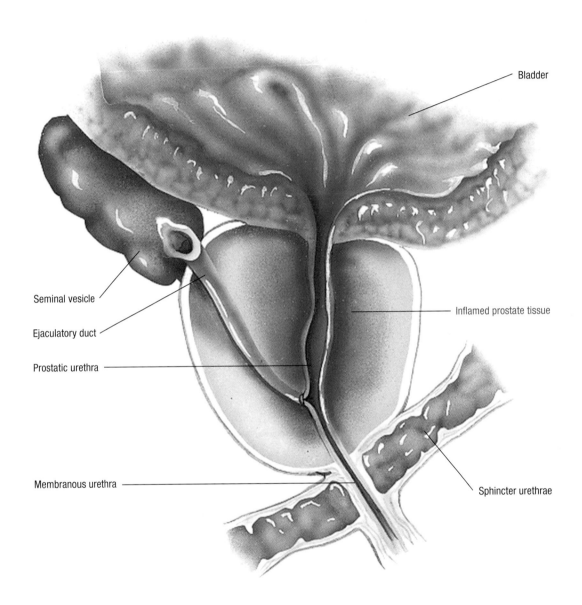

Bladder

Seminal vesicle

Ejaculatory duct

Prostatic urethra

Membranous urethra

Inflamed prostate tissue

Sphincter urethrae

SEXUALLY TRANSMITTED INFECTIONS

CHLAMYDIA

Chlamydial urethritis in men and chlamydial urethritis and cervicitis in women are a group of infections caused by the same organism. They are transmitted by orogenital contact or vaginal or rectal intercourse with an infected person. Chlamydial infections are the most common sexually transmitted diseases in the United States.

Causes

Chlamydia trachomatis.

Signs and symptoms

- Commonly asymptomatic
- Dysuria, urinary frequency, pyuria, pelvic or abdominal pain
- Chills, fever
- Genital discharge, genital pain
- Vaginal bleeding after intercourse; painful scrotal swelling.

Diagnostic tests

- Smears and cultures (urethra, cervix, rectum)
- Cultures of aspirated material establishes diagnosis of epididymitis.

Treatment

Doxycycline for 7 days or a single dose of azithromycin.

GONORRHEA

This infection of the genitourinary tract (most commonly the urethra or cervix), or, occasionally, the rectum, pharynx, or eyes almost always follows sexual contact with an infected person. An infected mother can transmit it during delivery.

Causes

Neisseria gonorrhoeae.

Signs and symptoms

In males:
- May be asymptomatic
- Three to six days after contact, urethritis, dysuria, purulent discharge, redness, and swelling at the site.
  In females:
- Generally asymptomatic
- Occasionally, inflammation, burning, itching, or greenish-yellow discharge.
  In either sex:
- Urinary frequency, incontinence, pelvic and lower abdominal pain or distention
- Nausea, vomiting, fever, tachycardia, polyarthritis (advanced disease).
  Gonococcal ophthalmia neonatorum:
- Lid edema, redness, abundant purulent discharge appearing 2 or 3 days postpartum.

Diagnostic tests

- Positive culture from infection site
- Smear showing gram-negative diplococci
- Conjunctival scrapings
- Gonococcal arthritis: Gram stain of smears from joint fluid and skin lesions.

Treatment

- Ceftriaxone plus doxycycline
- Alternative agents given with doxycycline:
- cefixime, olfloxacin, spectinomycin, ciprofloxacin, erythromycin.

GENITAL HERPES

Genital herpes is an acute inflammatory disease of the genitalia. It typically is transmitted through sexual intercourse, orogenital sexual activity, kissing, and hand-to-body contact. Pregnant women may transmit the infection to newborns during vaginal delivery if an active infection is present.

Causes

- Herpes simplex virus type 2 — most common
- Herpes simplex virus type 1 — increasing incidence.

Signs and symptoms

In both men and women after a 3- to 7-day incubation period:
- Appearance of genital vesicles:
- usually painless at first; rupture and develop into extensive, shallow, painful ulcers, with redness, marked edema, tender inguinal lymph nodes, and characteristic yellow, oozing centers
- Fever, malaise, dysuria, possible lesions on mouth or anus.
  In women:
- Cervix (primary site), labia, perianal skin, vulva, or vagina
- Leukorrhea.
  In men:
- Glans penis, foreskin, or penile shaft.

Diagnostic tests

- Virologic assay on cultured specimens
- Immunoassay for specific antigens.

Treatment

- Acyclovir:
- oral administration for new infection or recurrent outbreaks
- I.V. administration for patient hospitalized with severe genital herpes or immunocompromised patient with a potentially life-threatening herpes infection
- daily prophylaxis reduces the frequency of recurrences by at least 50%, but is only appropriate for patients with frequent outbreaks and may not decrease transmission rate
- Other antiviral agents, such as famciclovir, valacyclovir.

(Text continues on page 322.)

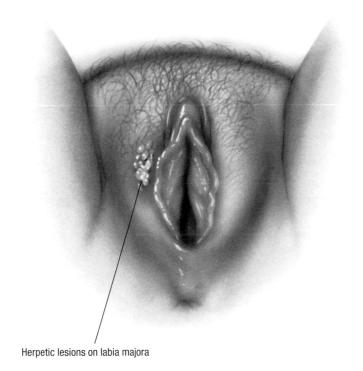

Herpetic lesions on labia majora

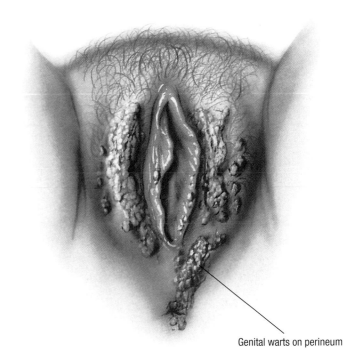

Genital warts on perineum

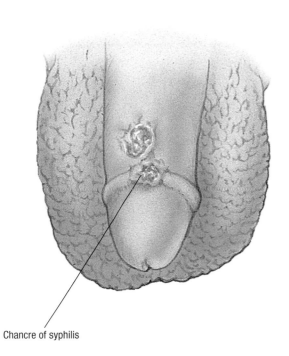

Chancre of syphilis

Trichomonal vaginitis

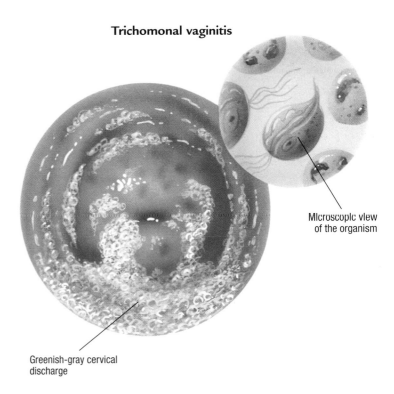

Microscopic view of the organism

Greenish-gray cervical discharge

Genital warts

Genital warts are also known as venereal warts or condylomata acuminata. The warts grow rapidly in the presence of immune suppression or pregnancy and can accompany other genital infections.

Causes

Human papilloma virus.

Signs and symptoms

● After a 1- to 6-month incubation period (usually 2 months), tiny, red or pink, painless swellings on moist surfaces:
– subpreputial sac, in urethral meatus and, less commonly, on penile shaft
– vulva and on vaginal and cervical walls
● Progressive disease:
– spread to perineum and perianal area
– large warts up to about 4" (10 cm) in diameter
– pedunculated; typical cauliflower-like appearance
● Resemble condylomata lata associated with second-stage syphilis.

Diagnostic tests

● Dark-field examination of scrapings
● Biopsy only if neoplasia is strongly suspected.

Treatment

● None to eradicate virus; relapse is common
● Small warts: topical 10% to 25% podophyllum in tincture of benzoin, trichloroacetic acid, or bichloroacetic acid
● Warts larger than 1" (2.5 cm): carbon dioxide laser treatment, cryosurgery, or electrocautery
● Podofilox (antimitotic), imiquimod (immune response modifier), interferon, combined laser and interferon therapy.

Syphilis

Syphilis is a contagious, systemic venereal or congenital disease caused by a spirochete. It begins in the mucous membranes and quickly spreads to nearby lymph nodes and the bloodstream. Transmission occurs primarily through sexual contact during the primary, secondary, and early latent stages of infection. Transmission from a mother to her fetus is possible.

Causes

The spirochete *Treponema pallidum.*

Signs and symptoms

Primary syphilis:
● Develops after 3-week incubation period
● One or more chancres erupt at site of infection, usually genitalia; or, possibly, on anus, fingers, lips, tongue, nipples, tonsils, eyelids.
  Secondary syphilis:
● Symptoms develop within a few days or up to 8 weeks after onset of primary chancres
● Symmetrical mucocutaneous lesions — of uniform size; well defined; macular, papular, pustular, or nodular:

– commonly between rolls of fat on the trunk and, proximally, on the arms, palms, soles, face, and scalp
– in warm, moist areas (perineum, scrotum, vulva, and between rolls of fat), lesions enlarge and erode becoming highly contagious, pink or grayish white lesions (condylomata lata)
● Headache, malaise, anorexia, weight loss, nausea, vomiting, sore throat and, possibly, slight fever, lymphadenopathy
● Alopecia, usually temporary; brittle, pitted nails.
  Latent tertiary syphilis:
● Absence of clinical symptoms
● Reactive serologic test for syphilis.
  Late syphilis:
● Final, destructive but noninfectious stage of the disease
● Any or all of three subtypes: late benign syphilis, cardiovascular syphilis, and neurosyphilis.

Diagnostic tests

● Dark-field examination for *T. pallidum*
● Fluorescent treponemal antibody-absorption test
● Venereal Disease Research Laboratories test
● Rapid plasma reagin test.

Treatment

● Primary, secondary, or early latent: single injection of penicillin G benzathine I.M.
● One year duration (latent): penicillin G benzathine I.M.
● Nonpregnant patients allergic to penicillin: oral tetracycline or doxycycline for 15 days for early syphilis, 30 days for late infections.

Trichomoniasis

A protozoal infection, trichomoniasis affects about 15% of sexually active females and 10% of sexually active males. Common sites of infection in females include the vagina, urethra and, possibly, the endocervix, bladder, Bartholin's glands, or Skene's glands; in males, the lower urethra and, possibly, the prostate gland, seminal vesicles, or epididymis.

Causes

Trichomonas vaginalis, a tetraflagellated, motile protozoan.

Signs and symptoms

● None in approximately 70% of females — including those with chronic infections — and most males
● In females with acute infection:
– gray or greenish-yellow and possibly profuse and frothy, malodorous vaginal discharge
– severe itching, redness, swelling, dyspareunia, dysuria; occasionally, postcoital spotting, menorrhagia, dysmenorrhea.

Diagnostic tests

● Microscopic examination of vaginal or seminal discharge or urine specimen for *T. vaginalis.*

Treatment

● Treatment of choice: metronidazole; or, metronidazole given twice daily for 7 days.

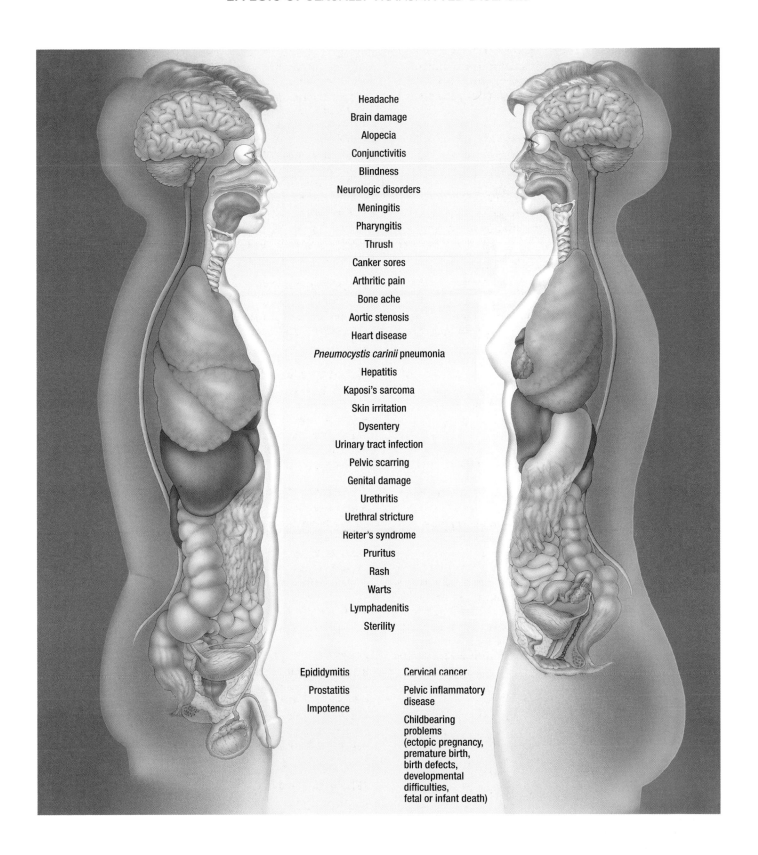

Headache
Brain damage
Alopecia
Conjunctivitis
Blindness
Neurologic disorders
Meningitis
Pharyngitis
Thrush
Canker sores
Arthritic pain
Bone ache
Aortic stenosis
Heart disease
Pneumocystis carinii pneumonia
Hepatitis
Kaposi's sarcoma
Skin irritation
Dysentery
Urinary tract infection
Pelvic scarring
Genital damage
Urethritis
Urethral stricture
Reiter's syndrome
Pruritus
Rash
Warts
Lymphadenitis
Sterility

Epididymitis

Prostatitis

Impotence

Cervical cancer

Pelvic inflammatory disease

Childbearing problems (ectopic pregnancy, premature birth, birth defects, developmental difficulties, fetal or infant death)

TESTICULAR CANCER

Most testicular tumors originate in gonadal cells. About 40% are seminomas — uniform, undifferentiated cells resembling primitive gonadal cells. The remainder are nonseminomas — tumor cells showing various degrees of differentiation. The prognosis varies with the cell type and disease stage. When treated with surgery and radiation, almost all patients with localized disease survive beyond 5 years.

 AGE ALERT
Malignant testicular tumors primarily affect young to middle-aged men and are the most common solid tumor in these age-groups. Incidence peaks between ages 20 and 40. Testicular tumors seldom occur in children.

Testicular cancer is rare in nonwhite males and accounts for fewer than 1% of male cancer deaths.

Causes
Primary cause unknown.
Associated conditions:
- Cryptorchidism (even if surgically corrected)
- Maternal use of diethylstilbestrol during pregnancy.

Pathophysiology
Testicular cancer may metastasize to the lungs, liver, viscera, or bone. It spreads through the lymphatic system to the iliac, para-aortic, and mediastinal lymph nodes.

Signs and symptoms
- Firm, painless, smooth testicular mass, varying in size and sometimes producing a sense of testicular heaviness
- Gynecomastia and nipple tenderness may result if tumor produces chorionic gonadotropin or estrogen may result.
In advanced stages:
- Ureteral obstruction
- Abdominal mass
- Cough, hemoptysis, shortness of breath
- Weight loss
- Fatigue, pallor, lethargy.

Diagnostic tests
- Excretory urography
- Urinary or serum luteinizing hormone levels
- Lymphangiography
- Ultrasonography
- Abdominal computed tomography scan
- Serum alpha-fetoprotein and beta-human chorionic gonadotropin
- Surgical excision and biopsy of the tumor and testis with inguinal exploration.

Treatment
Surgery:
- Orchiectomy and retroperitoneal node dissection
- Hormone replacement therapy after bilateral orchiectomy.
Postoperative radiation:
- Seminoma: retroperitoneal and homolateral iliac nodes
- Nonseminoma: all positive nodes
- Retroperitoneal extension: mediastinal and supraclavicular nodes prophylactically.
Combination chemotherapy:
- Essential for tumors beyond stage 0
- Agents include bleomycin, etoposide, and cisplatin; cisplatin, vindesine, and bleomycin; cisplatin, vinblastine, and bleomycin; cisplatin, vincristine, methotrexate, bleomycin, and leucovorin.
Unresponsive malignancy:
- Chemotherapy and radiation
- Autologous bone marrow transplantation.

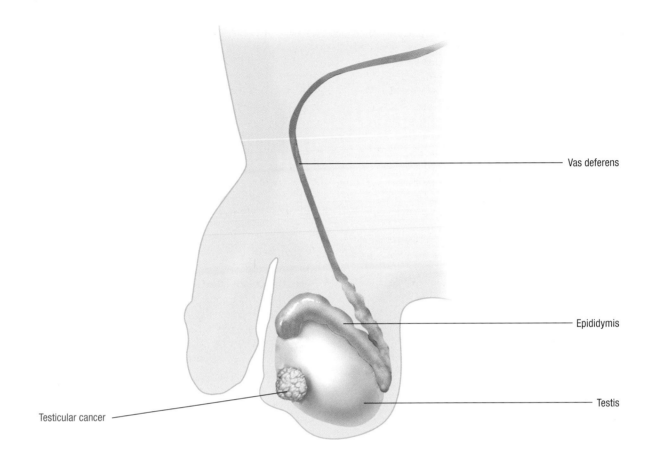

Vas deferens

Epididymis

Testis

Testicular cancer

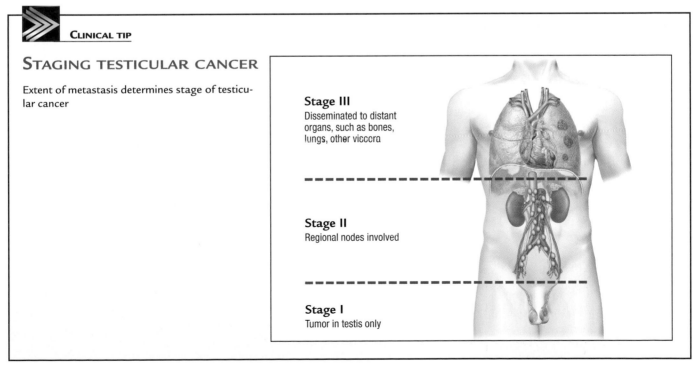

CLINICAL TIP

STAGING TESTICULAR CANCER

Extent of metastasis determines stage of testicular cancer

Stage III
Disseminated to distant organs, such as bones, lungs, other viscera

Stage II
Regional nodes involved

Stage I
Tumor in testis only

TESTICULAR TORSION

Testicular torsion is an abnormal twisting of the spermatic cord due to rotation of a testis or the mesorchium; it may occur inside or outside the tunica vaginalis. Intravaginal torsion is most common in adolescents, extravaginal, in neonates. Onset may be spontaneous or follow physical exertion or trauma. Potential outcomes range from strangulation to eventual infarction of the testis without treatment. This condition is almost always (90%) unilateral.

AGE ALERT
The greatest risk occurs during the neonatal period and again between ages 12 and 18 (puberty), but it may occur at any age. Infants with torsion of one testis have a greater incidence of torsion of the other testis later in life than do males in the general population. The prognosis is good with early detection and prompt treatment.

Causes
Intravaginal torsion:
● Abnormality of the coverings of the testis and abnormally positioned testis
● Incomplete attachment of the testis and spermatic fascia to the scrotal wall, leaving the testis free to rotate around its vascular pedicle.
Extravaginal torsion:
● Loose attachment of the tunica vaginalis to the scrotal lining causing spermatic cord rotation above the testis
● Sudden forceful contraction of the cremaster muscle due to physical exertion or irritation of the muscle.

Pathophysiology
Normally, the tunica vaginalis envelops the testis and attaches to the epididymis and spermatic cord. Normal contraction of the cremaster muscle causes the left testis to rotate counter-clockwise, and the right, clockwise. In testicular torsion, the testis rotates on its vascular pedicle and twists the arteries and vein in the spermatic cord, interrupting blood flow to the testis. Vascular engorgement and ischemia ensue, causing scrotal swelling unrelieved by rest or elevation of the scrotum. If manual reduction is unsuccessful, torsion must be surgically corrected within 6 hours after the onset of symptoms to preserve testicular function (70% salvage rate). After 12 hours, the testis becomes dysfunctional and necrotic.

Signs and symptoms
● Excruciating pain in the affected testis or iliac fossa of the pelvis
● Edematous, elevated, and ecchymotic scrotum
● Loss of the cremasteric reflex (stimulation of the skin on the inner thigh retracts the testis on the same side) on the affected side
● Abdominal pain; nausea and vomiting.

Diagnostic tests
Doppler ultrasonography to help distinguish testicular torsion from strangulated hernia, undescended testes, or epididymitis (absent blood flow and avascular testis in torsion).

Treatment
● Manual manipulation of the testis counterclockwise to improve blood flow before surgery (not always possible)
● Immediate surgical repair by:
– orchiopexy: fixation of a viable testis to the scrotum and prophylactic fixation of the contralateral testis
– orchiectomy: excision of a nonviable testis to limit risk for autoimmune response to necrotic testis and its contents, damage to unaffected testis, and subsequent infertility.

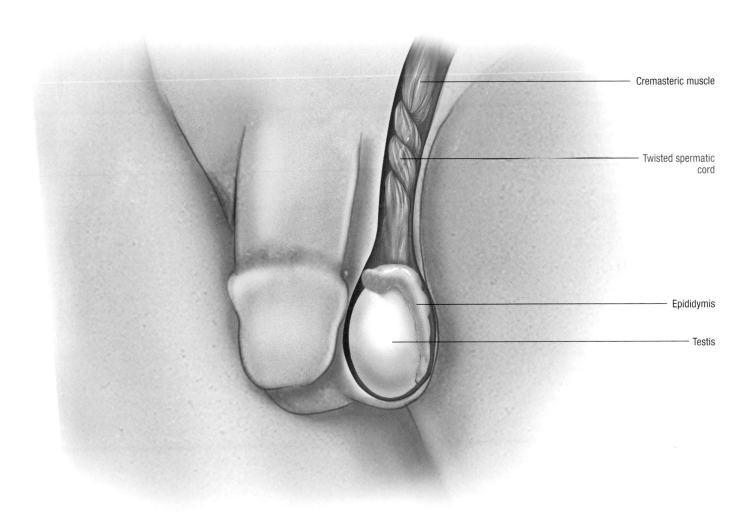

Cremasteric muscle

Twisted spermatic cord

Epididymis

Testis

VAGINITIS

Vaginitis is inflammation of the vulva (vulvitis) and vagina (vaginitis). Because of the proximity of these two structures, inflammation of one occasionally causes inflammation of the other. Vaginitis may occur at any age and affects most females at some time. The prognosis is excellent with treatment.

Causes
Vaginitis (with or without consequent vulvitis):
- *Trichomonas vaginalis*, a protozoan flagellate, usually transmitted through sexual intercourse
- *Candida albicans*, a fungus that requires glucose for growth.

CLINICAL TIP
Some women are at particular risk of infection with *C. albicans*. The incidence of candidal vaginitis rises during the secretory phase of the menstrual cycle and doubles during pregnancy. The infection is also common in women with diabetes and in those who use oral contraceptives. Incidence may reach 75% in patients receiving systemic therapy with broad-spectrum antibiotics.

- *Gardnerella vaginalis*, a gram-negative bacillus.
  Vulvitis:
- Parasite infestation, as with *Phthirus pubis* (crab louse)
- Trauma (skin breakdown may lead to secondary infection)
- Poor personal hygiene
- Chemical irritants, or allergic reactions to hygiene sprays, douches, detergents, clothing, or toilet paper
- Vulvar atrophy in menopausal women due to decreasing estrogen levels
- Retention of a foreign body, such as a tampon or diaphragm.

Pathophysiology
Bacterial vaginitis is caused by a disturbance of the normal vaginal flora. There is an overgrowth of anaerobic bacteria and of an organism, *Gardnerella*, with an associated loss of the normally dominant *Lactobacillus* species.

Candida albicans is normally found in small amounts in the vagina, mouth, digestive tract, and on the skin, without causing disease or symptoms. Symptoms appear when the balance between normal micro-organisms of the vagina is lost; the *C. albicans* population then becomes larger in relation to other micro-organism populations. This happens when the environment (vagina) has certain favorable conditions that allow for growth and nourishment of *C. albicans*. An environment that makes it difficult for other micro-organisms to survive may also cause an imbalance and lead to yeast infection.

Yeast infection may develop in reaction to antibiotics prescribed for another purpose. The antibiotics change the normal flora in the vagina and suppress the growth of the protective bacteria, *Lactobacillus*.

Infection is common among women who use estrogen-containing birth control pills and among women who are pregnant. This is due to the increased level of estrogen in the body, causing changes in the environment that make it perfect for fungal growth and nourishment.

Signs and symptoms
T. vaginitis:
- Thin, bubbly, green-tinged, malodorous discharge
- Irritation, itching; urinary symptoms, such as burning and frequency.
  C. albicans:
- Thick, white, cottage-cheese–like discharge
- Red, edematous mucous membranes, with white flecks adhering to the vaginal wall
- Intense itching.
  G. vaginalis:
- Gray, foul, "fishy" smelling discharge.
  Acute vulvitis:
- Mild to severe inflammatory reaction, including edema, erythema, burning, and pruritus
- Severe pain on urination, dyspareunia.
  Chronic vulvitis:
- Relatively mild inflammation
- Possibly, severe edema that may involve the entire perineum.

Diagnostic tests
- Vaginitis: microscopic examination of vaginal exudate on a wet slide preparation (a drop of vaginal exudate placed in normal saline solution)
- Vulvitis or suspected venereal disease:
  - complete blood count, urinalysis, cytology screening
  - biopsy of chronic lesions
  - culture of exudate from acute lesions
  - possibly, human immunodeficiency virus assay.

Treatment
- Trichomonal vaginitis: oral metronidazole
- Candidal infection:
  - topical miconazole or clotrimazole
  - single dose of oral fluconazole
- *Gardnerella* infection: oral or vaginal metronidazole
- Acute vulvitis:
  - cold compresses or cool sitz baths for pruritus
  - warm compresses for severe inflammation
  - topical corticosteroids to reduce inflammation
- Chronic vulvitis:
  - topical hydrocortisone or antipruritics
  - good hygiene, especially in elderly or incontinent patients
- Atrophic vulvovaginitis: topical estrogen ointment.

Candida infection

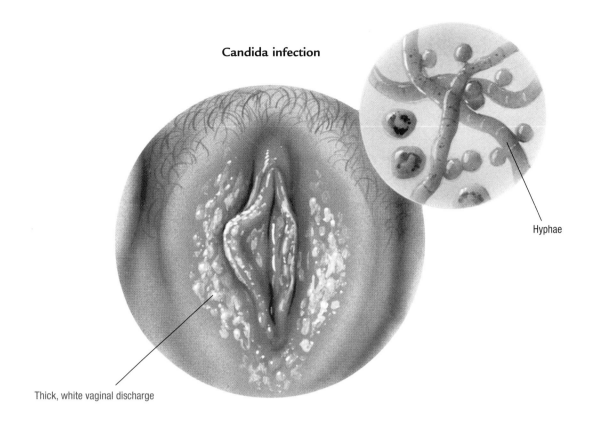

Hyphae

Thick, white vaginal discharge

Bacterial vaginosis

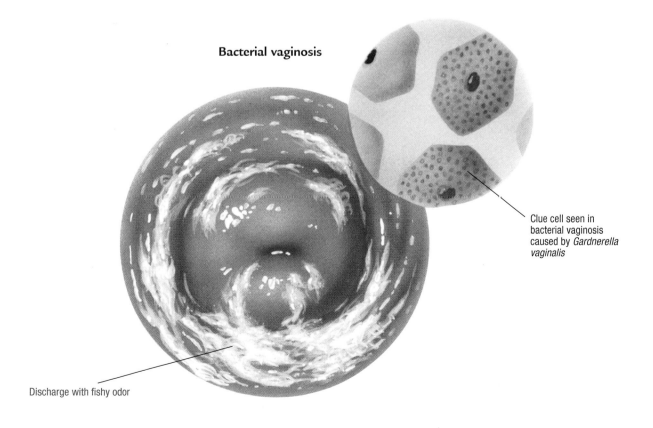

Clue cell seen in
bacterial vaginosis
caused by *Gardnerella
vaginalis*

Discharge with fishy odor

VARICOCELE

A mass of dilated and tortuous varicose veins in the spermatic cord is called a varicocele. It is classically described as a "bag of worms." Thirty percent of all men diagnosed with infertility have a varicocele; 95% of cases affect the left spermatic cord.

 AGE ALERT
Varicocele occurs in 10% to 15% of all males, usually between ages 13 and 18.

Causes
• Incompetent or congenitally absent valves in spermatic veins
• Tumor or thrombus obstructing inferior vena cava (unilateral left-sided varicocele).

Pathophysiology
As a result of a valvular disorder in the spermatic vein, blood pools in the pampiniform plexus of veins that drain each testis rather than flowing into the venous system. One function of the pampiniform plexus is to keep the testes slightly cooler than the body temperature, which is the optimum temperature for sperm production. Inadequate blood flow through the testis thus compromises spermatogenesis and may lead to testicular atrophy.

Signs and symptoms
• Usually asymptomatic
• Feeling of heaviness on the affected side
• Testicular pain and tenderness on palpation.

Diagnostic tests
None; physical examination only.

Treatment
• Mild varicocele, fertility not a concern: scrotal support to relieve discomfort
• To retain or restore fertility, surgical repair or removal by ligation of the spermatic cord at the internal inguinal ring.

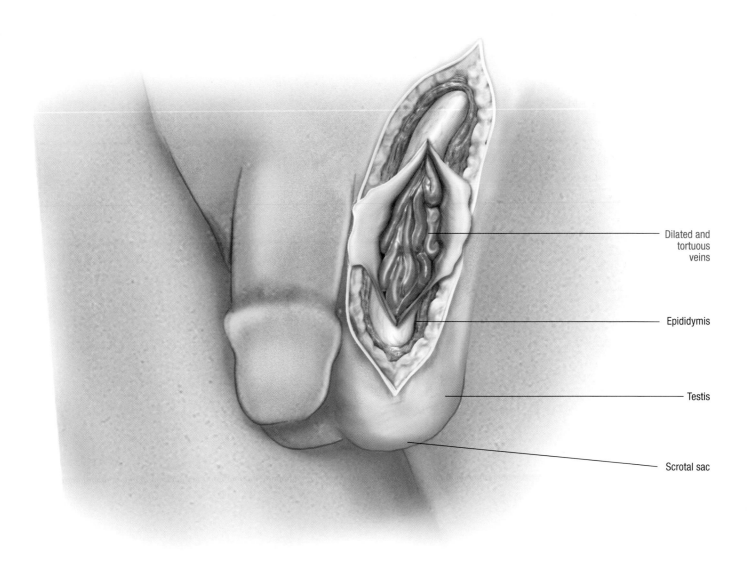

Dilated and tortuous veins

Epididymis

Testis

Scrotal sac

Vulvar cancer

Cancer of the vulva accounts for approximately 4% of all gynecologic malignancies.

 AGE ALERT
Vulvar cancer can occur at any age, even in infants, but its peak incidence is in the mid-60s.

The most common vulvar cancer is squamous cell carcinoma. Early diagnosis increases the chance of effective treatment and survival. If lymph node dissection reveals no positive nodes, 5-year survival rate is 85%; otherwise, less than 75%.

Causes
Primary cause unknown.
Predisposing factors:
• Leukoplakia (white epithelial hyperplasia), in about 25% of patients
• Chronic vulvar granulomatous disease
• Chronic pruritus of the vulva, with friction, swelling, and dryness
• Pigmented moles that are constantly irritated by clothing or perineal pads
• Irradiation of the skin such as nonspecific treatment for pelvic cancer
• Infection with human papilloma virus
• Obesity, hypertension, diabetes.

Pathophysiology
Vulvar neoplasms may arise from varying cell origins. Because much of the vulva is made of skin, any type of skin cancer can develop there. The majority of vulvar cancers arise from squamous epithelial cells.

Signs and symptoms
In 50% of patients:
• Vulvar pruritus, bleeding
• Small vulvar mass — may begin as small ulcer on the surface, which eventually becomes infected and painful.

Less common:
• Mass in the groin
• Abnormal urination or defecation.

Diagnostic tests
• Colposcopy and toluidine-blue staining to identify biopsy sites
• Histologic examination of biopsy samples
• Complete blood count
• X-ray, computed tomography scan.

Treatment
Small, confined lesions with no lymph node involvement:
• Simple vulvectomy or hemivulvectomy (without pelvic node dissection):
– personal considerations (young age of patient, active sexual life) may mandate such conservative management
– requires careful postoperative follow-up because it leaves the patient at risk for developing a new lesion.
For widespread tumor:
• Radical vulvectomy
• Radical wide local excision — can be as effective as more radical resection, but with much less morbidity
• Depending on extent of metastasis, resection may include the urethra, vagina, and bowel, leaving an open perineal wound until healing — about 2 to 3 months
• Plastic surgery, including mucocutaneous graft to reconstruct pelvic structures.
Extensive metastasis, advanced age, or fragile health:
• Rules out surgery
• Palliative treatment with irradiation of the primary lesion or chemotherapy.

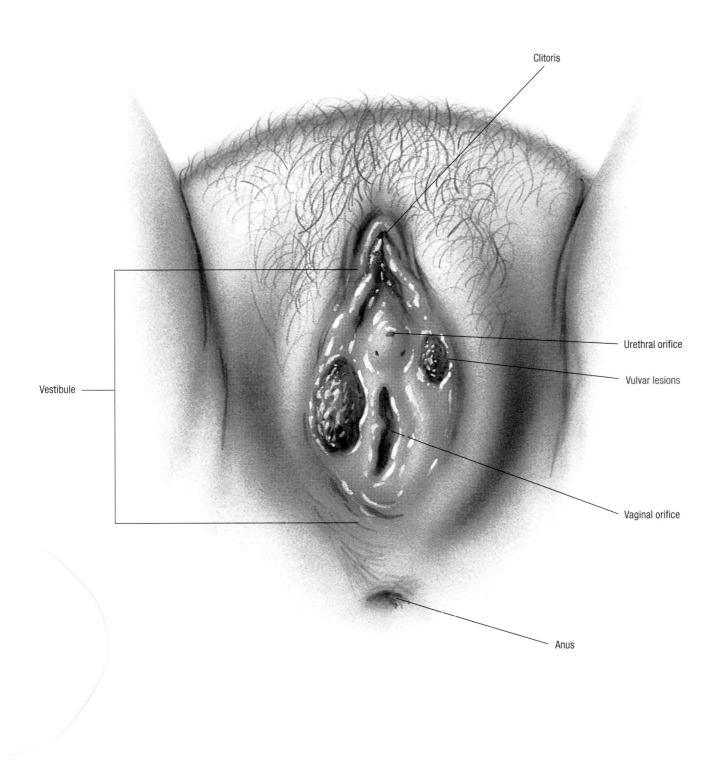

Clitoris

Urethral orifice

Vulvar lesions

Vaginal orifice

Vestibule

Anus

ACUTE TUBULAR NECROSIS

Acute tubular necrosis (ATN), also known as acute tubulointerstitial nephritis, accounts for about 75% of all cases of acute renal failure and is the most common cause of acute renal failure in critically ill patients. ATN injures the tubular segment of the nephron, causing renal failure and uremic syndrome. Mortality ranges from 40% to 70%, depending on complications from underlying diseases. Nonoliguric forms of ATN have a better prognosis.

Causes
• Diseased tubular epithelium, which permits leakage of glomerular filtrate across the membranes and reabsorption of filtrate into the blood
• Obstruction of urine flow by accumulated damaged cells, casts, red blood cells (RBCs), and other cellular debris in the lumen
• Ischemic injury to glomerular epithelial cells, resulting in cellular collapse and decreased glomerular capillary permeability
• Ischemic injury to vascular endothelium, eventually resulting in cellular swelling and obstruction.

Pathophysiology
ATN results from ischemic or nephrotoxic injury, most commonly in debilitated patients, such as the critically ill or those who have undergone extensive surgery. In ischemic injury, disruption of blood flow to the kidneys may result from circulatory collapse, severe hypotension, trauma, hemorrhage, dehydration, cardiogenic or septic shock, surgery, anesthetics, or reactions to transfusions. Nephrotoxic injury may follow ingestion of certain chemical agents or result from a hypersensitive reaction of the kidneys. Because nephrotoxic ATN doesn't damage the basement membrane of the nephron, it's potentially reversible. However, ischemic ATN can damage the epithelial and basement membranes and can cause lesions in the renal interstitium.

Signs and symptoms
• Early stages: effects of primary disease may mask symptoms of ATN
• Decreased urine output may be first recognizable effect
• Hyperkalemia

• Uremic syndrome, with oliguria (or, rarely, anuria) and confusion, which may progress to uremic coma
• Heart failure, uremic pericarditis
• Pulmonary edema, uremic lung
• Anemia
• Anorexia
• Intractable vomiting
• Poor wound healing.

CLINICAL TIP
Fever and chills may signal the onset of an infection, the leading cause of death in ATN.

Diagnostic tests
• Urinary sediment analysis; urine specific gravity, osmolality, sodium
• Blood urea nitrogen, serum creatinine, serum electrolyte levels
• Arterial blood gas analysis for metabolic acidosis
• Complete blood count
• Electrocardiogram.

Treatment
Acute phase:
• Vigorous supportive measures until normal kidney function resumes; initial treatment may include:
- diuretics
- intravenous fluids to flush tubules of cellular casts and debris and to replace fluid loss.
  Long-term fluid management:
• Daily replacement of projected and calculated losses (including insensible loss).
  Other measures to control complications:
• Packed RBCs for anemia; epoetin alfa to stimulate RBC production
• Antibiotics for infection
• Emergency I.V. administration of 50% glucose, regular insulin, and sodium bicarbonate for hyperkalemia
• Sodium polystyrene sulfonate with sorbitol by mouth or by enema to reduce extracellular potassium levels
• Peritoneal dialysis or hemodialysis if patient is catabolic.

TYPES OF ACUTE TUBULAR NECROSIS

Ischemic necrosis

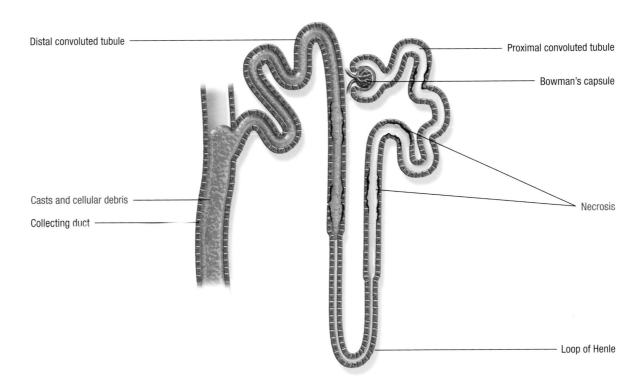

Distal convoluted tubule

Proximal convoluted tubule

Bowman's capsule

Casts and cellular debris

Collecting duct

Necrosis

Loop of Henle

Nephrotoxic injury

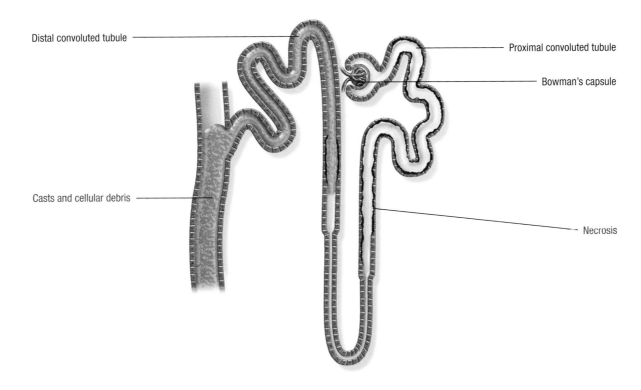

Distal convoluted tubule

Proximal convoluted tubule

Bowman's capsule

Casts and cellular debris

Necrosis

BLADDER CANCER

Cancer of the bladder is the most common cancer of the urinary tract.

Workers in certain industries (rubber workers, weavers and leather finishers, aniline dye workers, hairdressers, petroleum workers, and spray painters) are at high risk for bladder cancer. The period between exposure to the carcinogen and development of symptoms is about 18 years.

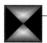 **AGE ALERT**
Bladder tumors are most prevalent in men over age 50 and are most common in densely populated industrial areas.

Causes
Primary cause unknown.
Predisposing factors:
- Transitional cell tumors: certain environmental carcinogens, including 2-naphthylamine, benzidine, tobacco, nitrates
- Squamous cell carcinoma of the bladder:
- schistosomiasis
- chronic bladder irritation or infection; for example, from kidney stones, indwelling urinary catheters, cystitis from cyclophosphamide.

Pathophysiology
Bladder tumors can develop on the surface of the bladder wall (benign or malignant papillomas) or grow within the bladder wall (generally more virulent) and quickly invade underlying muscles. Ninety percent of bladder tumors are transitional cell carcinomas, arising from the transitional epithelium of mucous membranes. Less common are adenocarcinomas, epidermoid carcinomas, squamous cell carcinomas, sarcomas, tumors in bladder diverticula, and carcinoma in situ.

Signs and symptoms
- In early stages, no symptoms in approximately 25% of patients
- First sign: gross, painless, intermittent hematuria (in many cases with clots in the urine)
- Invasive lesions: suprapubic pain after voiding
- Other signs and symptoms include:
- bladder irritability, urinary frequency
- nocturia
- dribbling.

Diagnostic tests
- Cystoscopy and biopsy confirm diagnosis.
Provide essential information about the tumor:
- Urinalysis, urine cytology
- Excretory urography
- Retrograde cystography.

Help to confirm the diagnosis:
- Pelvic arteriography
- Computed tomography scan
- Ultrasonography.

Treatment
Superficial bladder tumors:
- Transurethral cystoscopic resection and fulguration (electrical destruction); adequate when the tumor has not invaded the muscle
- Intravesicular chemotherapy; useful for multiple tumors (especially those that occur in many sites) and to prevent tumor recurrence
- If additional tumors develop:
- fulguration every 3 months
- more radical therapy if tumors penetrate the muscle layer or recur frequently.
Larger tumors:
- Segmental bladder resection to remove a full-thickness section of the bladder; only if tumor isn't near the bladder neck or ureteral orifices
- Instillation of thiotepa after transurethral resection.
Infiltrating bladder tumors:
- Radical cystectomy: removal of the bladder with perivesical fat, lymph nodes, urethra, and prostate and seminal vesicles or uterus and adnexa
- Possibly preoperative external beam therapy to bladder
- Urinary diversion, usually an ileal conduit; patient must then wear an external pouch continuously
- Possible later penile implant.
Advanced bladder cancer:
- Cystectomy to remove the tumor
- Radiation therapy
- Systemic chemotherapy:
- cyclophosphamide, fluorouracil, doxorubicin, cisplatin combination may arrest bladder cancer
- cisplatin most effective single agent.
Investigational treatments:
- Photodynamic therapy:
- I.V. injection of a photosensitizing agent such as hematoporphyrin ether, which malignant cells readily absorb, followed by cystoscopic laser treatment to kill malignant cells
- treatment also renders normal cells photosensitive; patient must totally avoid sunlight for about 30 days
- Intravesicular administration of interferon alfa and tumor necrosis factor.

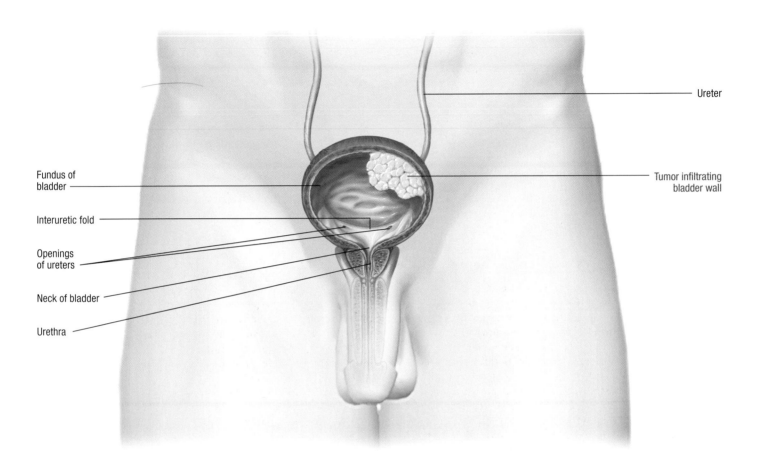

Fundus of
bladder

Interuretic fold

Openings
of ureters

Neck of bladder

Urethra

Ureter

Tumor infiltrating
bladder wall

CYSTITIS

Cystitis and urethritis, the two forms of lower urinary tract infection (UTI), are nearly 10 times more common in women than in men and affect approximately 10% to 20% of all women at least once. Lower UTI is also a prevalent bacterial disease in children, most commonly in girls. Men are less vulnerable because their urethras are longer and their prostatic fluid serves as an antibacterial shield. In both men and women, infection usually ascends from the urethra to the bladder. UTIs often respond readily to treatment, but recurrence and resistant bacterial flare-up during therapy are possible.

CLINICAL TIP
All children with proven UTI should receive a work-up to exclude an abnormality of the urinary tract that would predispose them to renal damage.

Causes

In women:
• Predisposition to infection by bacteria from vagina, perineum, rectum, or a sexual partner may result from short urethra.

  In men and children:
• Frequently related to anatomic or physiologic abnormalities.

  Recurrence:
• In 99% of patients, reinfection by the same organism or a new pathogen
• Persistent infection — usually from renal calculi, chronic bacterial prostatitis, or a structural anomaly that harbors bacteria.

AGE ALERT
As a person ages, progressive weakening of bladder muscles may result in incomplete bladder emptying and chronic urine retention — factors that predispose the older person to bladder infections.

Pathophysiology

Most lower UTIs result from ascending infection by a single, gram-negative, enteric species of bacteria, such as *Escherichia* (often *E. coli*), *Klebsiella, Proteus, Enterobacter, Pseudomonas,* or *Serratia.* However, in a patient with neurogenic bladder, an indwelling catheter, or a fistula between the intestine and bladder, lower UTI may result from simultaneous infection with multiple pathogens.

Recent studies suggest that infection results from a breakdown in local defense mechanisms in the bladder that allow bacteria to invade the bladder mucosa and multiply. These bacteria can't be readily eliminated by normal micturition.

Signs and symptoms
• Urgency, frequency, dysuria
• Cramps or spasms of the bladder
• Itching, feeling of warmth during urination
• Nocturia
• Urethral discharge in males
• Hematuria
• Fever, chills
• Other common features include:
– malaise
– nausea, vomiting
– low back pain, flank pain
– abdominal pain, tenderness over the bladder area.

Diagnostic tests
• Microscopic urinalysis
• Bacterial count in clean-catch midstream urine specimen; catheterization may reintroduce urethral bacteria into bladder
• Sensitivity testing to determine the appropriate therapeutic antimicrobial agent
• If warranted by patient history and physical examination, blood test or a stained smear of the discharge to rule out STD
• Voiding cystoureterography or excretory urography may detect congenital anomalies that predispose the patient to recurrent UTIs.

Treatment
• Appropriate antimicrobials:
– single-dose therapy with amoxicillin or co-trimoxazole may be effective in women with acute noncomplicated UTI
• If urine isn't sterile after 3 days:
– bacterial resistance likely
– use of a different antimicrobial necessary.

  Recurrent infections:
• Infected renal calculi, chronic prostatitis, or structural abnormality: possible surgery
• Prostatitis: long-term antibiotic therapy
• In absence of predisposing conditions: long-term, low-dose antibiotic therapy.

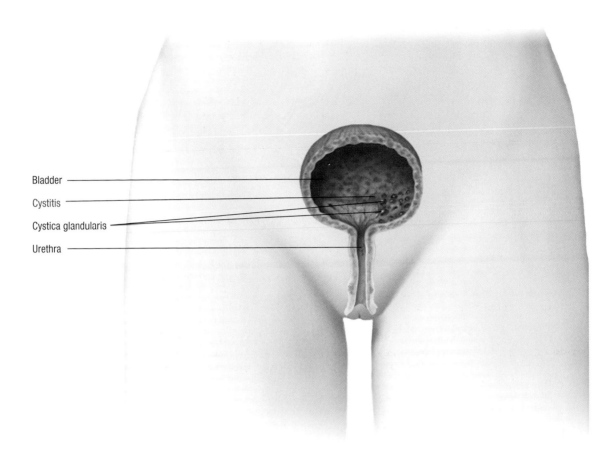

Bladder

Cystitis

Cystica glandularis

Urethra

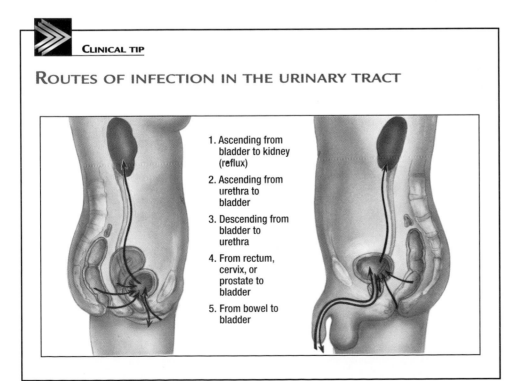

> **CLINICAL TIP**
>
> ## ROUTES OF INFECTION IN THE URINARY TRACT
>
> 1. Ascending from bladder to kidney (reflux)
> 2. Ascending from urethra to bladder
> 3. Descending from bladder to urethra
> 4. From rectum, cervix, or prostate to bladder
> 5. From bowel to bladder

Bladder wall — Endoscopic view

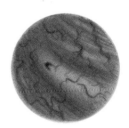

Normal wall

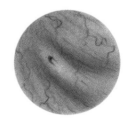

Acute cystitis

GLOMERULONEPHRITIS

Glomerulonephritis (GN) is a bilateral inflammation of the glomeruli, often following a streptococcal infection. Acute GN is also called acute poststreptococcal GN.

AGE ALERT
Acute GN is most common in boys aged 3 to 7, but can occur at any age. Rapidly progressive glomerulonephritis (RPGN) most commonly occurs between ages 50 and 60. Up to 95% of children and 70% of adults recover fully. Elderly patients may progress to chronic renal failure within months.

RPGN — also called subacute, crescentic, or extracapillary GN — may be idiopathic or associated with a proliferative glomerular disease, such as poststreptococcal GN.

Chronic GN is a slowly progressive disease characterized by inflammation, sclerosis, scarring, and, eventually, renal failure. It usually remains undetected until the progressive (irreversible) phase.

Causes
Acute or RPGN:
- Streptococcal infection of the respiratory tract
- Immunoglobulin A (IgA) nephropathy (Berger's disease)
- Impetigo
- Lipoid nephrosis.
  Chronic GN:
- Membranoproliferative GN
- Membranous glomerulopathy
- Focal glomerulosclerosis
- RPGN, poststreptococcal GN
- Systemic lupus erythematosus, Goodpasture's syndrome
- Hemolytic uremic syndrome.

Pathophysiology
In nearly all types of GN, the epithelial or podocyte layer of the glomerular membrane is damaged.

Acute poststreptococcal GN results from the entrapment and collection of antigen-antibody complexes, also known as immune complexes, in the glomerular capillary membranes, after infection with a group A beta-hemolytic streptococcus. The antigens, which are endogenous or exogenous, stimulate the formation of antibodies, which form immune complexes. Circulating immune complexes become lodged in the glomerular capillaries. The severity of glomerular damage and consequent renal insufficiency is related to the size, number, location (focal or diffuse), duration of exposure, and type of immune complexes.

In the glomerular capillary wall, immune complexes activate biochemical mediators of inflammation — complement, leukocytes, and fibrin. Activated complement attracts neutrophils and monocytes, which release lysosomal enzymes that damage the cell walls and cause a proliferation of the extracellular matrix, affecting glomerular blood flow. Those events increase membrane permeability, which causes a loss of negative charge across the glomerular membrane and enhanced protein filtration. Membrane damage also leads to platelet aggrega-

tion, and platelet degranulation releases substances that increase glomerular permeability.

Protein molecules and red blood cells can now pass into the urine, resulting in proteinuria or hematuria. Activation of the coagulation system leads to fibrin deposits in Bowman's space. The result is formation of crescent-shaped blood cells and diminished renal blood flow and glomerular filtration rate (GFR). The presence of crescents signifies severe, often irreversible kidney damage. Glomerular bleeding acidifies the urine and thereby transforms hemoglobin to methemoglobin; the result is brown urine without clots.

The inflammatory response decreases GFR, which causes fluid retention and decreased urine output, extracellular fluid (ECF) volume expansion, and hypertension. Gross proteinuria is associated with nephrotic syndrome. After 10 to 20 years, renal insufficiency develops and is followed by nephrotic syndrome and end-stage renal failure.

RPGN may be idiopathic or associated with proliferative glomerular disease, such as poststreptococcal GN.

Chronic GN can slowly progress to the point of requiring renal dialysis. Conditions that can lead to chronic GN include poststreptococcal GN, RPGN, membranous GN, focal glomerulosclerosis, and membranoproliferative GN.

Signs and symptoms
- Decreased urination, smoky or coffee-colored urine
- Shortness of breath, dyspnea, orthopnea, bibasilar crackles
- Periorbital edema
- Mild to severe hypertension

AGE ALERT
An elderly patient with GN may report vague symptoms — nausea, malaise, or arthralgia.

Diagnostic tests
- Electrolyte, blood urea nitrogen, and creatinine
- Serum protein, serum complement, hemoglobin
- Antistreptolysin-O, streptozyme, and anti-DNAase B titers
- Urinalysis
- Fibrin-degradation products and C3 protein.
  Other tests:
- Throat culture for group A beta-hemolytic streptococcus
- Kidney-ureter-bladder X-ray , renal biopsy.

Treatment
- Treatment for primary disease, antibiotics for infections
- Bed rest to reduce metabolic demands
- Fluid and dietary sodium restriction, correction of electrolyte imbalances
- Loop diuretics, metolazone or furosemide, for ECF overload
- Vasodilators, hydralazine or nifedipine, for hypertension
- Corticosteroids to decrease antibody synthesis and suppress inflammatory response
- In RPGN, anticoagulants to control fibrin crescent formation; plasmapheresis to suppress rebound antibody production, possibly combined with corticosteroids and cyclophosphamide
- In chronic GN, dialysis or kidney transplantation.

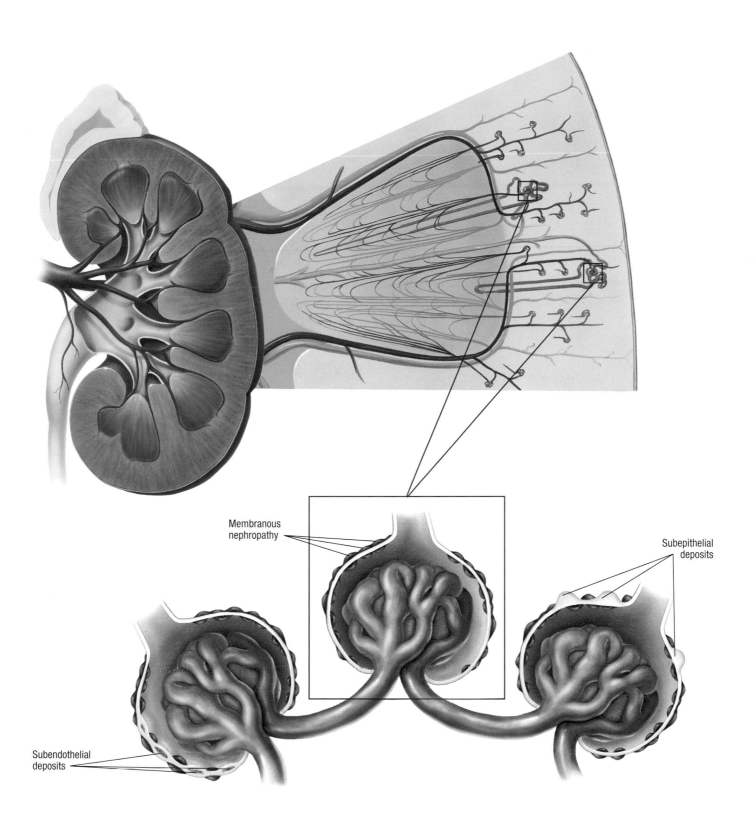

Membranous
nephropathy

Subepithelial
deposits

Subendothelial
deposits

HYDRONEPHROSIS

Hydronephrosis is an abnormal dilation of the renal pelvis and the calyces of one or both kidneys, caused by an obstruction of urine flow in the genitourinary tract. Although partial obstruction and hydronephrosis may not produce symptoms initially, the pressure built up behind the area of obstruction eventually results in symptomatic renal dysfunction.

Causes
- Almost any type of obstructive uropathy
- Most common:
- benign prostatic hyperplasia
- urethral strictures
- calculi
- Less common causes:
- strictures or stenosis of the ureter or bladder outlet congenital abnormalities
- trauma
- abdominal tumors
- blood clots
- neurogenic bladder.

Pathophysiology
If obstruction is in the urethra or bladder, hydronephrosis is usually bilateral; if obstruction is in a ureter, it's usually unilateral. Obstructions distal to the bladder cause the bladder to dilate and act as a buffer zone, delaying hydronephrosis. Total obstruction of urine flow with dilation of the collecting system ultimately causes complete cortical atrophy and cessation of glomerular filtration.

Signs and symptoms
Clinical features of hydronephrosis vary with the cause of the obstruction.
- No symptoms or mild pain and slightly decreased urinary flow
- Severe, colicky renal pain or dull flank pain that may radiate to the groin
- Gross urinary abnormalities, such as hematuria, pyuria, dysuria, alternating oliguria and polyuria, complete anuria
- Nausea, vomiting, abdominal fullness, pain on urination, dribbling, hesitancy.

Diagnostic tests
- Excretory urography
- Renal ultrasonography
- Renal function studies.

Treatment
- Surgical removal of the obstruction:
- dilation for stricture of the urethra
- prostatectomy for benign prostatic hyperplasia
- With renal damage: diet low in protein, sodium, and potassium to slow progression before surgery
- Inoperable obstructions: decompression and drainage of kidney through temporary or permanent nephrostomy tube in the renal pelvis
- Concurrent infection: appropriate antibiotic therapy.

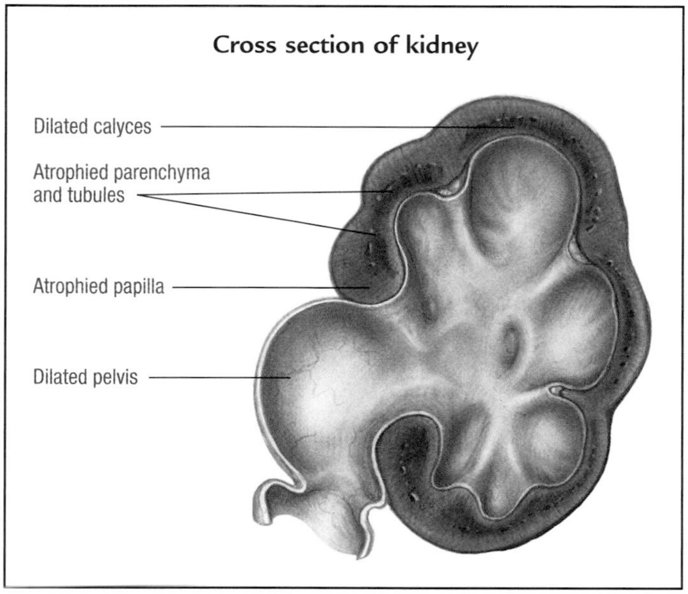

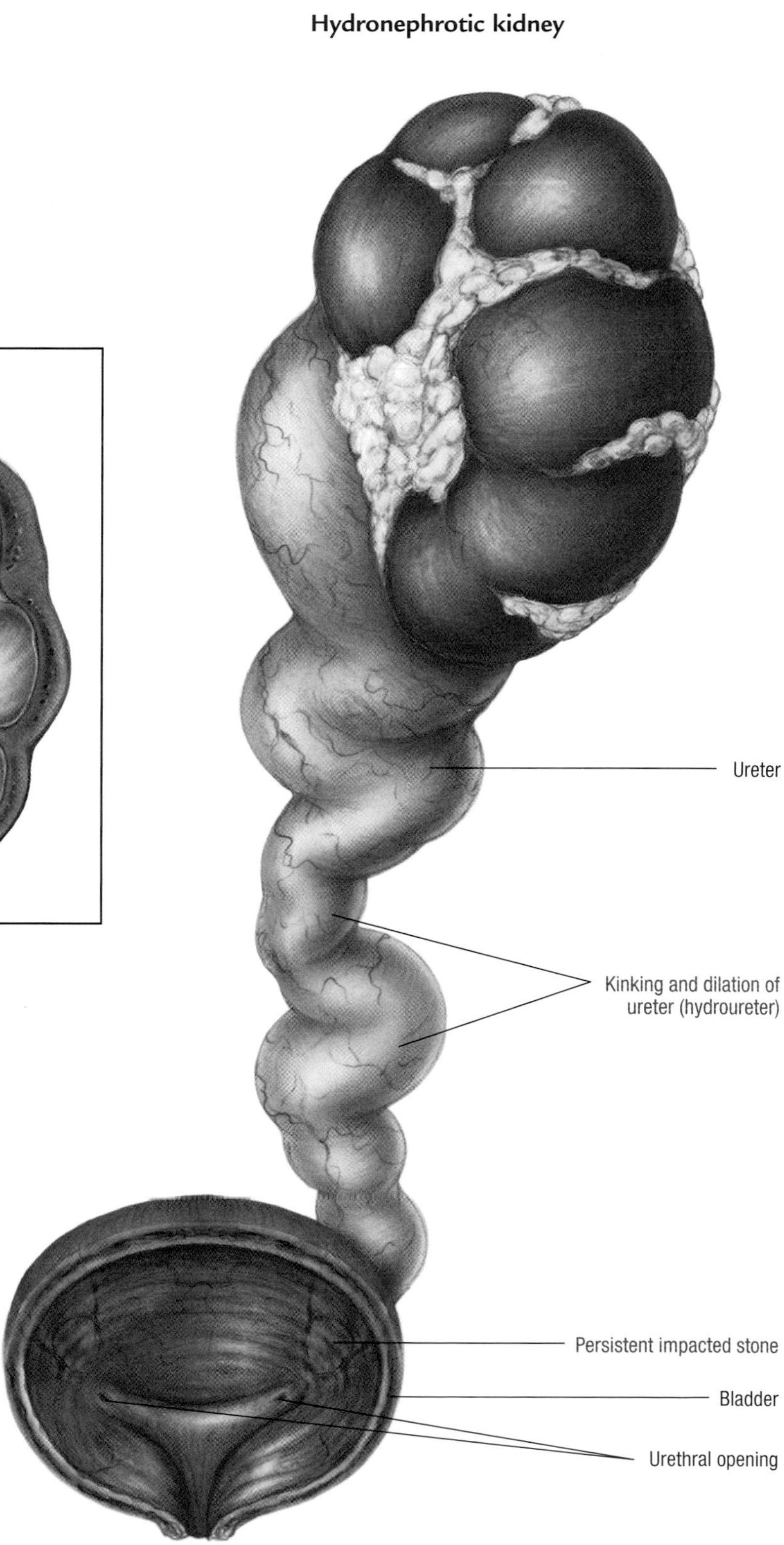

Hydronephrotic kidney

Cross section of kidney

Dilated calyces

Atrophied parenchyma
and tubules

Atrophied papilla

Dilated pelvis

Ureter

Kinking and dilation of
ureter (hydroureter)

Persistent impacted stone

Bladder

Urethral opening

POLYCYSTIC KIDNEY DISEASE

Polycystic kidney disease is an inherited disorder characterized by multiple, bilateral, grapelike clusters of fluid-filled cysts that enlarge the kidneys, compressing and eventually replacing functioning renal tissue. The disease affects males and females equally and appears in distinct infantile and adult-onset forms. The adult form, autosomal dominant polycystic kidney disease (ADPKD) occurs in 1 in 1,000 to 1 in 3,000 persons and accounts for about 10% of end-stage renal disease in the United States. Autosomal recessive polycystic kidney disease occurs in 1 in 10,000 to 1 in 40,000 live births. Renal deterioration is more gradual in adults than infants, but in both age-groups, the disease progresses relentlessly to fatal uremia.

AGE ALERT

The rare infantile form causes stillbirth or early neonatal death due to pulmonary hypoplasia. The adult form has an insidious onset. It usually becomes obvious between ages 30 and 50; rarely, it remains asymptomatic until the patient is in his 70s.

The prognosis in adults is extremely variable. Progression may be slow, even after symptoms of renal insufficiency appear. Once uremia symptoms develop, polycystic disease usually is fatal within 4 years, unless the patient receives dialysis.

Causes

● Autosomal dominant trait (adult type); 3 genetic variants identified
● Autosomal recessive trait (infantile type).

Pathophysiology

Grossly enlarged kidneys are caused by multiple spherical cysts, a few millimeters to centimeters in diameter, that contain straw-colored or hemorrhagic fluid. The cysts are distributed evenly throughout the cortex and medulla. Hyperplastic polyps and renal adenomas are common. Renal parenchyma may have varying degrees of tubular atrophy, interstitial fibrosis, and nephrosclerosis. The cysts cause elongation of the pelvis, flattening of the calyces, and indentations in the kidney.

Accompanying hepatic fibrosis and intrahepatic bile duct abnormalities may cause portal hypertension and bleeding varices. In most cases, about 10 years after symptoms appear, progressive compression of kidney structures by the enlarging mass causes renal failure.

Cysts also form on the liver, spleen, pancreas, or ovaries. Intracranial aneurysms, colonic diverticula, and mitral valve prolapse also occur.

Signs and symptoms

In neonates:
● Potter facies: pronounced epicanthic folds; pointed nose; small chin; floppy, low-set ears
● Huge, bilateral, symmetrical masses on the flanks that are tense and can't be transilluminated
● Signs of respiratory distress, heart failure, and, eventually, uremia and renal failure.
In adults:
● Hypertension
● Lumbar pain
● Widening abdominal girth
● Swollen or tender abdomen, worsened by exertion and relieved by lying down
● Grossly enlarged kidneys on palpation.

Diagnostic tests

● Excretory or retrograde urography
● Ultrasonography, tomography, and radioisotope scans
● Computed tomography scan, magnetic resonance imaging
● Urinalysis, creatinine clearance.

Treatment

● Antibiotics for infections
● Analgesics for abdominal pain
● Adequate hydration to maintain fluid balance
● Surgical drainage of cystic abscess or retroperitoneal bleeding
● Nephrectomy not recommended (polycystic kidney disease occurs bilaterally, and infection could recur in the remaining kidney)
● Dialysis or kidney transplantation for progressive renal failure.

Cross section

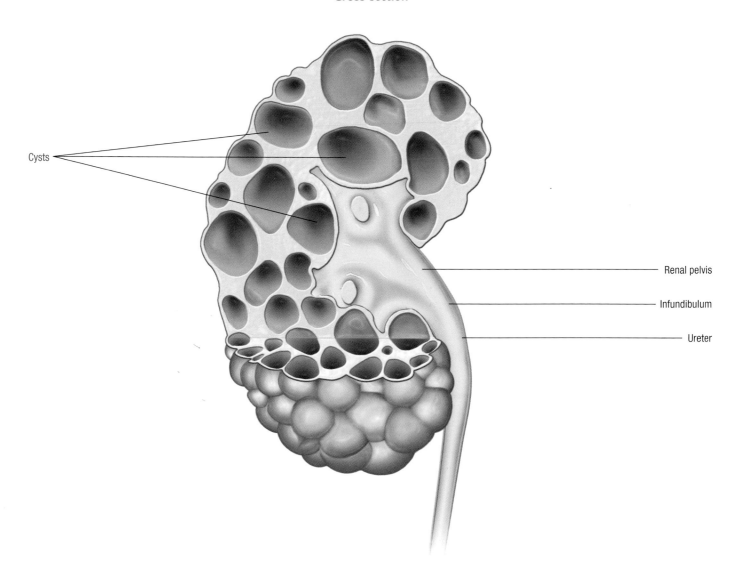

Cysts

Renal pelvis

Infundibulum

Ureter

PYELONEPHRITIS

Acute pyelonephritis (also known as acute infective tubulointerstitial nephritis) is a sudden inflammation caused by bacterial infection; it primarily affects the interstitial area and the renal pelvis or, less often, the renal tubules. It's one of the most common renal diseases. Symptoms characteristically develop rapidly over a few hours or a few days and may disappear within days, even without treatment. However, residual bacterial infection is likely and may cause symptoms to recur later. With treatment and continued follow-up care, the prognosis is good and extensive permanent damage is rare.

Causes

● Vesicoureteral reflux, which may result from congenital weakness at the junction of the ureter and the bladder
● Instrumentation, such as catheterization, cystoscopy, urologic surgery
● Hematogenic infection, as in septicemia or endocarditis
● Lymphatic infection
● Inability to empty the bladder, as in neurogenic bladder
● Urinary stasis
● Urinary obstruction due to tumor, stricture, or benign prostatic hyperplasia.

CLINICAL TIP

Pyelonephritis occurs more often in females, probably because bacteria reach the bladder more easily through the short female urethra; the urinary meatus is in close proximity to the vagina and the rectum, and women lack the male's antibacterial prostatic secretions.
Incidence increases with age and is higher in the following groups:
● *Sexually active women:* intercourse increases the risk of bacterial contamination.
● *Pregnant women:* about 5% develop asymptomatic bacteriuria; if untreated, about 40% develop pyelonephritis.
● *Persons with diabetes:* neurogenic bladder causes incomplete emptying and urinary stasis; glycosuria may support bacterial growth in the urine.
● *Persons with other renal diseases:* compromised renal function increases susceptibility.

Pathophysiology

Acute pyelonephritis results from bacterial infection of the kidneys. Infecting bacteria usually are normal intestinal and fecal flora that grow readily in urine. The most common causative organism is *Escherichia coli,* but *Proteus* or *Pseudomonas* species, *Staphylococcus aureus,* or *Enterococcus faecalis* (formerly *Streptococcus faecalis*) may also cause this infection.

Signs and symptoms

● Urgency, frequency, nocturia
● Burning during urination, dysuria
● Hematuria, usually microscopic but may be gross
● Cloudy urine, ammonia-like or fishy odor
● Fever of 102° F (38.9° C) or higher, shaking chills
● Flank pain
● Anorexia
● General fatigue.

AGE ALERT
Elderly patients may exhibit GI or pulmonary symptoms rather than the usual febrile responses to pyelonephritis.

In children younger than age 2, fever, vomiting, nonspecific abdominal complaints, or failure to thrive may be the only signs of acute pyelonephritis.

Diagnostic tests

● Urinalysis and culture
● Computed tomography scan of the kidney-ureter-bladder
● Excretory urography.

Treatment

Antibiotic therapy appropriate to the specific infecting organism after identification by urine culture and sensitivity studies:
● *Enterococcus* — ampicillin, penicillin G, vancomycin
● *Staphylococcus* — penicillin G; if resistance develops, a semisynthetic penicillin, such as nafcillin, or a cephalosporin
● *E. coli* — sulfisoxazole, nalidixic acid, nitrofurantoin
● *Proteus* — ampicillin, sulfisoxazole, nalidixic acid, a cephalosporin
● *Pseudomonas* — gentamicin, tobramycin, or carbenicillin
● Not identified — broad-spectrum antibiotic, such as ampicillin or cephalexin
● Pregnancy or renal insufficiency — antibiotics must be prescribed cautiously.
    Follow-up:
● Repeat urine culture 1 week after drug therapy stops, then periodically for the next year.
    Infection from obstruction or vesicoureteral reflux:
● Antibiotics may be less effective
● Surgery to relieve the obstruction or correct the anomaly.
    Patients at high risk of recurring urinary tract and kidney infections:
● Prolonged use of an indwelling catheter or maintenance antibiotic therapy
● Long-term follow-up to prevent chronic pyelonephritis.

3. End phase

Progressive
scarring

Atrophied
parenchyma

2. Progressive phase

**Acute pyelonephritis
and progressive scarring
from repeated infection**

Focal
parenchyma
scarring

Narrowed
calyx neck

1. Early phase
(edematous)

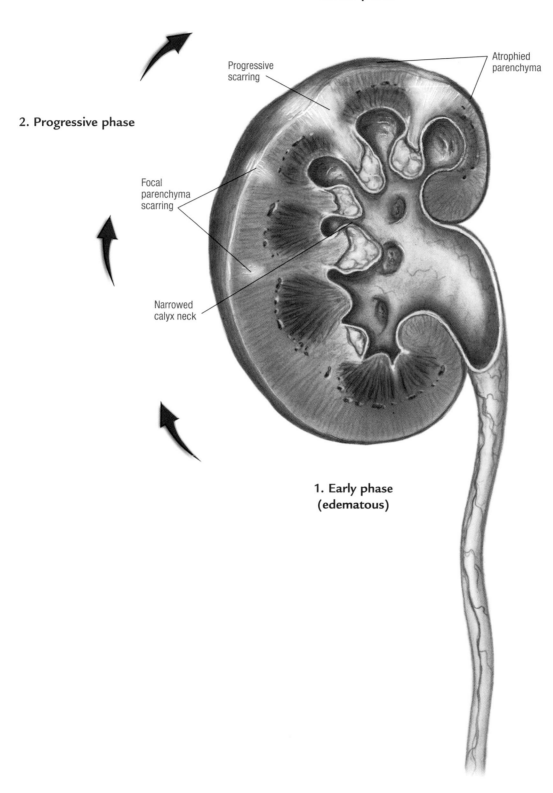

RENAL CALCULI

Renal calculi, or stones (nephrolithiasis), can form anywhere in the urinary tract, although they most commonly develop on the renal pelves or calyces. They may vary in size and may be single or multiple.

 AGE ALERT
Renal calculi are more common in men than in women and rarely occur in children. Calcium stones generally occur in middle-aged men with a familial history of stone formation.

Causes
Exact cause unknown.
Predisposing factors:
- Dehydration
- Infection
- Changes in urine pH (calcium carbonate stones, high pH; uric acid stones, lower pH)
- Obstruction to urine flow leading to stasis in the urinary tract
- Immobilization causing bone reabsorption
- Metabolic factors, such as hyperparathyroidism, renal tubular acidosis, elevated uric acid, defective oxalate metabolism
- Dietary factors, such as increased intake of calcium or of oxalate-rich foods
- Renal disease.

Pathophysiology
Calcium oxalate and calcium phosphate account for 75% to 80% of stones; struvite (magnesium, ammonium, and phosphate), 15%; uric acid, 7%; and cystine, 1% of all renal stones.

Calculi form when substances that are normally dissolved in the urine, such as calcium oxalate and calcium phosphate, precipitate. Dehydration may lead to renal calculi as calculus-forming substances concentrate in urine.

Stones form around a nucleus or nidus in the appropriate environment. A stone-forming substance (calcium oxalate, calcium carbonate, magnesium, ammonium, phosphate, uric acid, or cystine) forms a crystal that becomes trapped in the urinary tract, where it attracts other crystals to form a stone. A high urine saturation of these substances encourages crystal formation and results in stone growth. The pH of the urine affects the solubility of many stone-forming substances. Formation of calcium oxalate and cystine stones is independent of urine pH. Most stones are calcium oxalate or a combination of oxalate and phosphate.

Stones may form in the papillae, renal tubules, calyces, renal pelves, ureter, or bladder. Most are less than 5 mm in diameter and are usually passed in the urine. Staghorn calculi (casts of the calyceal and pelvic collecting system) can continue to grow in the pelvis, extending to the calyces, forming a branching stone, and ultimately resulting in renal failure if not surgically removed.

Calcium stones are the smallest. Although 80% are idiopathic, they frequently occur in patients with hyperuricosuria. Prolonged immobilization can lead to bone demineralization, hypercalciuria, and stone formation. In addition, hyperparathyroidism, renal tubular acidosis, and excessive intake of vitamin D or dietary calcium may predispose to renal calculi.

Struvite (magnesium, ammonium, and phosphate) stones are often precipitated by an infection, particularly with *Pseudomonas* or *Proteus* species. These urea-splitting organisms are more common in women. Struvite calculi can destroy renal parenchyma.

Signs and symptoms
- Severe pain from obstruction
- Nausea and vomiting
- Fever and chills from infection
- Hematuria when calculi abrade a ureter
- Abdominal distention
- Anuria from bilateral obstruction, or obstruction of only kidney.

Diagnostic tests
- Kidney-ureter-bladder radiography
- Excretory urography
- Kidney ultrasonography
- Urine culture
- 24-hour urine collection, for calcium oxalate, phosphorus, and uric acid excretion levels
- Calculus analysis for mineral content
- Serial blood calcium and phosphorus levels
- Serum protein level.

Treatment
- Fluid intake greater than 3 L/day to promote hydration
- Antimicrobial agents; vary with the cultured organism
- Analgesics, such as meperidine or morphine
- Diuretics to prevent urinary stasis and further calculus formation; thiazides to decrease calcium excretion
- Methenamine mandelate to suppress calculus formation when infection is present
- Cystoscopy and manipulation of calculus to remove stones too large for natural passage
- Percutaneous ultrasonic lithotripsy and extracorporeal shock wave lithotripsy or laser therapy to shatter the calculus into fragments for removal by suction or natural passage
- Surgical removal of cystine calculi or large stones
- Placement of urinary diversion around the stone.
Type specific treatment:
- Low-calcium diet
- Oxalate-binding cholestyramine
- Parathyroidectomy
- Allopurinol for uric acid calculi
- Daily small doses of ascorbic acid to acidify urine.

TYPES OF RENAL CALCULI

Uric acid stones

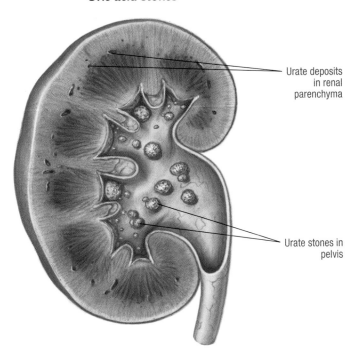

Urate deposits
in renal
parenchyma

Urate stones in
pelvis

Ammoniomagnesium phosphate (struvite) stones

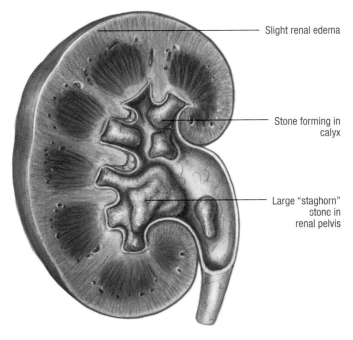

Slight renal edema

Stone forming in
calyx

Large "staghorn"
stone in
renal pelvis

Calcium stones

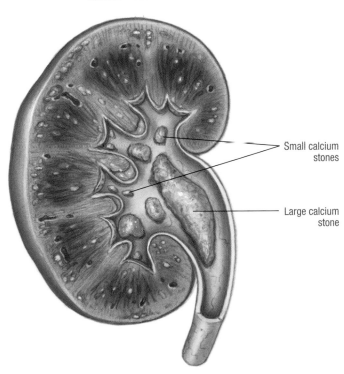

Small calcium
stones

Large calcium
stone

RENAL CANCER

Renal cancer (nephrocarcinoma, renal cell carcinoma, hyper-nephroma, Grawitz's tumor) usually occurs in older adults. Although the incidence of this malignancy is rising, it accounts for only about 2% of all adult cancers. Most renal tumors are metastases from primary cancer sites. Renal pelvic tumors and Wilms' tumor occur primarily in children. Kidney tumors are large, firm, nodular, encapsulated, unilateral, and solitary; they are classified histologically as clear-cell, granular, or spindle-cell tumors.

Causes
Primary cause unknown.
Predisposing factors:
- Tobacco use
- Environmental toxins
- Advancing age.

 AGE ALERT
Kidney cancer is more common in men than women and peaks in incidence between ages 50 and 70.

Pathophysiology
Renal cancers arise from tubular epithelium and can occur anywhere in the kidney. The tumor margins are usually clearly defined, and the tumors can include areas of ischemia, necrosis, and focal hemorrhage. Tumor cells vary from well differentiated to very anaplastic.

Signs and symptoms
Classic clinical triad:
- Hematuria — microscopic or gross; may be intermittent; suggests spread to renal pelvis
- Pain — constant abdominal or flank pain; may be dull; if cancer causes bleeding or blood clots, acute and colicky
- Palpable mass — generally smooth, firm, and nontender
- All three coexist in only about 10% of patients.
  Other signs:
- Fever
- Hypertension
- Rapidly progressing hypercalcemia
- Urine retention, edema in the legs
- Nausea, vomiting, weight loss.

Diagnostic tests
- Computed tomography scans
- I.V. and retrograde pyelography
- Ultrasonography
- Cystoscopy to rule out associated bladder cancer
- Nephrotomography or renal angiography
- Liver function studies: alkaline phosphatase, bilirubin, alanine aminotransferase, aspartate aminotransferase, prothrombin time
- Routine laboratory tests: urinalysis, complete blood count, serum calcium, erythrocyte sedimentation rate.

Treatment
- Radical nephrectomy, with or without regional lymph node dissection — the only chance of cure
- High-dose radiation — used only if the cancer spreads to the perinephric region or the lymph nodes or if the primary tumor or metastatic sites can't be fully excised
- Chemotherapy — results usually poor against kidney cancer
- Biotherapy (interferon and interleukins) — often used in advanced disease; has produced few durable remissions.

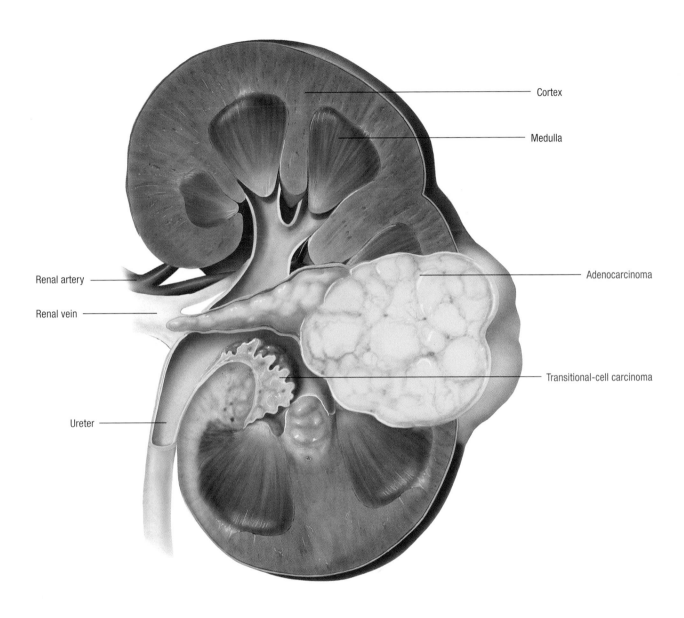

Cortex

Medulla

Renal artery

Renal vein

Adenocarcinoma

Transitional-cell carcinoma

Ureter

RENAL FAILURE

Acute renal failure, the sudden interruption of renal function, can be caused by obstruction, poor circulation, or underlying kidney disease. It may be prerenal, intrarenal, or postrenal in origin; it usually passes through three distinct phases: oliguric, diuretic, and recovery.

Causes

Prerenal failure:
- Arrhythmias, cardiac tamponade, cardiogenic shock, heart failure, myocardial infarction
- Burns, trauma, sepsis, tumor
- Dehydration, hypovolemic shock
- Diuretic overuse, antihypertensive drugs
- Hemorrhage, arterial embolism, arterial or venous thrombosis, vasculitis
- Disseminated intravascular coagulation
- Eclampsia, malignant hypertension.
  Intrarenal failure:
- Poorly treated prerenal failure
- Nephrotoxins
- Obstetric complications
- Crush injuries
- Myopathy
- Transfusion reaction
- Acute glomerulonephritis, acute interstitial nephritis, acute pyelonephritis, bilateral renal vein thrombosis, malignant nephrosclerosis, papillary necrosis
- Polyarteritis nodosa
- Renal myeloma
- Sickle cell disease
- Systemic lupus erythematosus
- Vasculitis.
  Postrenal failure:
- Bladder, ureteral, or urethral obstruction.

Pathophysiology

Prerenal failure ensues when a condition that diminishes blood flow to the kidneys causes hypoperfusion. Examples include hypovolemia, hypotension, vasoconstriction, or inadequate cardiac output. When renal blood flow is interrupted, so is oxygen delivery. The ensuing hypoxemia and ischemia can rapidly and irreversibly damage the kidney. The tubules are most susceptible to the effects of hypoxemia. Azotemia develops in 40% to 80% of all cases of acute renal failure.

Intrarenal failure, also called intrinsic or parenchymal renal failure, results from damage to the filtering structures of the kidneys. Causes of intrarenal failure are classified as nephrotoxic, inflammatory, or ischemic. When the damage is caused by nephrotoxicity or inflammation, the delicate layer under the epithelium (the basement membrane) becomes irreparably damaged, often leading to chronic renal failure. Severe or prolonged lack of blood flow by ischemia may lead to renal damage (ischemic parenchymal injury) and excess nitrogen in the blood (intrinsic renal azotemia).

Postrenal failure is a consequence of bilateral obstruction of urine outflow. The cause may be in the bladder, ureters, or urethra.

Signs and symptoms

Acute renal failure:
- Oliguria
- Tachycardia and hypotension
- Dry mucous membranes and flat neck veins
- Lethargy
- Cool, clammy skin.
  Progressive disease:
- Edema
- Confusion
- GI symptoms
- Crackles
- Infection
- Seizures and coma
- Hematuria, petechiae, ecchymosis.

Diagnostic tests

- Blood studies: BUN, serum creatinine, potassium, bicarbonate, hematocrit, and hemoglobin, pH, serum osmolality
- Urinalysis; protein, osmolality, sodium
- Creatinine clearance
- Electrocardiogram
- Ultrasonography
- X-ray of abdomen; kidney-ureter-bladder radiography
- Excretory urography, retrograde pyelography
- Renal scan, computed tomographic scan, nephrotomography.

Treatment

- High-calorie diet low in protein, sodium, and potassium
- Electrolyte imbalance: I.V. fluids and electrolytes; hemodialysis or peritoneal dialysis if needed
- Edema: fluid restriction
- Oliguria: diuretic therapy
- With mild hyperkalemic symptoms (malaise, anorexia, muscle weakness): sodium polystyrene sulfonate by mouth or enema
- With severe hyperkalemic symptoms (numbness and tingling and electrocardiogram changes): hypertonic glucose, insulin, and sodium bicarbonate I.V.

 CLINICAL TIP
Chronic renal failure is usually the end result of gradual tissue destruction and loss of kidney function. It can also result from a rapidly progressing disease of sudden onset that destroys the nephrons and causes irreversible kidney damage.

Few symptoms develop while more than 25% of glomerular filtration remains. The normal parenchyma then deteriorates rapidly, and symptoms worsen as renal function decreases. This syndrome is fatal without treatment, but maintenance on dialysis or a kidney transplant can sustain life.

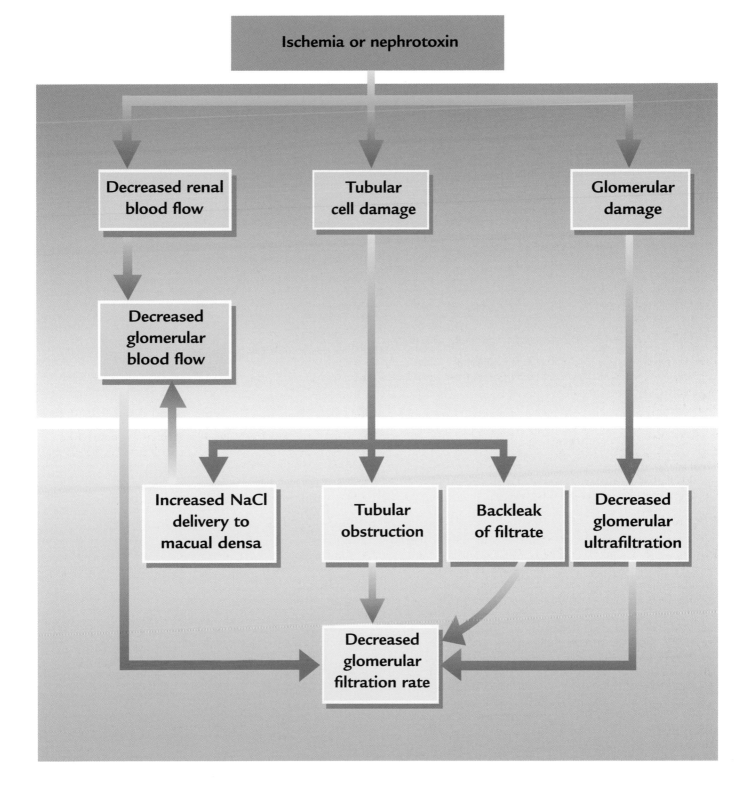

RENOVASCULAR HYPERTENSION

Renovascular hypertension is a rise in systemic blood pressure resulting from stenosis of the major renal arteries or their branches or from intrarenal atherosclerosis. The narrowing or sclerosis may be partial or complete, and the resulting blood pressure elevation, benign or malignant. Approximately 5% to 10% of patients with high blood pressure display renovascular hypertension; it's most common in persons under age 30 or over age 50.

Causes

In 95% of all patients with renovascular hypertension:
- Atherosclerosis (especially in older men)
- Fibromuscular diseases of the renal artery wall layers, such as medial fibroplasia and, less commonly, intimal or subadventitial fibroplasia.

   Other causes:
- Arteritis
- Anomalies of renal arteries
- Embolism
- Trauma
- Tumor
- Dissecting aneurysm.

Pathophysiology

Stenosis or occlusion of the renal artery stimulates the affected kidney to release the enzyme renin, which converts the plasma protein angiotensinogen to angiotensin I. As angiotensin I circulates through the lungs and liver, it is converted to angiotensin II, which causes peripheral vasoconstriction, increased arterial pressure and aldosterone secretion and, eventually, hypertension.

Signs and symptoms

- Elevated systemic blood pressure
- Headache, light-headedness
- Palpitations, tachycardia
- Anxiety, mental sluggishness
- Decreased tolerance of temperature extremes
- Retinopathy
- Significant complications: heart failure, myocardial infarction, cerebrovascular accident, renal failure.

Diagnostic tests

- Arterial digital subtraction angiography (DSA); when stenosis is significant, concurrent transluminal angioplasty
- Venous renin assay
- Gandolitium enhanced magnetic resonance angiography (MRA)
- Duplex Doppler ultrasonography
- Oral captopril renography.

Treatment

- Surgery to restore adequate circulation and to control severe hypertension or severely impaired renal function:
  - renal artery bypass, endarterectomy, arterioplasty
  - as a last resort, nephrectomy
- Balloon catheter renal artery dilation in selected cases to correct renal artery stenosis without risks and morbidity of surgery
- Symptomatic measures: antihypertensives, diuretics, and a sodium-restricted diet.

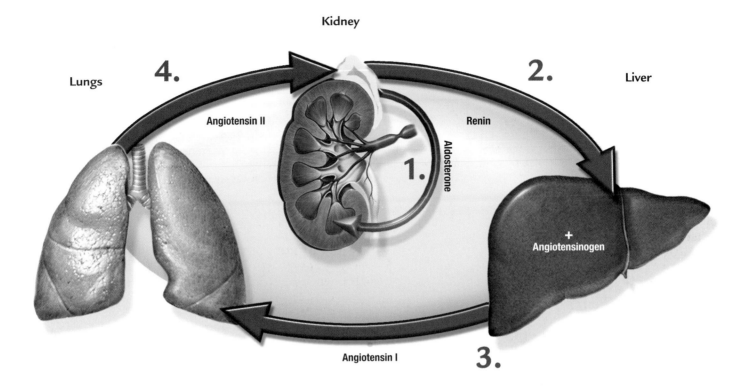

Kidney

Lungs **4.**

Angiotensin II

Renin

2. Liver

Aldosterone

1.

+
Angiotensinogen

Angiotensin I **3.**

Mechanism of renovascular hypertension

1. Renal artery stenosis causes reduction of blood flow to kidneys.
2. Kidneys secrete renin in response.
3. Renin combines with angiotensinogen in the liver to form angiotensin I.
4. In the lungs, angiotensin I is converted to angiotensin II, a vasoconstrictor.

ACNE

Acne is an inflammatory disease of the pilosebaceous units (hair follicles). It occurs on areas of the body that have sebaceous glands, such as the face, neck, chest, back, and shoulders and is associated with a high rate of sebum secretion. When sebum blocks a hair follicle, one of two types of acne ensues. In *inflammatory* acne, bacterial growth in the blocked follicle leads to inflammation and eventual rupture of the follicle; in *noninflammatory* acne, the follicle remains dilated by accumulating secretions but doesn't rupture.

 AGE ALERT
Acne occurs in both males and females. *Acne vulgaris* develops in 80% to 90% of adolescents or young adults, primarily between ages 15 and 18, although the lesions can appear as early as age 8.

Causes
- Multifactorial; diet not believed to be a factor.
  Predisposing factors:
- Heredity
- Androgen stimulation
- Certain drugs, including corticosteroids, corticotropin, androgens, iodides, bromides, trimethadione, phenytoin, isoniazid, lithium, halothane
- Exposure to heavy oils, greases, tars, cosmetics
- Cobalt irradiation
- Hyperalimentation
- Trauma; skin friction from tight clothing
- Emotional stress
- Oral contraceptive use may exacerbate acne in some women.

Pathophysiology
Androgens stimulate sebaceous gland growth, sebum production, and shedding of the epithelial cells that line sebaceous follicles. The stimulated follicles become dilated, and sebum and keratin from the epithelial cells form a plug that seals the follicle, creating a favorable environment for bacterial growth. The bacteria, usually *Propionibacterium acne* or *Staphylococcus epidermis,* are normal skin flora that secrete lipase. This enzyme interacts with sebum to produce free fatty acids, which provoke inflammation and formation of open or closed comedos, which may rupture.

Signs and symptoms
- Closed comedo, or whitehead; does not protrude from follicle, covered by epidermis
- Open comedo, or blackhead; protrudes from the follicle, not covered by epidermis; melanin or pigment of the follicle causes the black color
- Rupture or leakage of comedo into the epidermis:
- inflammation
- pustules, papules
- in severe forms, cysts or abscesses (chronic, recurring lesions producing acne scars).

Diagnostic tests
Acne vulgaris is confirmed by characteristic acne lesions, especially in adolescents.

Treatment
- Gentle cleansing with a sponge to dislodge superficial comedones.
  Topical agents for mild acne:
- Antibacterial agents, such as benzyl peroxide gels (2%, 5% or 10%), clindamycin, or erythromycin
- Keratolytic agents:
- dry and peel the skin to open blocked follicles and release sebum
- benzyl peroxide, tretinoin.
  Systemic therapy for moderate to severe acne:
- Tetracycline or minocycline
- Oral isotretinoin to inhibit sebaceous gland function and abnormal keratinization; has severe adverse effects, which limit its use to patients with severe papulopustular or cystic acne not responding to conventional therapy
- For females, antiandrogens: birth control pills, such as norgestimate/ethinyl estradiol or spironolactone.
  For severe acne:
- Surgery (usually outpatient) to remove comedones and to open and drain pustules
- For severe scarring: dermabrasion or laser resurfacing to smooth the skin
- Bovine collagen injections into dermis beneath scarred area to fill in pitted areas and smooth skin surface (not recommended by all dermatologists).

HOW ACNE DEVELOPS

Excessive sebum production

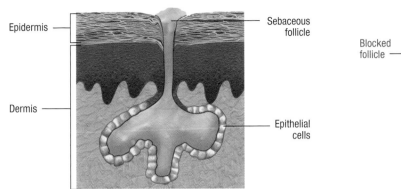

Epidermis

Dermis

Sebaceous follicle

Epithelial cells

Increased shedding of epithelial cells

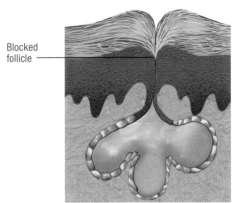

Blocked follicle

Inflammatory response in follicle

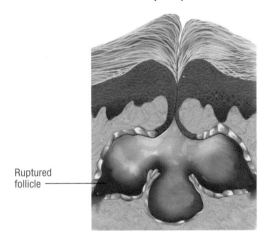

Ruptured follicle

COMEDONES OF ACNE

Closed comedo (whitehead)   ### Open comedo (blackhead)

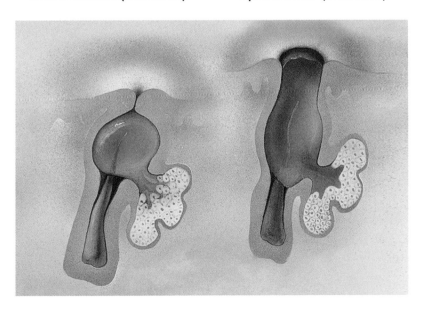

ATOPIC DERMATITIS

Atopic (allergic) dermatitis (also called atopic or infantile eczema) is a chronic or recurrent inflammatory response often associated with other atopic diseases, such as bronchial asthma and allergic rhinitis. It usually develops in infants and toddlers between ages 1 month and 1 year, usually in those with a strong family history of atopic disease. These children often develop other atopic disorders as they grow older.

Typically, this form of dermatitis flares and subsides repeatedly before finally resolving during adolescence, but it can persist into adulthood.

Causes

Exact etiology unknown; genetic predisposition likely.
Possible contributing factors:
- Food allergy
- Infection
- Chemical irritants
- Extremes of temperature and humidity
- Psychological stress or strong emotions.

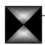

AGE ALERT
About 10% of childhood cases of atopic dermatitis are caused by allergy to certain foods, especially eggs, peanuts, milk, or wheat.

Pathophysiology

The allergic mechanism of hypersensitivity results in a release of inflammatory mediators through sensitized antibodies of the immunoglobulin E (IgE) class. Histamine and other cytokines induce acute inflammation. Abnormally dry skin and a decreased threshold for itching set up the "itch-scratch-itch" cycle, which eventually causes lesions (excoriations, lichenification).

Signs and symptoms

- Erythematous areas on excessively dry skin; in children, typically on the forehead, cheeks, and extensor surfaces of the arms and legs; in adults, at flexion points (antecubital fossa, popliteal area, and neck)
- Edema, crusting, scaling due to pruritus and scratching
- Multiple areas of dry, scaly skin, with white dermatographia, blanching, and lichenification with chronic atrophic lesions
- Pinkish, swollen upper eyelid and double fold under lower lid
- Viral, fungal, or bacterial infections and ocular disorders can be secondary conditions.

Diagnostic tests

Diagnosis of atopic dermatitis involves careful history and physical exam. Elevated serum IgE levels are not diagnostic.

Treatment

- Eliminating allergens and avoiding irritants (strong soaps, cleansers, and other chemicals), extreme temperature changes, and other precipitating factors
- Preventing excessive dryness of the skin (critical to successful therapy)
- Topical tar preparations in a lubricating base (contraindicated on intensely inflamed or open lesions)
- Topical corticosteroid ointment, especially after bathing, to alleviate inflammation; moisturizing cream between steroid doses to help retain moisture.

AGE ALERT
Chronic use of potent fluorinated corticosteroids may cause striae or skin atrophy in children.

- Systemic antihistamines, such as diphenhydramine
- Systemic corticosteroid therapy during extreme exacerbations
- Ultraviolet B (UVB) or psoraten plus ultraviolet A (PUVA) therapy
- In severe adult-onset disease, cyclosporine A may work if other treatments fail
- Antibiotics if skin culture positive for bacteria.

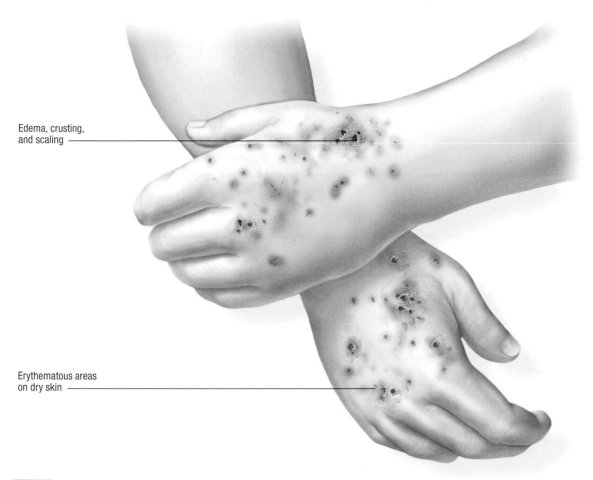

Edema, crusting, and scaling

Erythematous areas on dry skin

 CLINICAL TIP

RECOGNIZING ATOPIC DERMATITIS

In children with atopic dermatitis, severe pruritis leads to characteristic pink pigmentation and swelling of upper eyelid and a double fold under the lower lid (Morgan's line, Dennie's sign, or mongolian fold).

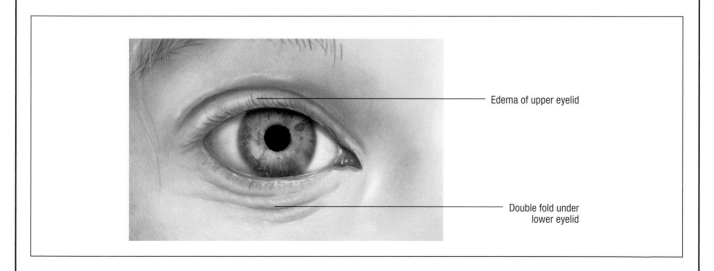

Edema of upper eyelid

Double fold under lower eyelid

Burns

Burns are classified into four degrees according to the extent of skin and tissue damage.

Causes
- Thermal: residential fires, automobile accidents, playing with matches, improper handling of firecrackers, scalds caused by kitchen or bathroom accidents
- Chemical: contact, ingestion, inhalation, or injection of acids, alkalis, or vesicants
- Electrical: contact with faulty electrical wiring, electrical cords or high-voltage power lines
- Friction or abrasion
- Ultraviolet radiation: sunburn.

Pathophysiology
The injuring agent denatures all cellular proteins. Some cells die because of traumatic or ischemic necrosis. Denaturation also disrupts collagen cross-links in connective tissue. The consequent abnormal osmotic and hydrostatic pressure gradients force intravascular fluid into interstitial spaces. Cellular injury triggers the release of mediators of inflammation, further contributing to local or systemic increases in capillary permeability.

First-degree burns. Localized injury to or destruction of epidermis by direct (such as chemical spill) or indirect (such as sunlight) contact. This type of burn is not life-threatening.

Second-degree superficial partial-thickness burns. Destruction of epidermis and some of the upper area of the dermis. Thin-walled, fluid-filled blisters develop within minutes of the injury. As these blisters break, the nerve endings become exposed to air. Pain and tactile responses remain intact; treatments can be painful. The barrier function of the skin is lost.

Second-degree deep partial-thickness burns. Destruction of epidermis and more of the dermis, producing blisters and mild to moderate edema and pain. Hair follicles are still intact, so hair will grow again. Less pain sensation with this burn because sensory neurons have been extensively destroyed. Areas around injury remain sensitive to pain. The barrier function of skin is lost.

Third- and fourth-degree burns. Affect every body system and organ. A third-degree burn extends through the epidermis and dermis and into the subcutaneous tissue layer; a fourth-degree burn damages muscle, bone, and interstitial tissues. Within hours, fluids and protein shift from capillary to interstitial spaces, causing edema. An immediate immunologic response to injury makes wound sepsis a potential threat. An increase in metabolic rate after a burn injury mandates aggressive nutritional support.

Signs and symptoms
- First-degree burn — localized pain and erythema, usually without blisters in the first 24 hours
- More severe first-degree burn — chills, headache, localized edema, nausea, vomiting
- Second-degree superficial partial-thickness burn — thin-walled, fluid-filled blisters appear within minutes of injury; mild to moderate edema and pain

- Second-degree deep partial-thickness burn — white, waxy appearance of damaged area
- Third- and fourth-degree burns — white, brown, or black leathery tissue; visible thrombosed vessels; no blisters
- Electrical burn — silver-colored, raised area, usually at the site of electrical contact
- Smoke inhalation and pulmonary damage — singed nasal hairs, mucosal burns, voice changes, coughing, wheezing, soot in mouth or nose, and darkened sputum.

Clinically, burn damage is estimated by using the Rule of Nines chart to calculate the percentage of damaged body surface area (BSA) and the Lund-Browder chart to estimate severity by correlating a burn's depth and size.

Minor burns:
- Third-degree burns on less than 2% of BSA
- Second-degree burns on less than 15% of adult BSA (less than 10% in children).

Moderate burns:
- Third-degree burns on 2% to 10% of BSA
- Second-degree burns on 15% to 25% of adult BSA (10% to 20% in children).

Major burns:
- Third-degree burns on more than 10% of BSA
- Second-degree burns on more than 25% of adult BSA (over 20% in children)
- Burns of hands, face, feet, or genitalia
- Burns complicated by fractures or respiratory damage
- Electrical burns
- All burns in poor-risk patients.

Diagnostic tests
- Complete blood count, electrolytes, glucose, blood urea nitrogen, serum creatinine levels
- Arterial blood gas analysis
- Blood type and cross-matching
- Urinalysis for myoglobin and hemoglobin.

Treatment
- Minor burns — immersion of burned area in cool water (55°F [12.8°C]) or application of cool compresses
- First immediate treatment for moderate and major burns — maintain an open airway, endotracheal intubation, 100% oxygen
- Immediate I.V. therapy to prevent hypovolemic shock and maintain cardiac output (lactated Ringer's solution or a fluid replacement formula; additional I.V. lines may be needed)
- Partial-thickness burns over 30% of BSA or full-thickness burns over 5% of BSA — cover patient with a clean, dry, sterile bed sheet to help preserve body temperature; *do not* cover large burns with saline-soaked dressings
- Debridement followed by application of antimicrobial and nonstick bulky dressing; tetanus prophylaxis if needed
- Pain or anti-inflammatory medication as needed
- Major burns — systemic antimicrobial therapy.

CLASSIFICATION OF BURNS BY DEPTH OF INJURY

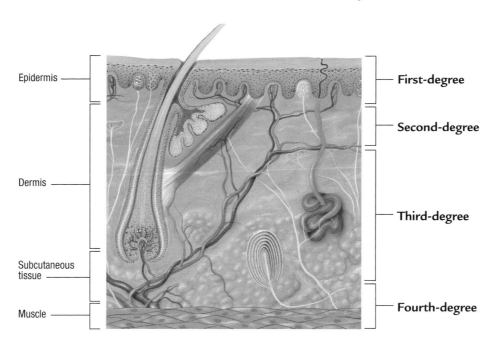

Epidermis — First-degree

Dermis — Second-degree

— Third-degree

Subcutaneous tissue — Fourth-degree

Muscle

⟩⟩⟩ CLINICAL TIP

ESTIMATING THE EXTENT OF BURNS

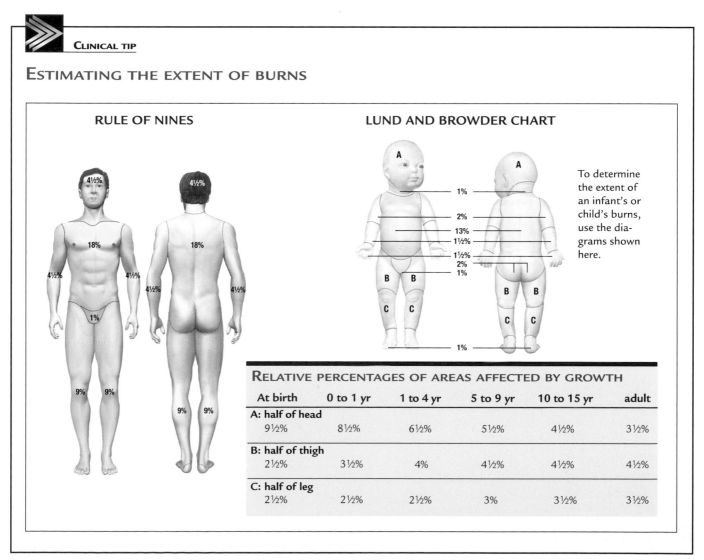

RULE OF NINES

LUND AND BROWDER CHART

To determine the extent of an infant's or child's burns, use the diagrams shown here.

RELATIVE PERCENTAGES OF AREAS AFFECTED BY GROWTH

	At birth	0 to 1 yr	1 to 4 yr	5 to 9 yr	10 to 15 yr	adult
A: half of head	9½%	8½%	6½%	5½%	4½%	3½%
B: half of thigh	2½%	3½%	4%	4½%	4½%	4½%
C: half of leg	2½%	2½%	2½%	3%	3½%	3½%

CELLULITIS

Cellulitis is an acute, spreading infection of the dermis or subcutaneous layer of the skin. It may follow damage to the skin, such as a bite or wound. As the cellulitis spreads, fever, erythema, and lymphangitis may occur. Persons with contributing health problems, such as diabetes, immunodeficiency, or impaired circulation, have an increased risk. If treated promptly, the prognosis is usually good.

 AGE ALERT
Cellulitis of the lower extremity is more likely to develop into thrombophlebitis in an elderly patient.

Causes
- Bacterial infections, commonly with group A streptococcus or *Staphylococcus aureus*
- Uncommonly, fungal infections.

Pathophysiology
As the offending organism invades the compromised area, it overwhelms the normal defensive cells (neutrophils, eosinophils, basophils, and mast cells) that normally contain and localize inflammation, and cellular debris accumulates. As cellulitis progresses, the organism invades tissue around the initial wound site.

Signs and symptoms
- Classic signs: erythema and edema due to inflammatory response
- Pain at site and possibly in surrounding area
- Fever and warmth.

Diagnostic tests
- White blood cell count
- Erythrocyte sedimentation rate
- Gram stain and culture of fluid from abscesses and bulla
- Culture of primary lesion by biopsy or aspiration
- "Touch" preparation — skin lesion specimen touched to microscope slide; application of KOH; examination for yeast and mycelial forms of fungus.

Treatment
- Oral or I.V. penicillin (drug of choice for initial treatment) unless patient has known penicillin allergy; antifungal medications if necessary
- Warm soaks to the site to help relieve pain and decrease edema by increasing vasodilation
- Pain medication as needed
- Elevation of infected extremity.

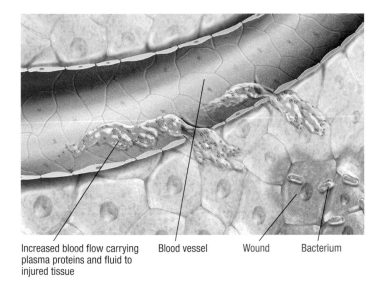

Increased blood flow carrying plasma proteins and fluid to injured tissue   Blood vessel   Wound   Bacterium

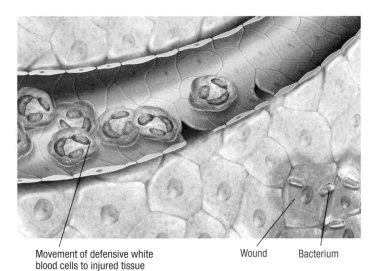

Movement of defensive white blood cells to injured tissue   Wound   Bacterium

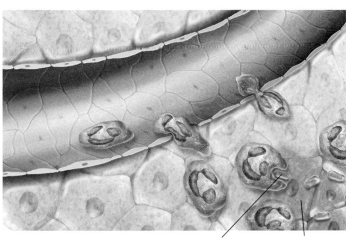

Phagocyte engulfing bacterium   Wound

CLINICAL TIP

RECOGNIZING CELLULITIS

The classic signs of cellulitis, a spreading soft tissue infection, are erythema and edema surrounding the initial wound. The tissue is warm to the touch.

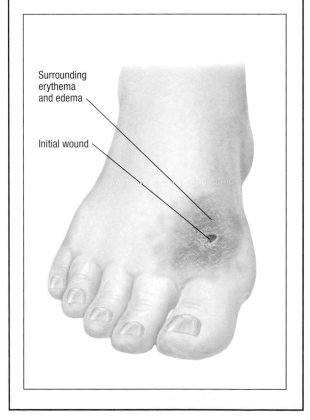

Surrounding erythema and edema

Initial wound

FOLLICULITIS, FURUNCLES, CARBUNCLES

Folliculitis is a bacterial infection in the upper portion of a hair follicle that causes a pustule to form. The infection can be superficial (follicular impetigo or Bockhart's impetigo) or deep (sycosis barbae). Furuncles, also known as boils, are another form of deep folliculitis. Carbuncles are a group of interconnected furuncles.

With appropriate treatment, the prognosis for patients with folliculitis is good. The disorder usually resolves within 2 to 3 weeks. The prognosis for patients with carbuncles depends on the severity of the infection and the patient's physical condition and ability to resist infection.

Causes
- Coagulase-positive *Staphylococcus aureus* (most common)
- *Klebsiella*, *Enterobacter*, or *Proteus* organisms (gram-negative folliculitis in patients on long-term antibiotic therapy, such as for acne)
- *Pseudomonas aeruginosa* (thrives in warm environment with high pH and low chlorine content—"hot-tub folliculitis").
    Predisposing risk factors include:
- Infected wound, poor hygiene
- Chronic staphylococcus carrier state in nares, axillae, perineum, bowel
- Diabetes
- Debilitation
- Immunosuppressive therapy, defects in chemotaxis, hyper-IgE syndrome
- Tight clothes, friction.

Pathophysiology
The affecting organism enters the body, usually at a break in the skin barrier (such as a wound site). The organism then causes an inflammatory reaction within the hair follicle.

Signs and symptoms
Folliculitis:
- In children: pustules on scalp, arms, legs
- In adults: pustules on trunk, buttocks, legs.
    Furuncles:

- Hard, painful nodules, commonly on neck, face, axillae, buttocks
- Nodules enlarge for several days, then rupture, discharging pus and necrotic material
- After rupture, pain subsides; erythema and edema persist for days or weeks.
    Carbuncles (now rare):
- Extremely painful, deep abscesses draining through multiple openings onto the skin surface, usually around several hair follicles
- Fever and malaise.

Diagnostic tests
- Wound cultures
- White blood cell count.

Treatment
- Thorough cleaning of infected area with antibacterial soap and water
- Warm, wet compresses to promote vasodilation and drainage
- Topical antibiotics, such as mupirocin ointment or clindamycin or erythromycin solution.
    Specific treatments:
- Extensive folliculitis: systemic antibiotics, such as a cephalosporin or dicloxacillin
- Furuncles (ripe lesions):
- warm, wet compresses
- incision and drainage
- systemic antibiotic
- Carbuncles:
- incision and drainage
- systemic antibiotic therapy.

DISTINGUISHING FOLLICULITIS, FURUNCLES, AND CARBUNCLES

Superficial folliculitis
- Erythema
- Pustule
- Single-follicle involvement

Deep folliculitis
- Extensive follicular involvement

Furuncle
- Red, tender nodule surrounding a follicle
- Single draining point

Carbuncle
- Deep follicular abscesses of several follicles
- Several draining points

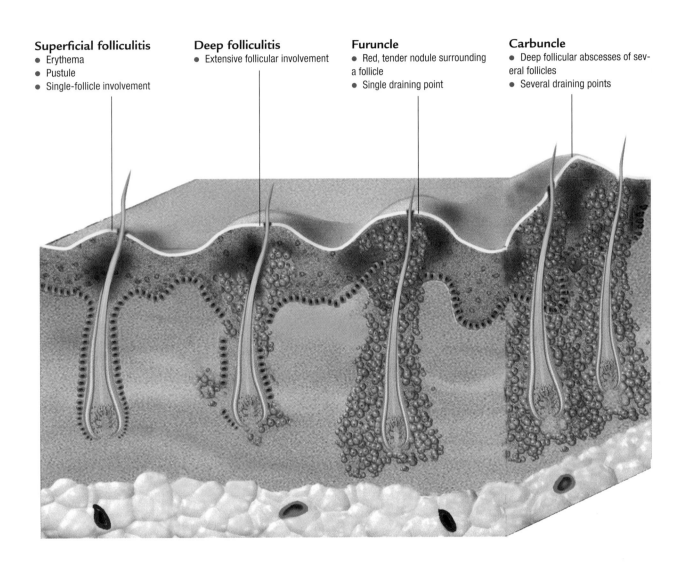

Fungal infections

Fungal infections of the skin are often regarded as superficial infections affecting the hair, nails, and stratum corneum (the dead top layer of the skin). Fungi infect and survive only on the nonviable keratin within these structures. The most common fungal infections are dermatophyte infections (tineas) and candidiasis.

Tinea infections are classified by the body location in which they occur; for example:
- *capitis*, scalp
- *corporis*, body
- *pedis*, foot
- *cruris*, groin.

Some forms infect one gender more commonly than the other. For example, tinea cruris is more common in males. Obesity and diabetes predispose to tinea infection.

 AGE ALERT
Tinea commonly infects children and adolescents. Elderly patients are also at greater risk for these infections.

Candidiasis of the skin or mucous membranes is also classified according to the infected site or area:
- intertrigo — axilla or inner aspect of thigh
- balanoposthities — glans penis and prepuce
- vulvitis
- diaper dermatitis
- paronychia, folds of skin at margin of a nail
- onychia — nailbed
- thrush — mouth.

Candida organisms may be normal flora of the skin, mouth, GI tract, or genitalia.

Candidiasis usually occurs in children and immunosuppressed individuals. Infection rates are also higher in pregnant women, in patients with diabetes mellitus, and in those with indwelling catheters or I.V. lines.

The prognoses for tinea infection and candidiasis are very good. They usually respond well to appropriate drug therapy and resolve completely. It's important to reduce risk factors to obtain a good outcome from the infection. Antifungal therapy usually resolves candidiasis, but if risk factors aren't avoided, a chronic condition can develop.

Causes
- *Tinea* or *Candida* fungus

Risk factors for *Tinea (Microsporum, Trichophyton,* or *Epidermophyton)* infection:
- Obesity
- Softened skin from prolonged water contact, as in water sports or diaphoresis
- Atopy, immunosuppression
- Antibiotic therapy with suppression of normal flora

Risk factors for *Candida* infection:
- Depletion of normal flora (such as after antibiotic therapy)
- Neutropenia and bone marrow suppression in immunocompromised patients (at greater risk for the disseminating form).

Pathophysiology
Tinea infection: The fungi attack the outer, dead skin layers. They grow best in a dark, warm, moist environment. Tinea infections can spread from human to human, animal to human, or soil to human. Tinea corporis, for example, can be contracted from animals infected with *Microsporium canis* or *Trichophyton mentagrophytes* or from humans infected with *Trichophyton rubrum*.

Candidiasis: The organism penetrates the epidermis after binding to integrin receptors and adhesion molecules and then secreting proteolytic enzymes, which facilitate tissue invasion. An inflammatory response results from the attraction of neutrophils to the area and from activation of the complement cascade.

Signs and symptoms
Tinea infection:
- Erythema, scaling, pustules, vesicles, bullae
- Itching, stinging, and burning
- Circular lesions with erythema and a collarette of scale (central clearing).

Candidiasis:
- Superficial papules and pustules; later, erosions
- Erythema and edema of epidermis or mucous membrane
- As inflammation progresses, a white-yellow, curd-like crust over the infected area
- In thrush: white coating of tongue; possibly, lesions in mouth
- Severe pruritus and pain at the lesion sites (common).

Diagnostic tests
- Microscopic examination of a KOH-treated skin scraping
- Culture to determine the causative organism and suggest mode of transmission.

Treatment
Tinea infection:
- Topical fungicidal agents, such as an allylamine product
- If no response to topical treatment — oral agents such as griseofulvin, diflucan, sporonox, ketoconazole.

Candidiasis:
- Intertrigo, balanitis, vulvitis, diaper dermatitis, paronychia — nystatin, or imidazoles
- Oral candidiasis (thrush) — azoles, imidazoles
- Systemic infections — I.V. amphotericin B or oral ketonazole.

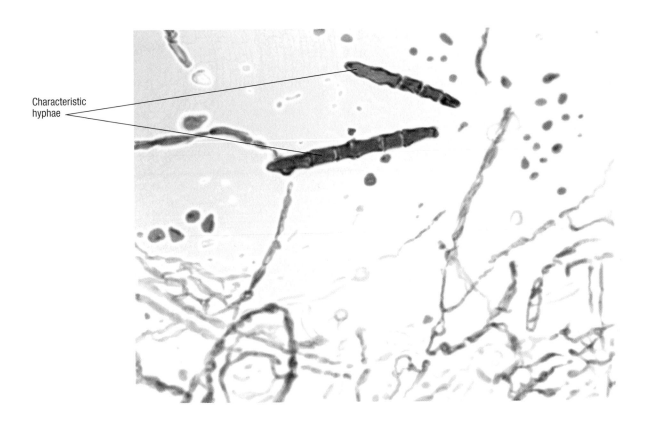

Characteristic hyphae

FUNGAL INFECTION OF NAIL

Onycholysis

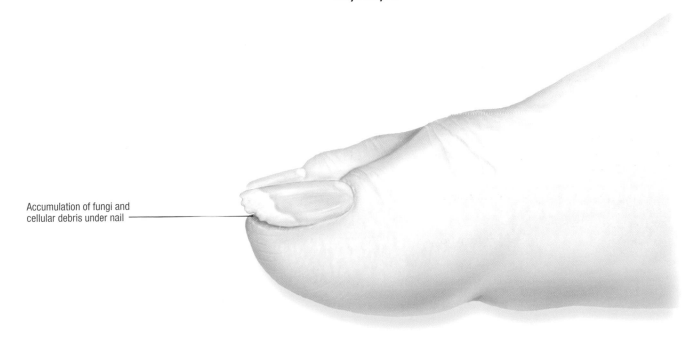

Accumulation of fungi and cellular debris under nail

LYME DISEASE

A multisystemic disorder, Lyme disease is caused by the spirochete *Borrelia burgdorferi*, which is carried by the minute tick *Ixodes dammini* or another tick in the Ixodidae family. It commonly begins in the summer with a papule that becomes red and warm but isn't painful. This classic skin lesion is called erythema chronicum migrans (ECM). Weeks or months later, cardiac or neurologic abnormalities sometimes develop, possibly followed by arthritis of the large joints.

Causes

Borrelia burgdorferi.

Pathophysiology

Lyme disease begins when a tick injects spirochete-laden saliva into the bloodstream or deposits fecal matter on the skin. After incubating for 3 to 32 days, the spirochetes migrate out to the skin, causing ECM. Then they disseminate to other skin sites or organs by the bloodstream or lymph system. The spirochetes' life cycle isn't completely clear. They may survive for years in the joints or they may trigger an inflammatory response in the host and then die.

Signs and symptoms

Stage one:
● Persistent sore throat and dry cough, may appear several days before ECM
● Red macule or papule (ECM) that resembles a bull's eye or target:
– commonly at the site of a tick bite
– typically feels hot and itchy and may grow to over 20" (50 cm) in diameter
● Within a few days:
– possibly, more lesions
– a migratory, ringlike rash, conjunctivitis, or diffuse urticaria
● In 3 to 4 weeks:
– lesions replaced by small red blotches, which persist for several more weeks
– constant malaise and fatigue

– intermittent headache, neck stiffness, fever, chills, achiness, regional lymphadenopathy
– less commonly meningeal irritation, mild encephalopathy, migrating musculoskeletal pain, hepatitis, splenomegaly.
  Stage two:
● Neurologic abnormalities — fluctuating meningoencephalitis with peripheral and cranial neuropathy; facial palsy especially noticeable; usually resolve after days or months
● Cardiac abnormalities — such as a brief, fluctuating atrioventricular heart block, left ventricular dysfunction, or cardiomegaly; last only a few weeks but may be fatal.
  Stage three:
● Begins weeks or years later
● Migrating musculoskeletal pain leads to frank arthritis with marked swelling, especially in the large joints
● Recurrent attacks may precede chronic arthritis with severe cartilage and bone erosion.

Diagnostic tests

● Usually based on the characteristic ECM lesion and related clinical findings, especially in endemic areas:
– attempted isolation of *B. burgdorferi* seldom successful in humans
– indirect immunofluorescent antibody tests marginally sensitive
● Diagnosis supported by complete blood count, elevated erythrocyte sedimentation rate, serum immunoglobulin M and aspartate aminotransferase.

Treatment

Early stage:
● 28-day course of doxycycline, treatment of choice for adults
● Oral penicillin usually prescribed for children
● Can minimize later complications.
  Late stage:
● High-dose I.V. ceftriaxone may be successful.

LYME DISEASE ORGANISM AND LESION

Borrelia burgdorferi **spirochete — Darkfield microscopic view**

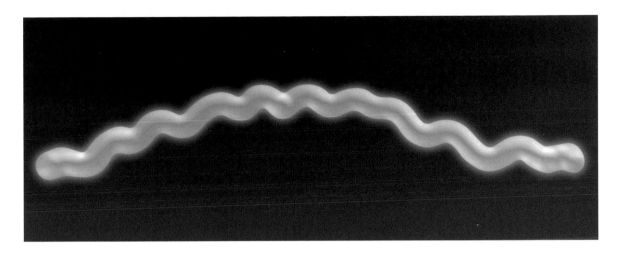

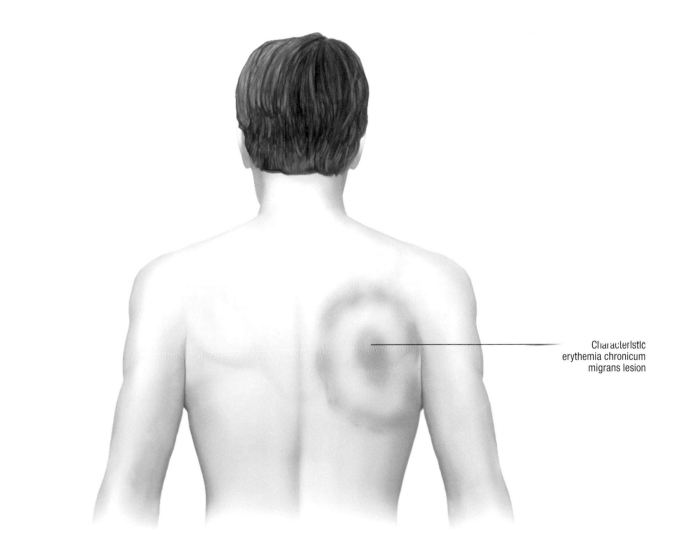

Characteristic erythemia chronicum migrans lesion

PRESSURE ULCERS

Pressure ulcers, commonly called pressure sores or bedsores, are localized areas of cellular necrosis that occur most commonly in the skin and subcutaneous tissue over bony prominences. These ulcers may be superficial, caused by local skin irritation with subsequent surface maceration, or deep, originating in underlying tissue. Deep lesions often go undetected until they penetrate the skin, and by then they've usually caused subcutaneous damage.

Five body locations together account for 95% of all pressure ulcer sites: sacral area, greater trochanter, ischial tuberosity, heel, and lateral malleolus. Patients who have contractures are at an increased risk for developing pressure ulcers because the abnormal position adds pressure on the tissue and the alignment of the bones.

 AGE ALERT
Age also has a role in the incidence of pressure ulcers. Muscle and subcutaneous tissue are lost with aging, and skin elasticity decreases. Both factors increase the risk for developing pressure ulcers.

A *stage 1* pressure ulcer is an observable pressure-related alteration of intact skin. The ulcer appears as a defined area of persistent redness in lightly pigmented skin; in darker skin, the ulcer may appear with persistent red, blue, or purple hues.

A *stage 2* pressure ulcer is characterized by partial-thickness skin loss involving the epidermis or dermis. The ulcer is superficial and appears as an abrasion, blister, or shallow crater. These wounds heal within a few weeks.

A *stage 3* pressure ulcer is characterized by full-thickness skin loss involving damage or necrosis of subcutaneous tissue, which may extend down to, but not through, the underlying fascia. The ulcer appears as a deep crater with or without undermining of adjacent tissue.

Full-thickness skin loss with extensive destruction, tissue necrosis, or damage to muscle, bone, or support structures (for example, tendon or joint capsule) characterize a *stage 4* pressure ulcer. Tunneling and sinus tracts also may be associated with these ulcers.

Ulcers of the subcutaneous tissue and muscle may require several months to heal. If the damage has affected the bone in addition to the skin layers, osteomyelitis may occur, which will prolong healing times.

Causes
- Immobility and decreased level of activity
- Friction and shear causing damage to the epidermal and upper dermal skin layers
- Constant moisture on the skin causing tissue maceration
- Impaired hygiene, as with fecal incontinence, leading to skin breakdown.
    Contributing conditions:
- Malnutrition
- Medical conditions such as diabetes, orthopedic injuries
- Psychological factors such as depression, chronic emotional stresses.

Pathophysiology
A pressure ulcer is caused by an injury to the skin and its underlying tissues. The pressure exerted on the area restricts blood flow to the site and causes ischemia and hypoxemia. As the capillaries collapse, thrombosis occurs and leads to tissue edema and necrosis. Ischemia also adds to an accumulation of waste products, which produce toxins. The toxins further break down the tissue and also contribute to tissue necrosis.

Signs and symptoms
- First clinical sign — blanching erythema, varying from pink to bright red depending on the patient's skin color; in dark-skinned people, purple discoloration or a darkening of normal skin color; when the examiner presses a finger on the reddened area, the pressed on area whitens and color returns within 1 to 3 seconds if capillary refill is good
- Pain at the site and surrounding area
- Localized edema and increased body temperature due to initial inflammatory response; in more severe cases, cool skin due to severe damage or necrosis
- In more severe cases with deeper dermal involvement — non-blanching erythema, ranging from dark red to purple or cyanotic
- As ulcer progresses — skin deterioration, blisters, crusts, or scaling
- Deep ulcer originating at the bony prominence below the skin surface — usually dusky-red, possibly mottled appearance, doesn't bleed easily, warm to the touch.

Diagnostic tests
- White blood cell count, erythrocyte sedimentation rate
- Total serum protein and serum albumin.

Treatment
Stage I:
- For immobile patients, repositioning by the caregiver every 2 hours or more often if indicated, with support of pillows; for those able to move, a pillow and encouragement to change position
- Foam, gel, or air mattress to aid in healing by reducing pressure on the ulcer site and reducing the risk for more ulcers
- Foam, gel, or air mattress on chairs and wheelchairs as indicated
- Nutritional supplements, such as vitamin C and zinc, for the malnourished patient
- Adequate fluid intake (I.V. if indicated) and increased fluids for a dehydrated patient
- Meticulous skin care and hygiene practices, particularly for incontinent patients.
    Stage II:
- Transparent film, polyurethane foam, or hydrocolloid dressing.
    Stage III or IV:
- Loosely fill wound with saline- or gel-moistened gauze; manage exudate with absorbent dressing (moist gauze or foam); cover with secondary dressing
- Surgical debridement.

Stage I

Reddened area

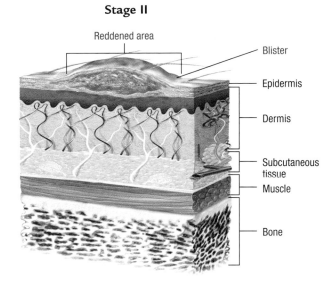

Epidermis

Dermis

Subcutaneous tissue

Muscle

Bone

Stage II

Reddened area

Blister

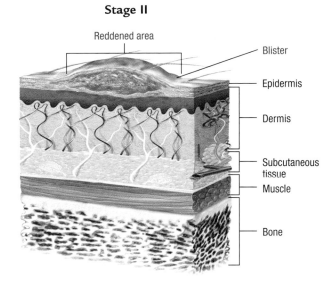

Epidermis

Dermis

Subcutaneous tissue

Muscle

Bone

Stage III

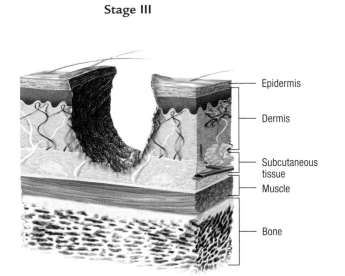

Epidermis

Dermis

Subcutaneous tissue

Muscle

Bone

Stage IV

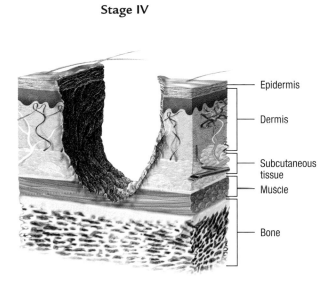

Epidermis

Dermis

Subcutaneous tissue

Muscle

Bone

PSORIASIS

Psoriasis is a chronic, recurrent disease marked by epidermal proliferation and characterized by remissions and exacerbations. Flare-ups are often related to specific systemic and environmental factors, but may be unpredictable. Widespread involvement is called *exfoliative* or *erythrodermic* psoriasis.

Although this disorder often affects young adults, it may strike at any age, including infancy. Genetic factors predetermine the incidence of psoriasis; affected families have a significantly greater incidence of human leukocyte antigens (HLA) B13, B17, and CW6.

Flare-ups can usually be controlled with therapy. Appropriate treatment depends on the type of psoriasis, extent of the disease, the patient's response, and the effect of the disease on the patient's lifestyle. No permanent cure exists, and all methods of treatment are palliative.

Causes
Etiology unknown.
Possible causes:
- Genetically determined tendency to develop psoriasis
- Possible immune disorder, as suggested by HLA type in families
- Flare-up of guttate (drop-shaped) lesions from infections, especially beta-hemolytic streptococci.

Other contributing factors:
- Pregnancy
- Endocrine changes
- Climate (cold weather tends to exacerbate psoriasis)
- Emotional stress or physical illness
- Infection.

Pathophysiology
A skin cell normally takes 14 days to move from the basal layer to the stratum corneum, where it is sloughed off after 14 days of normal wear and tear. Thus, the life-cycle of a normal skin cell is 28 days.

In psoriasis, the immune system sends signals that speed up the normal process from 28 days to just 4 days. This markedly shortened cycle doesn't allow time for the cell to mature. Consequently, the stratum corneum becomes thick with extra skin cells. On the surface, the skin cells pile up and the dead cells create a white, flaky layer, the cardinal manifestation of psoriasis.

Signs and symptoms
- Erythematous papules and plaques with thick silver scales, most commonly on the scalp, chest, elbows, knees, back, and buttocks
- Plaques with characteristic silver scales that either flake off easily or thicken, covering the lesion; scale removal can produce fine bleeding (Auspitz's sign)
- Itching and occasional pain from dry, cracked, encrusted lesions
- Occasional small guttate lesions (usually thin and erythematous, with few scales), either alone or with plaques.

Diagnostic tests
Diagnosis is based on patient history, appearance of the lesions, and, if needed, the results of skin biopsy.

Treatment
- Low-dose antihistamines, oatmeal baths, emollients, and open wet dressings to help relieve pruritus
- Aspirin and local heat to help alleviate the pain of psoriatic arthritis; nonsteroidal anti-inflammatory drugs in severe cases
- Ultraviolet B (UVB) or natural sunlight exposure to retard rapid cell production to the point of minimal erythema
- Tar preparations or crude coal tar applications to the affected areas about 15 minutes before exposure to UVB or at bedtime and wiped off the next morning
- Steroid creams and ointments applied twice daily, preferably after bathing to facilitate absorption, and overnight use of occlusive dressings to control symptoms of psoriasis
- Intralesional steroid injection for small, stubborn plaques
- Anthralin ointment or paste mixture for well-defined plaques (because anthralin injures and stains normal skin, apply petroleum jelly around affected skin before applying it)
- Anthralin at night and steroids during the day
- Calcipotriene ointment, a vitamin D analogue; best when alternated with a topical steroid
- Ingram technique (variation of the Goeckerman regimen) using anthralin instead of tar with ultraviolet light
- Tazarotene, a topical retinoid
- Topical administration of psoralens (plant extracts that accelerate exfoliation) followed by exposure to high-intensity UVA (PUVA therapy)
- Extensive psoriasis — acitretin, a retinoid compound
- Resistant disease — cyclosporine
- Last-resort treatment for refractory psoriasis — cytotoxin, usually methotrexate
- Psoriasis of scalp — tar shampoo followed by a steroid lotion
- Psoriasis of the nails — no effective topical treatment.

PSORIATIC LESION

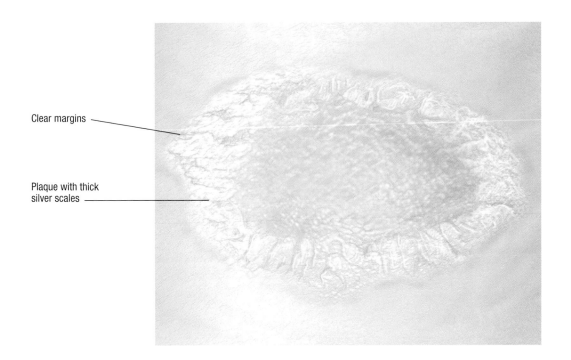

Clear margins

Plaque with thick
silver scales

DIFFUSE PSORIATIC PLAQUES

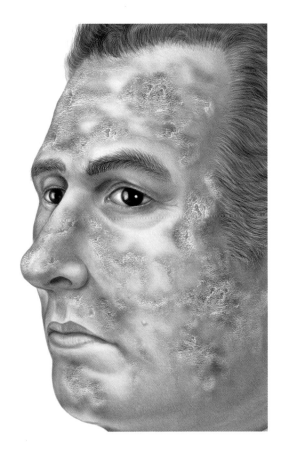

SKIN CANCERS

BASAL CELL CARCINOMA

Basal cell carcinoma, also known as basal cell epithelioma, is a slow-growing, destructive skin tumor.

Causes
- Prolonged sun exposure (most common)
- Arsenic, radiation, burns, immunosuppression.

Pathophysiology
The pathogenesis is uncertain, but it is thought to originate when undifferentiated basal cells become carcinomatous instead of differentiating into sweat glands, sebum, and hair.

Signs and symptoms
Noduloulcerative lesions:
- Usually occur on the face, particularly the forehead, eyelid margins, and nasolabial folds
- Early lesions are small, smooth, pinkish, and translucent papules; telangiectatic vessels cross the surface; occasionally pigmented
- Lesions enlarge; centers become depressed and borders become firm and elevated
- Local invasion and ulceration, "rodent ulcers," eventually occur; these rarely metastasize, but can spread to vital areas and become infected or cause massive hemorrhage.
  Superficial basal cell carcinoma:
- Often multiple; commonly occur on chest and back
- Oval or irregularly shaped, lightly pigmented plaques, with sharply defined, slightly elevated threadlike borders:
  – superficial erosion appears scaly; small, atrophic areas in center resemble psoriasis or eczema
  – usually chronic and unlikely to invade other areas.
  Sclerosing basal cell carcinoma (morphea-like carcinoma):
- Waxy, sclerotic, yellow to white plaques; no distinct borders
- Occur on head and neck.

Diagnostic tests
- Incisional or excisional biopsy
- Histologic study.

Treatment
- Curettage and electrodesiccation
- Topical 5-fluorouracil
- Microscopically controlled surgical excision (Mohs' surgery)
- Irradiation
- Cryotherapy with liquid nitrogen
- Chemosurgery — for persistent or recurrent lesions.

SQUAMOUS CELL CARCINOMA

Squamous cell carcinoma of the skin is an invasive tumor with metastatic potential that arises from the keratinizing epidermal cells.

Causes
- Overexposure to the sun's ultraviolet rays
- Premalignant lesions, such as actinic keratosis or Bowen's disease
- X-ray therapy
- Ingested herbicides containing arsenic
- Chronic skin irritation and inflammation
- Local carcinogens, such as tar and oil
- Hereditary diseases, such as xeroderma pigmentosum, albinism.

Signs and symptoms
- Induration and inflammation of a preexisting lesion
- Slowly growing nodule on a firm, indurated base; eventual ulceration and invasion of underlying tissues
- Metastasis to regional lymph nodes — characteristic systemic symptoms of pain, malaise, fatigue, weakness, and anorexia.

Diagnostic tests
- Excisional biopsy
- Laboratory tests depending on systemic symptoms.

Treatment
- Wide surgical excision
- Electrodesiccation and curettage
- Radiation therapy
- Chemosurgery.

MALIGNANT MELANOMA

A malignant neoplasm that arises from melanocytes, malignant melanoma is relatively rare and accounts for only 1% to 2% of all malignancies. However, the incidence is rapidly increasing, 300% in the past 40 years. The four types of melanomas are *superficial spreading* melanoma, *nodular malignant* melanoma, *lentigo maligna*, and *acral lentiginous* melanoma.

Melanoma spreads through the lymphatic and vascular systems and metastasizes to the regional lymph nodes, skin, liver, lungs, and central nervous system. Its course is unpredictable, and recurrence and metastases may not appear for more than 5 years after resection of the primary lesion. The prognosis varies with tumor thickness. Generally, superficial lesions are curable, whereas deeper lesions tend to metastasize.

Causes
- Excessive exposure to sunlight.
  Contributing factors:
- Skin type — most common in persons with blonde or red hair, fair skin, and blue eyes; are prone to sunburn; and are of Celtic or Scandinavian ancestry; rare among people of African ancestry
- Hormonal factors — pregnancy may exacerbate growth
- Family history — slightly more common within families
- Past history of melanoma.

(Text continues on page 376.)

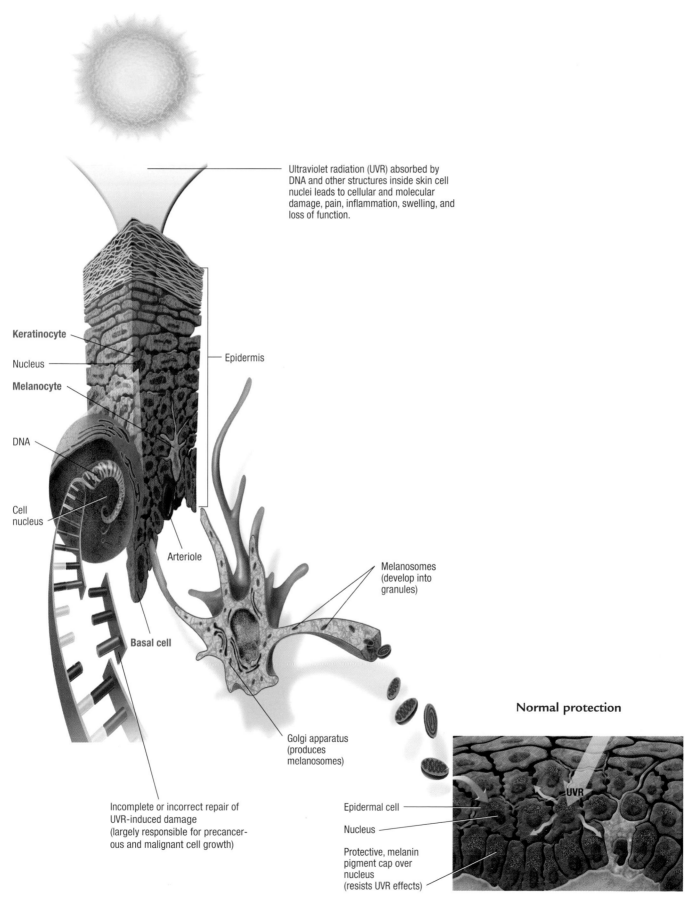

Ultraviolet radiation (UVR) absorbed by DNA and other structures inside skin cell nuclei leads to cellular and molecular damage, pain, inflammation, swelling, and loss of function.

Keratinocyte

Nucleus

Melanocyte

DNA

Cell nucleus

Epidermis

Arteriole

Basal cell

Melanosomes (develop into granules)

Golgi apparatus (produces melanosomes)

Incomplete or incorrect repair of UVR-induced damage (largely responsible for precancerous and malignant cell growth)

Normal protection

Epidermal cell

Nucleus

Protective, melanin pigment cap over nucleus (resists UVR effects)

UVR

Skin cancers   **375**

SKIN CANCERS *(continued)*

Signs and symptoms

Melanoma, if any skin lesion or nevus:
- Enlarges, becomes inflamed or sore, itches, ulcerates, bleeds, undergoes textural changes
- Changes color or shows signs of surrounding pigment regression (halo nevus or vitiligo).

Superficial spreading melanoma:
- Arises on an area of chronic irritation
- In women, most common between the knees and ankles; in Blacks and Asians, on the toe webs and soles — lightly pigmented areas subject to trauma
- Red, white, and blue color over a brown or black background and an irregular, notched margin
- Irregular surface with small elevated tumor nodules that may ulcerate and bleed.

Nodular melanoma:
- Usually a polypoidal nodule, with uniformly dark or grayish coloration — resembles a blackberry
- Occasionally, flesh-colored, with flecks of pigment around its base; possibly inflamed.

Lentigo maligna melanoma:
- Resembles a large (3- to 6-cm) flat freckle of tan, brown, black, whitish, or slate color
- Irregularly scattered black nodules on the surface
- Develops slowly, usually over many years, and eventually may ulcerate
- Commonly develops under fingernail, on face, or on back of hand.

Diagnostic tests
- Skin biopsy with histologic examination
- Baseline laboratory studies:
- complete blood count with differential, erythrocyte sedimentation rate, platelet count, liver function studies
- urinalysis
- Chest X-ray
- Bone scan; computed tomography (CT) scan of chest and abdomen; CT scan of brain.

Treatment
- Surgical resection to remove the tumor
- Regional lymphadenectomy
- Adjuvant chemotherapy and biotherapy
- Radiation therapy.

CLINICAL TIP

Regardless of the treatment method, melanomas require close long-term follow-up to detect metastasis and recurrences. Statistics show that 13% of recurrences develop more than 5 years after primary surgery.

TYPES OF SKIN CANCER

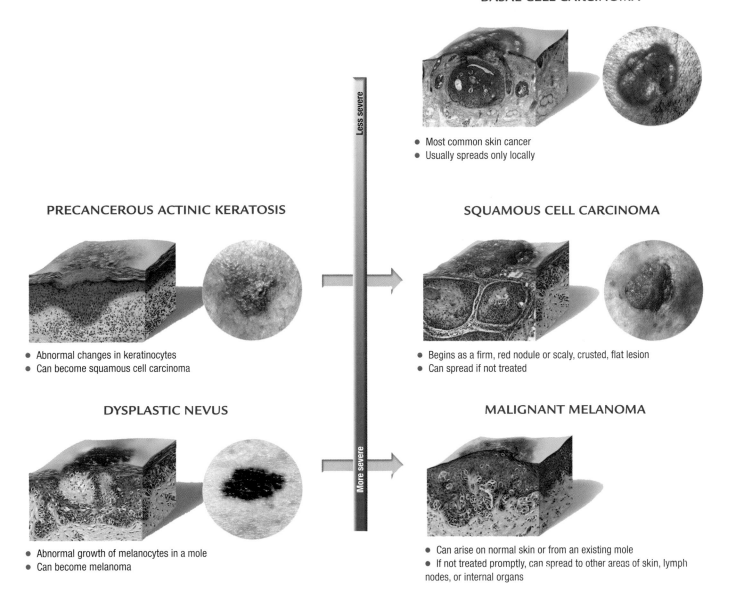

BASAL CELL CARCINOMA

- Most common skin cancer
- Usually spreads only locally

PRECANCEROUS ACTINIC KERATOSIS

- Abnormal changes in keratinocytes
- Can become squamous cell carcinoma

SQUAMOUS CELL CARCINOMA

- Begins as a firm, red nodule or scaly, crusted, flat lesion
- Can spread if not treated

DYSPLASTIC NEVUS

- Abnormal growth of melanocytes in a mole
- Can become melanoma

MALIGNANT MELANOMA

- Can arise on normal skin or from an existing mole
- If not treated promptly, can spread to other areas of skin, lymph nodes, or internal organs

Less severe

More severe

ABCDs OF MALIGNANT MELANOMA

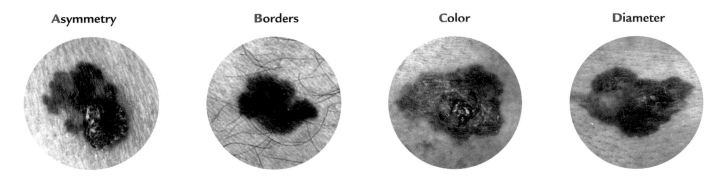

Asymmetry

Borders

Color

Diameter

WARTS

Warts, also known as verrucae, are common, benign, viral infections of the skin and adjacent mucous membranes. The prognosis varies; some warts disappear readily with treatment, and others need vigorous and prolonged treatment.

 AGE ALERT
Although their incidence is highest in children and young adults, warts may occur at any age.

Causes
- Human papilloma virus (HPV)
- Probably transmitted through direct contact; autoinoculation.

Pathophysiology
HPV replicates in the epidermal cells, causing irregular thickening of the stratum corneum in the infected areas. People who lack virus-specific immunity are susceptible.

Signs and symptoms
- *Common (verruca vulgaris):* rough, elevated, rounded surface; appears most frequently on extremities, particularly hands and fingers; most prevalent in children and young adults
- *Filiform:* single, thin, threadlike projection; commonly occurs around the face and neck
- *Periungual:* rough, irregularly shaped, elevated surface; occurs around edges of fingernails and toenails; when severe, may extend under the nail and lift it off the nail bed, causing pain
- *Flat (juvenile):* multiple groupings of up to several hundred slightly raised lesions with smooth, flat, or slightly rounded tops; common on the face, neck, chest, knees, dorsa of hands, wrists, and flexor surfaces of the forearms; usually occur in children but can affect adults; distribution is often linear because these can spread from scratching or shaving
- *Plantar:* slightly elevated or flat; occurs singly or in large clusters (mosaic warts), primarily at pressure points of the feet
- *Digitate:* fingerlike, horny projection arising from a pea-shaped base; occurs on scalp or near hairline

- *Condyloma acuminatum (moist wart):* usually small, pink to red, moist, and soft; may occur singly or in large cauliflower-like clusters on penis, scrotum, vulva, or anus; may be transmitted through sexual contact; not always venereal in origin.

Diagnostic tests
Sigmoidoscopy when anal warts are recurrent to rule out internal involvement necessitating surgery.

Treatment
Electrodesiccation and curettage:
- High-frequency electric current to destroy the wart, surgical removal of dead tissue at the base
- Effective for common, filiform and, occasionally, plantar warts
- More effective than cryosurgery.
  Cryotherapy:
- Liquid nitrogen kills the wart; resulting dried blister peeled off several days later
- If initial treatment unsuccessful, can be repeated at 2- to 4-week intervals
- Useful for periungual warts or for common warts on face, extremities, penis, vagina, or anus.
  Acid therapy (primary or adjunctive):
- Applications of plaster patches impregnated with acid (such as 40% salicylic acid plasters) or acid drops (such as 5% to 16.7% salicylic acid in flexible collodion) every 12 to 24 hours for 2 to 4 weeks
- Hyperthermia for *verruca plantaris.*
  For genital warts:
- Podophyllin in tincture of benzoin; avoid using this drug on pregnant patients: may be repeated every 3 to 4 days
- 25% to 50% trichloroacetic acid applied to wart and neutralized with baking soda or water when wart turns white
- Carbon dioxide laser therapy.
  Other:
- Antiviral drugs under investigation
- If immunity develops, warts may resolve without treatment.

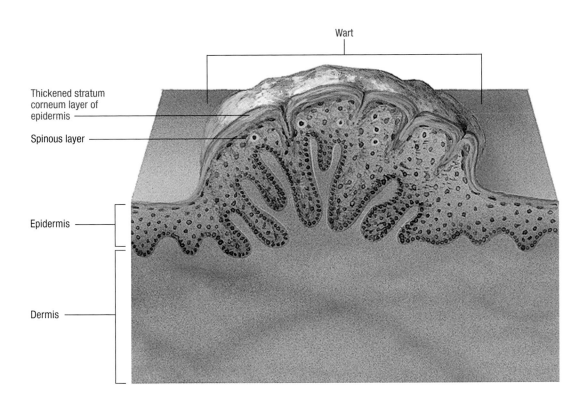

Wart

Thickened stratum corneum layer of epidermis

Spinous layer

Epidermis

Dermis

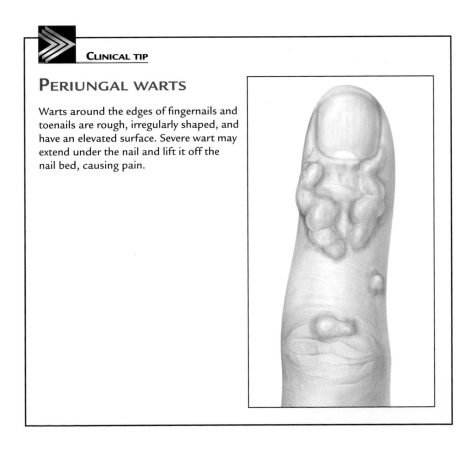

CLINICAL TIP

PERIUNGAL WARTS

Warts around the edges of fingernails and toenails are rough, irregularly shaped, and have an elevated surface. Severe wart may extend under the nail and lift it off the nail bed, causing pain.

CATARACT

A cataract is a gradually developing opacity of the lens or lens capsule. Light shining through the cornea is blocked by this opacity, and a blurred image is cast onto the retina. As a result, the brain interprets a hazy image. Cataracts commonly occur bilaterally, and each progresses independently. Exceptions are traumatic cataracts, which are usually unilateral, and congenital cataracts, which may remain stationary.

 AGE ALERT
Cataracts are most prevalent in people older than age 70. The prognosis is generally good; surgery improves vision in 95% of affected people.

Causes
- Aging
- Trauma, foreign body injury
- Exposure to ionizing radiation or infrared rays
- Exposure to ultraviolet radiation
- Drugs that are toxic to the lens, such as prednisone, ergot alkaloids, dinitrophenol, naphthalene, phenothiazines, pilocarpine
- Genetic abnormalities
- Infection, such as maternal rubella during first trimester of pregnancy
- Maternal malnutrition
- Metabolic disease, such as diabetes mellitus, hypothyroidism
- Myotonic dystrophy
- Uveitis, glaucoma, retinitis pigmentosa, retinal detachment
- Atopic dermatitis.

Pathophysiology
Pathophysiology may vary with each form of cataract. Congenital cataracts are particularly challenging. They may result from chromosomal abnormalities, metabolic disease, intrauterine nutritional deficiencies, or infection during pregnancy (such as rubella). Senile cataracts show evidence of protein aggregation, oxidative injury, and increased pigmentation in the center of the lens. In traumatic cataracts, phagocytosis of the lens or inflammation may occur when a lens ruptures. The mechanism of a complicated cataract varies with the disease process; for example, in diabetes, increased glucose in the lens causes it to absorb water.

Typically, cataract development goes through the following four stages:
- *immature* — partially opaque lens
- *mature* — completely opaque lens; significant vision loss
- *tumescent* — water-filled lens; may lead to glaucoma
- *hypermature* — lens proteins deteriorate; peptides leak through the lens capsule; glaucoma may develop if intraocular fluid outflow is obstructed.

Signs and symptoms
- Gradual painless blurring and loss of vision
- Milky white pupil
- Blinding glare from headlights at night
- Poor reading vision caused by reduced clarity of images
- In central opacity — vision improves in dim light; as pupils dilate, patients can see around the opacity.

 AGE ALERT
Elderly patients with reduced vision may become depressed and withdraw from social activities rather than complain about reduced vision.

Diagnostic tests
- Indirect ophthalmoscopy and slit-lamp examination
- Visual acuity test.

Treatment
- Extracapsular cataract extraction of anterior lens capsule and cortex:
  - phacoemulsification to fragment the lens with ultrasonic vibrations
  - aspiration of pieces
- Intracapsular cryoextraction of entire lens; rarely performed today
- Laser surgery to restore visual acuity if a secondary membrane forms in the intact posterior lens capsule after an extracapsular cataract extraction
- Discission (an incision) and aspiration may still be used in children with soft cataracts
- Contact lenses or lens implantation after surgery to improve visual acuity, binocular vision, and depth perception.

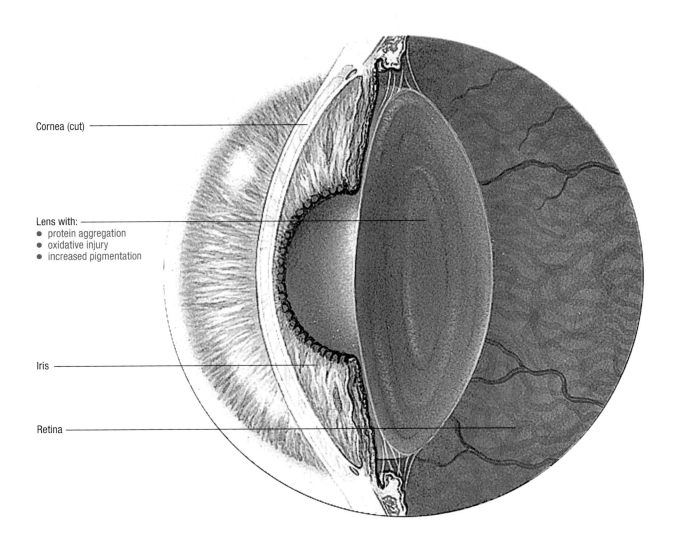

Cornea (cut)

Lens with:
- protein aggregation
- oxidative injury
- increased pigmentation

Iris

Retina

CLEFT LIP AND CLEFT PALATE

Cleft lip and cleft palate — an opening in the lip or palate — may occur separately or in combination. Cleft lip and cleft palate are twice as common in males as in females; isolated cleft palate is more common in females.

Causes
• Isolated birth defect — normal development of orofacial structures disrupted by a combination of genetic and environmental factors
• Part of a chromosomal or mendelian syndrome (cleft defects are associated with over 300 syndromes)
• Exposures to specific teratogens during fetal development.

CLINICAL TIP
A family history of cleft defects increases the risk that a couple may have a child with a cleft defect. Likewise, an individual with a cleft defect is at an increased risk to have a child with a cleft defect. Children with cleft defects and their parents or adult individuals should be referred for genetic counseling for accurate diagnosis of cleft type and recurrence-risk counseling. Recurrence-risk is based on family history, the presence or absence of other physical or cognitive traits within a family, and prenatal exposure information.

Pathophysiology
Cleft deformities originate in the second month of pregnancy, when the front and sides of the face and the palatine shelves fuse imperfectly. Cleft deformities usually occur unilaterally or bilaterally, rarely midline.

Signs and symptoms
• *Cleft lip* may range from a simple notch in the upper lip to a complete cleft from the lip edge through the floor of the nostril.
• *Cleft palate* may be partial or complete, involving only the soft palate or extending from the soft palate completely through the hard palate into the upper jaw or nasal cavity.

CLINICAL TIP
The constellation of U-shaped cleft palate, mandibular hypoplasia, and glossoptosis (downward displacement and retraction of the tongue) is known as Pierre Robin sequence, or Robin sequence. It can occur as an isolated defect or one feature of many different syndromes; therefore, a comprehensive genetic evaluation is suggested for infants with Robin sequence. Because of the mandibular hypoplasia and glossoptosis, careful evaluation and management of the airway are mandatory for infants with Robin sequence.

Diagnostic tests
Prenatal ultrasonography.

Treatment
Surgical correction, timing varies:
• Cleft lip:
– within the first few days of life to make feeding easier
– delay lip repairs for 2 to 8 months to minimize surgical and anesthesia risks, rule out associated congenital anomalies, and allow time for parental bonding
• Cleft palate — performed only after the infant is gaining weight and infection-free:
– usually completed by age 12 to 18 months
– two steps: soft palate between ages 6 and 18 months; hard palate as late as age 5 years.
   Speech therapy:
• Palate essential to speech formation; structural changes, even in a repaired cleft, can permanently affect speech patterns
• Hearing difficulties common in children with cleft palate because of middle ear damage or infections.

VARIATIONS OF CLEFT DEFORMITY

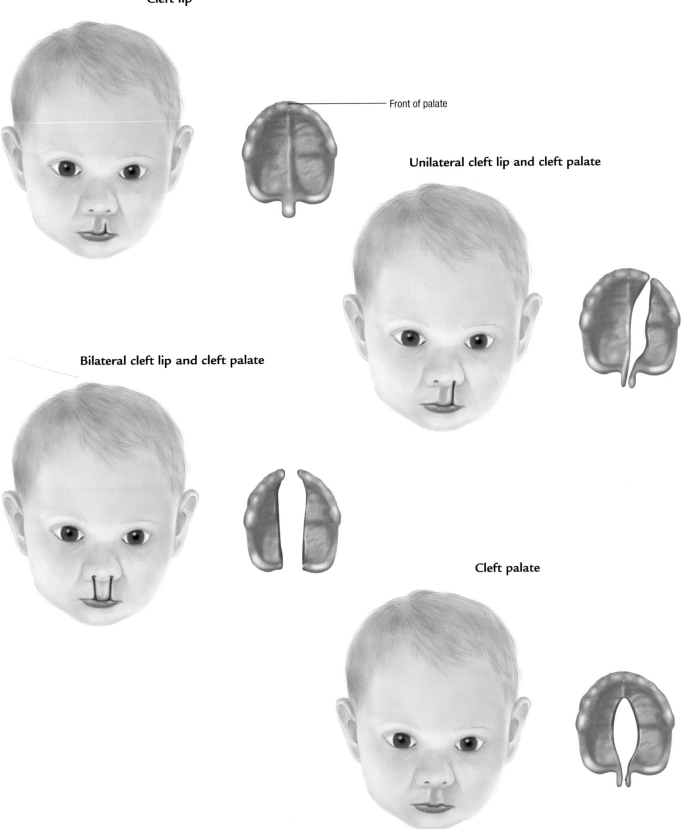

Cleft lip

Front of palate

Unilateral cleft lip and cleft palate

Bilateral cleft lip and cleft palate

Cleft palate

Conjunctivitis

Conjunctivitis is characterized by hyperemia of the conjunctiva. The three main types of conjunctivitis are infectious (called pinkeye), allergic, and chemical. This disorder usually occurs as benign, self-limiting pinkeye; it may also be chronic, possibly indicating degenerative changes or damage from repeated acute attacks. Epidemic keratoconjunctivitis is an acute, highly contagious viral conjunctivitis. Careful handwashing is essential to prevent the spread of this disease.

Causes

Infectious conjunctivitis — most commonly by:
- Bacterial: *Staphylococcus aureus, Streptococcus pneumoniae, Neisseria gonorrhoeae, Neisseria meningitidis*
- Chlamydial: *Chlamydia trachomatis* (inclusion conjunctivitis)
- Viral: adenovirus types 3, 7, and 8; herpes simplex 1.
    Allergic conjunctivitis — hypersensitivity to:
- Pollen, grass, unknown seasonal allergens (vernal conjunctivitis), animals
- Topical medications, cosmetics, fabrics
- Air pollutants, smoke
- Contact lenses or solutions.
    Chemical conjunctivitis — chemical reaction to:
- Environmental irritants (wind, dust, smoke, swimming pool chlorine)
- Occupational irritants (acids, alkalies).

Pathophysiology

Conjunctivitis is an inflammation of the conjunctiva, the transparent layer covering the surfaces in the inner eyelid and the front of the eyeball. It usually begins in one eye and rapidly spreads to the other by contamination of towels, washcloths, or the patient's own hands.

Vernal conjunctivitis (so-called because symptoms tend to be worse in the spring) is a severe form of IgE-mediated mast cell hypersensitivity reaction. This form of conjunctivitis is bilateral. It usually begins between ages 3 and 5 and persists for about 10 years. It's sometimes associated with other signs of allergy commonly related to pollens, asthma, or allergic rhinitis.

Signs and symptoms

- Hyperemia of the conjunctiva
- Discharge, tearing
- Pain, photophobia.

Acute bacterial conjunctivitis (pinkeye):
- Usually lasts only 2 weeks
- Itching, burning, and the sensation of a foreign body in the eye
- Crust of sticky, mucopurulent discharge on eyelids.
    N. gonorrhoeae conjunctivitis:
- Itching, burning, foreign body sensation
- Profuse, purulent discharge.
    Viral conjunctivitis:
- Copious tearing, minimal exudate
- Enlargement of the preauricular lymph node
- In children, sore throat or fever if cause is adenovirus
- Variable time course, depending on the virus:
- some are self-limiting, lasting 2 to 3 weeks
- others follow a chronic course, producing a severe disabling disease.

Diagnostic tests

- Stained smears of conjunctival scrapings
- Culture and sensitivity tests.

Treatment

- Bacterial conjunctivitis — topical appropriate broad-spectrum antibiotic
- Viral conjunctivitis:
- resists treatment; the most important aspect of treatment is preventing transmission
- herpes simplex infection generally responds to treatment with trifluridine drops, vidarabine ointment, oral acyclovir
- sulfonamide or broad-spectrum antibiotic eyedrops may prevent secondary infection
- Vernal (allergic) conjunctivitis:
- corticosteroid drops followed by cromolyn sodium
- cold compresses to relieve itching
- occasionally, oral antihistamines.

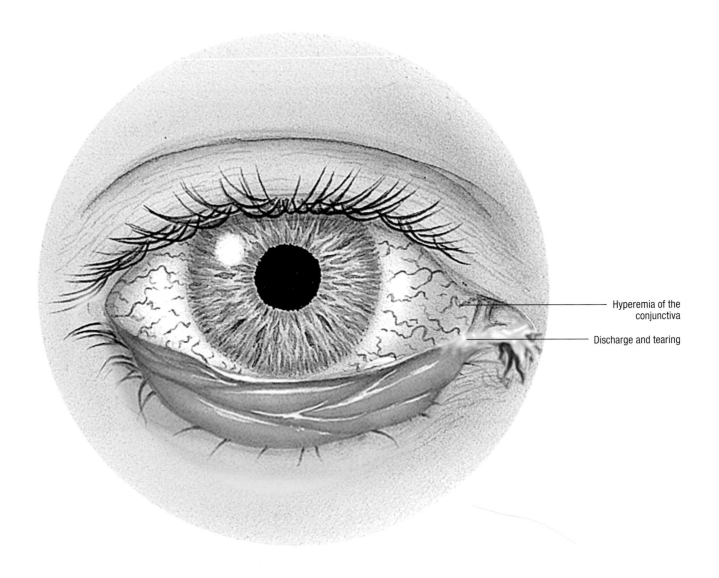

Hyperemia of the conjunctiva

Discharge and tearing

GLAUCOMA

Glaucoma is a group of disorders characterized by an abnormally high intraocular pressure (IOP) that damages the optic nerve and other intraocular structures. Untreated, it leads to a gradual loss of vision and, ultimately, blindness. Glaucoma occurs in several forms: chronic open-angle (primary), acute angle-closure, congenital (inherited as an autosomal recessive trait), and secondary to other causes. Chronic open-angle glaucoma is usually bilateral, with insidious onset and a slowly progressive course. Acute angle-closure glaucoma typically has a rapid onset, constituting an ophthalmic emergency. Unless treated promptly, this acute form of glaucoma causes blindness in 3 to 5 days.

Causes

Chronic open-angle glaucoma — risk factors include:
- genetics
- hypertension
- diabetes mellitus
- aging
- black ethnicity
- severe myopia.

  Acute angle-closure glaucoma — precipitating factors include:
- drug-induced mydriasis (extreme dilation of the pupil)
- excitement or stress, which can lead to hypertension.

  Secondary glaucoma may result from:
- uveitis
- trauma
- steroids
- diabetes
- infections
- surgery.

Pathophysiology

Chronic open-angle glaucoma results from overproduction or obstruction of the outflow of aqueous humor through the trabecular meshwork or the canal of Schlemm, causing IOP and damage to the optic nerve. In secondary glaucoma, conditions such as trauma and surgery increase the risk for obstruction of intraocular fluid outflow caused by edema or other abnormal processes.

Acute angle-closure glaucoma results from obstruction to the outflow of aqueous humor. Obstruction may be caused by anatomically narrow angles between the anterior iris and the posterior corneal surface, shallow anterior chambers, a thickened iris that causes angle closure on pupil dilation, or a bulging iris that presses on the trabeculae, closing the angle (peripheral anterior synechiae). Any of these may cause IOP to increase suddenly.

 AGE ALERT
In older patients, partial closure of the angle may also occur, so that two forms of glaucoma may coexist.

Signs and symptoms

Chronic open-angle glaucoma:
- Typically bilateral
- Mild aching in the eyes
- Loss of peripheral vision
- Images of halos around lights
- Reduced visual acuity, especially at night, not correctable with glasses.

  Acute angle-closure glaucoma:
- Rapid onset; usually unilateral
- Inflammation; red, painful eye
- Sensation of pressure over the eye
- Moderate papillary dilation nonreactive to light
- Cloudy cornea
- Blurring and decreased visual acuity; halos around lights
- Photophobia
- Nausea and vomiting.

Diagnostic tests

- Pressure measurement with applanation, Schiotz, or pneumatic tonometer
- Slit-lamp examination of anterior structures, including cornea, iris, and lens
- Gonioscopy to determine the angle of the anterior chamber of the eye
- Ophthalmoscopy to examine optic disk
- Perimetry or visual field tests
- Fundus photography.

Treatment

Chronic open-angle glaucoma:
- Beta-blockers, such as timolol or betaxolol (a beta 1-receptor antagonist)
- Alpha agonists, such as brimonidine or apraclonidine
- Carbonic anhydrase inhibitors, such as dorzolamide or acetazolamide
- Epinephrine
- Prostaglandins, such as latanoprost
- Miotic eye drops, such as pilocarpine
- Surgical procedures if medical therapy fails to reduce IOP:
- argon laser trabeculoplasty of the trabecular meshwork of an open angle, to produce a thermal burn that changes the surface of the meshwork and increases the outflow of aqueous humor
- trabeculectomy, to remove scleral tissue, followed by a peripheral iridectomy, to produce an opening for aqueous outflow under the conjunctiva, creating a filtering bleb.

  Acute angle-closure glaucoma:
- Ocular emergency, requiring immediate intervention, including:
- I.V. mannitol (20%) or oral glycerin (50%)
- steroid drops
- acetazolamide, a carbonic anhydrase inhibitor
- pilocarpine, to constrict the pupil, forcing the iris away from the trabeculae and allowing fluid to escape
- timolol, a beta-blocker
- narcotic analgesics
- laser iridotomy or surgical peripheral iridectomy
- cycloplegic drops, such as apraclonidine, in the affected eye (only after laser peripheral iridectomy).

Normal optic disk

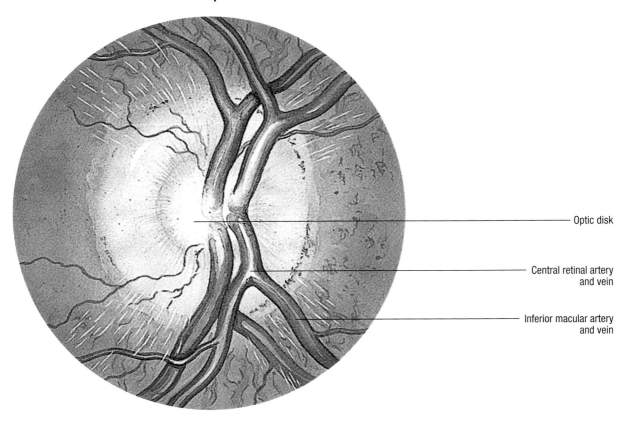

Optic disk

Central retinal artery
and vein

Inferior macular artery
and vein

Disk changes

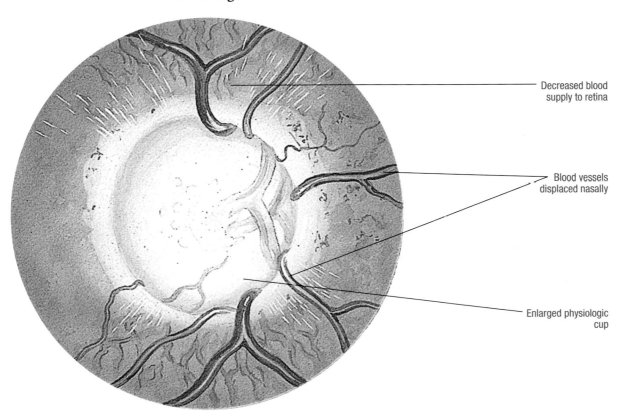

Decreased blood
supply to retina

Blood vessels
displaced nasally

Enlarged physiologic
cup

HEARING LOSS

Hearing loss, or deafness, results from a mechanical or nervous impediment to the transmission of sound waves and is the most common pathologic process associated with hearing alteration. Hearing loss is further defined as an inability to perceive the normal range of sounds audible to an individual with normal hearing. Types of hearing loss include congenital hearing loss, sudden deafness, noise-induced hearing loss, and presbycusis.

Causes
Congenital hearing loss:
- Dominant, autosomal dominant, autosomal recessive, or sex-linked recessive trait
- Maternal exposure to rubella or syphilis during pregnancy
- Use of ototoxic drugs during pregnancy
- Trauma or prolonged fetal anoxia during delivery
- Congenital abnormalities of ears, nose, or throat
- Prematurity or low-birth-weight
- Serum bilirubin levels above 20 mg/dl.
  Sudden deafness:
- Mumps; most common cause of unilateral sensorineural hearing loss in children
- Other bacterial and viral infections, such as rubella, rubeola, influenza, herpes zoster, infectious mononucleosis, mycoplasma
- Metabolic disorders — diabetes mellitus, hypothyroidism, hyperlipoproteinemia
- Vascular disorders — such as hypertension, arteriosclerosis
- Head trauma or brain tumors
- Ototoxic drugs — tobramycin, streptomycin, quinine, gentamicin, furosemide, ethacrynic acid
- Neurologic disorders — multiple sclerosis, neurosyphilis
- Blood dyscrasias — leukemia, hypercoagulation.
  Noise-induced hearing loss:
- Prolonged exposure to loud noise (85 to 90 dB)
- Brief exposure to extremely loud noise (greater than 90 dB).
  Presbycusis:
- Loss of hair cells in the organ of Corti.

Pathophysiology
The major forms of hearing loss are classified as *conductive loss,* interrupted passage of sound from the external ear to the junction of the stapes and oval window; *sensorineural loss,* impaired cochlea or acoustic (eighth cranial) nerve dysfunction, causing failure of transmission of sound impulses within the inner ear or brain; or *mixed loss,* combined dysfunction of conduction and sensorineural transmission.

Signs and symptoms
- Deficient response to auditory stimuli
- Impaired speech development
- Loss of perception of certain frequencies (around 4,000 Hz)
- Tinnitus
- Inability to understand the spoken word.

 AGE ALERT
A deaf infant's behavior can appear normal and mislead the parents as well as the professional, especially if the infant has autosomal recessive deafness and is the first child of carrier parents.

Diagnostic tests
- Complete audiologic examination
- Weber or Rinne tuning fork test
- Specialized audiologic tests to differentiate between conductive and sensorineural hearing loss.

Treatment
Congenital hearing loss:
- Surgery, if correctable
- Sign language, speech reading, or other effective means of developing communication
- Phototherapy and exchange transfusions for hyperbilirubinemia
- Appropriate childhood immunizations.
  Sudden deafness:
- Prompt identification of underlying cause, such as acoustic neuroma or noise and appropriate treatment.
  Noise-induced hearing loss:
- Overnight rest usually restores normal hearing after several hours' exposure to noise levels greater than 90 dB
- Reduction of exposure to loud noises generally prevents high-frequency hearing loss
- Repeated exposure to such noise may require speech and hearing rehabilitation, because hearing aids are seldom helpful.
  Presbycusis:
- Amplifying sound, as with a hearing aid, helps some patients
- Many patients are intolerant of loud noise and are not helped by a hearing aid.

CAUSES OF CONDUCTIVE HEARING LOSS

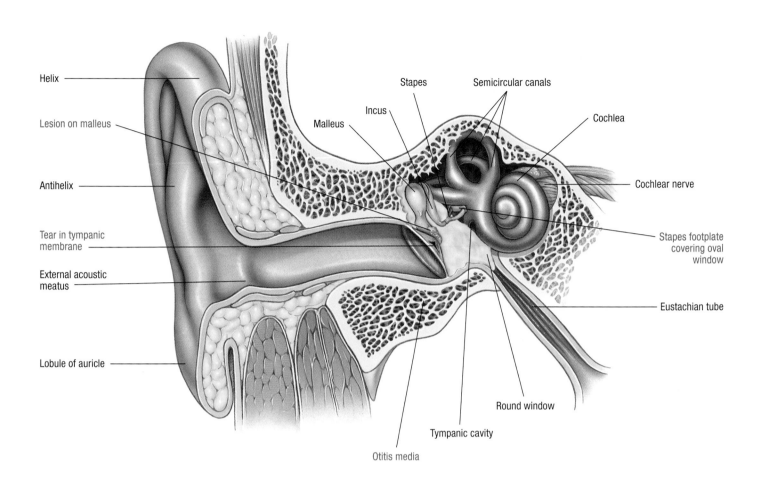

- Helix
- Lesion on malleus
- Antihelix
- Tear in tympanic membrane
- External acoustic meatus
- Lobule of auricle

- Stapes
- Incus
- Malleus
- Semicircular canals
- Cochlea
- Cochlear nerve
- Stapes footplate covering oval window
- Eustachian tube
- Round window
- Tympanic cavity
- Otitis media

CLINICAL TIP

HOW HEARING OCCURS

- Sound vibrations strike the tympanic membrane (eardrum)
- The auditory ossicles vibrate and the footplate of the stapes moves at the oval window
- Movement of the oval window causes the fluid inside the scala vestibuli and scala tympani to move
- Fluid movement against the cochlear duct sets off nerve impulses, which are carried to the brain via the cochlear nerve

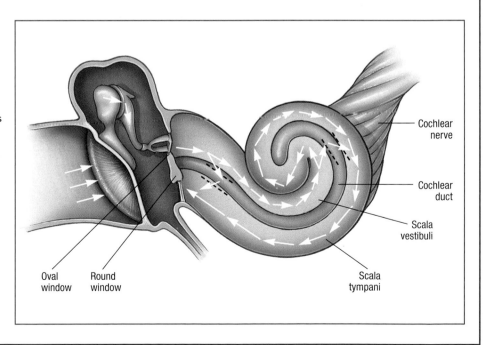

- Oval window
- Round window
- Cochlear nerve
- Cochlear duct
- Scala vestibuli
- Scala tympani

LARYNGEAL CANCER

The most common form of laryngeal cancer is squamous cell carcinoma (95%); rare forms include adenocarcinoma, sarcoma, and others.

Causes
- Smoking
- Alcoholism
- Chronic inhalation of noxious fumes
- Familial tendency.

Pathophysiology
Laryngeal cancer may be intrinsic or extrinsic. An *intrinsic* tumor is on the true vocal cord and does not tend to spread because underlying connective tissues lack lymph nodes. An *extrinsic* tumor is on some other part of the larynx and tends to spread early. Laryngeal cancer is further classified according to the following locations:
- *supraglottis* (false vocal cords)
- *glottis* (true vocal cords)
- *subglottis* (downward extension from vocal cords [rare]).

Signs and symptoms
Intrinsic laryngeal cancer:
- Hoarseness that persists longer than 3 weeks.
  Extrinsic cancer:
- Lump in the throat
- Pain or burning in the throat when drinking citrus juice or hot liquid.
  Later clinical effects of metastases:
- Dysphagia
- Dyspnea
- Cough
- Enlarged cervical lymph nodes
- Pain radiating to the ear.

Diagnostic tests
- Laryngoscopy
- Laryngeal tomography
- Computed tomography scan
- Laryngography
- Chest X-ray
- Biopsy.

Treatment
Precancerous lesions:
- Laser surgery.
  Early lesions:
- Surgery or radiation.
  Advanced lesions:
- Surgery; procedures vary with tumor size and can include cordectomy, partial or total laryngectomy, supraglottic laryngectomy, or total laryngectomy with laryngoplasty
- Laser surgery to help relieve obstruction caused by tumor growth
- Radiation and chemotherapy.
  Speech rehabilitation:
- If speech preservation isn't possible, may include:
- esophageal speech
- prosthetic devices
- experimental surgical techniques to construct a new voice box.

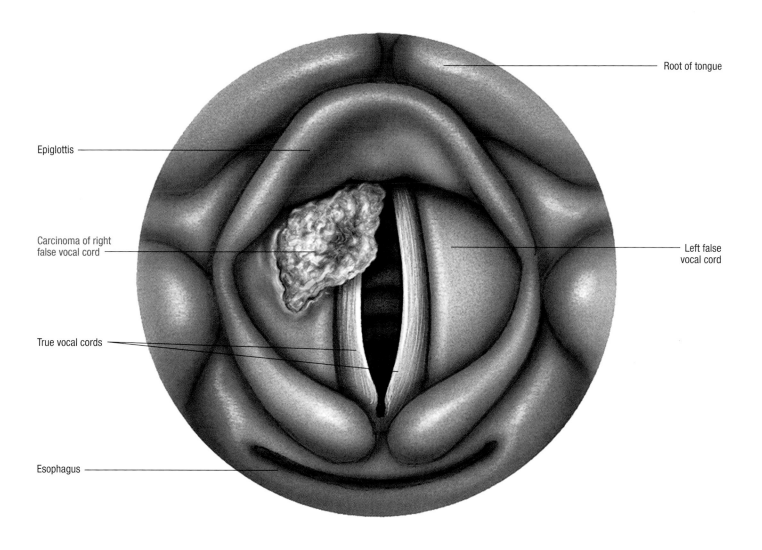

Root of tongue

Epiglottis

Carcinoma of right
false vocal cord

Left false
vocal cord

True vocal cords

Esophagus

MACULAR DEGENERATION

Macular degeneration — atrophy or degeneration of the macular disk — is the most common cause of legal blindness in adults. Commonly affecting both eyes, it accounts for about 12% of blindness in the United States and for about 17% of new blindness. It's one of the causes of severe, irreversible, and unpreventable loss of central vision in the elderly.

 AGE ALERT
Two types of age-related macular degeneration occur:
- Dry, or atrophic — characterized by atrophic pigment epithelial changes; most often causes mild, gradual visual loss
- Wet, or exudative — characterized by subretinal formation of new blood vessels (neovascularization) that cause leakage, hemorrhage, and fibrovascular scar formation; causes severe, rapid vision loss.

Causes
Primary cause unknown.
Possible contributing factors:
- Aging
- Inflammation
- Trauma
- Infection
- Poor nutrition.

Pathophysiology
Age-related macular degeneration results from hardening and obstruction of retinal arteries, which probably reflect normal degenerative changes. The formation of new blood vessels in the macular area obscures central vision. Underlying pathologic changes occur primarily in the retinal pigment epithelium, Bruch's membrane, and choriocapillaries in the macular region.

The dry form develops as yellow extracellular deposits, or drusen, accumulate beneath the pigment epithelium of the retina; they may be prominent in the macula. Drusen are common in the elderly. Over time, drusen grow and become more numerous. Visual loss occurs as the retinal pigment epithelium detaches and becomes atrophic.

Exudative macular degeneration develops as new blood vessels in the choroid project through abnormalities in Bruch's membrane and invade the potential space underneath the retinal pigment epithelium. As these vessels leak, fluid in the retinal pigment epithelium is increased, resulting in blurry vision.

Signs and symptoms
- Changes in central vision due to neovascularization, such as a blank spot (scotoma) in the center of a page when reading
- Distorted appearance of straight lines caused by relocation of retinal receptors.

Diagnostic tests
- Indirect ophthalmoscopy, to show gross macular changes, opacities, hemorrhage, neovascularization, retinal pallor, or retinal detachment
- I.V. fluorescein angiography sequential photographs, to show leaking vessels as fluorescein dye flows into the tissues from the subretinal neovascular net
- Amsler's grid test, to show central visual field loss.

Treatment
- Exudative form (subretinal neovascularization): laser photocoagulation
- Atrophic form: currently no cure.

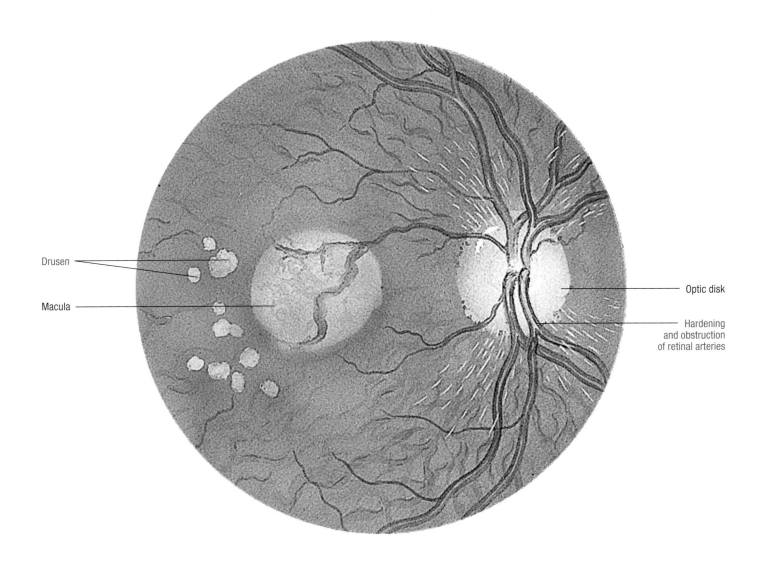

Drusen

Macula

Optic disk

Hardening
and obstruction
of retinal arteries

MÉNIÈRE'S DISEASE

Ménière's disease, a labyrinthine dysfunction also known as endolymphatic hydrops, causes severe vertigo, sensorineural hearing loss, and tinnitus.

 AGE ALERT
It usually affects adults between ages 30 and 60, men slightly more often than women. It rarely occurs in children.

Usually, only one ear is involved. After multiple attacks over several years, residual tinnitus and hearing loss can be incapacitating.

Causes

Cause unknown.
Possible associations:
- Positive family history
- Immune disorder
- Migraine headaches
- Middle ear infection
- Head trauma
- Autonomic nervous system dysfunction
- Premenstrual edema.

Pathophysiology

Ménière's disease may result from overproduction or decreased absorption of endolymph — the fluid contained in the labyrinth of the ear. Accumulated endolymph dilates the semicircular canals, utricle, and saccule and causes degeneration of the vestibular and cochlear hair cells. Overstimulation of the vestibular branch of cranial nerve VIII impairs postural reflexes and stimulates the vomiting reflex. This excessive cranial nerve stimulation and injury to sensory receptors for hearing may impair auditory acuity.

Signs and symptoms

- Sudden, severe spinning, whirling vertigo, lasting from 10 minutes to several hours, due to increased endolymph (attacks may occur several times a year, or remissions may last as long as several years)
- Tinnitus caused by altered firing of sensory auditory neurons; possibly residual tinnitus between attacks
- Hearing impairment due to sensorineural loss:
 - hearing may be normal between attacks
 - repeated attacks may progressively cause permanent hearing loss
- Feeling of fullness or blockage in the ear before an attack, a result of changing sensitivity of pressure receptors
- Severe nausea, vomiting, sweating, and pallor during an acute attack due to autonomic dysfunction

- Nystagmus due to asymmetry and intensity of impulses reaching the brain stem
- Loss of balance and falling to the affected side due to vertigo.

Diagnostic tests

- Audiometric testing
- Electronystagmography
- Cold caloric testing
- Electrocochleography
- Brain stem evoked response audiometry
- Computed tomography scan, magnetic resonance imaging.

Treatment

During an acute attack:
- Lying down to minimize head movement
- Avoiding sudden movements and glaring lights to reduce dizziness
- Promethazine or prochlorperazine to relieve nausea and vomiting
- Atropine to control an attack by reducing autonomic nervous system function
- Dimenhydrinate to control vertigo and nausea
- Central nervous system depressants, such as lorazepam or diazepam, to reduce excitability of vestibular nuclei
- Antihistamines, such as meclizine or diphenhydramine, to reduce dizziness and vomiting.

Long-term management:
- Diuretics, such as triamterene or acetazolamide, to reduce endolymph pressure
- Betahistine, to alleviate vertigo, hearing loss, and tinnitus
- Vasodilators, to dilate blood vessels supplying the inner ear
- Sodium restriction, to reduce endolymphatic hydrops
- Antihistamines or mild sedatives, to prevent attacks
- Systemic streptomycin, to produce chemical ablation of the sensory neuroepithelium of the inner ear, and thereby control vertigo in patients with bilateral disease for whom no other treatment can be considered.

Disease that persists, despite medical treatment, or produces incapacitating vertigo:
- Endolymphatic drainage and shunt placement, to reduce pressure on the hair cells of the cochlea and prevent further sensorineural hearing loss
- Vestibular nerve resection in patients with intact hearing, to reduce vertigo and prevent further hearing loss
- Labyrinthectomy to relieve vertigo in patients with incapacitating symptoms and poor or no hearing; destruction of the cochlea results in a total loss of hearing in the affected ear
- Cochlear implantation, to improve hearing in patients with profound deafness.

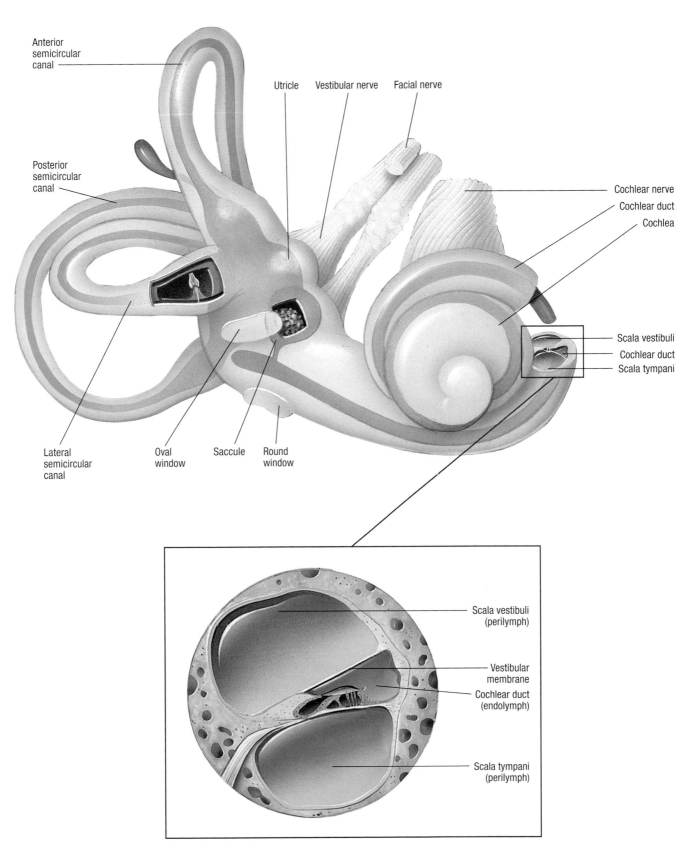

Anterior semicircular canal

Posterior semicircular canal

Utricle

Vestibular nerve

Facial nerve

Cochlear nerve

Cochlear duct

Cochlea

Scala vestibuli

Cochlear duct

Scala tympani

Lateral semicircular canal

Oval window

Saccule

Round window

Scala vestibuli (perilymph)

Vestibular membrane

Cochlear duct (endolymph)

Scala tympani (perilymph)

OTITIS MEDIA

Otitis media, inflammation of the middle ear, may be suppurative or secretory, acute, persistent, unresponsive, or chronic.

Acute otitis media is common in children; its incidence rises during the winter months, paralleling the seasonal rise in nonbacterial respiratory tract infections. With prompt treatment, the prognosis for acute otitis media is excellent; however, prolonged accumulation of fluid within the middle ear cavity causes chronic otitis media and, possibly, perforation of the tympanic membrane.

Chronic suppurative otitis media may lead to scarring, adhesions, and severe structural or functional ear damage. Chronic secretory otitis media, with its persistent inflammation and pressure, may cause conductive hearing loss. It most often occurs in children with tympanostomy tubes or those with a perforated tympanic membrane.

Recurrent otitis media is defined as three near-acute otitis media episodes within six months or four episodes of acute otitis media within one year.

Otitis media with complications involves damage, such as adhesions, retraction, pockets, cholesteatoma, and intratemporal and intracranial complications, to middle ear structures.

Causes

Suppurative otitis media (bacterial infection):
- Pneumococci
- *Haemophilus influenzae*, most common cause in children under age 6 years
- *Moraxella catarrhalis*
- Beta-hemolytic streptococci
- Staphylococci, most common cause in children age 6 or older
- Gram-negative bacteria.
  Chronic suppurative otitis media:
- Inadequate treatment of acute otitis episodes
- Infection by resistant strains of bacteria
- Tuberculosis (rare).
  Secretory otitis media:
- Obstruction of eustachian tube secondary to eustachian tube dysfunction from viral infection or allergy
- Barotrauma — pressure injury caused by inability to equalize pressures between the environment and the middle ear:
- during rapid aircraft descent in a person with an upper respiratory tract infection
- during rapid underwater ascent in scuba diving (barotitis media).
  Chronic secretory otitis media:
- Mechanical obstruction — adenoidal tissue overgrowth, tumors
- Edema — allergic rhinitis, chronic sinus infection
- Inadequate treatment of acute suppurative otitis media.

Pathophysiology

Otitis media results from disruption of eustachian tube patency. In the *suppurative form*, respiratory tract infection, allergic reaction, nasotracheal intubation, or positional changes allow nasopharyngeal flora to reflux through the eustachian tube and colonize the middle ear.

Signs and symptoms

Acute suppurative otitis media:
- Severe, deep, throbbing pain from pressure behind the tympanic membrane
- Signs of upper respiratory tract infection (sneezing, coughing)
- Mild to very high fever
- Hearing loss — usually mild and conductive
- Tinnitus, dizziness, nausea, vomiting
- Bulging, erythematous tympanic membrane; purulent drainage in the ear canal if tympanic membrane ruptures.
  Acute secretory otitis media:
- Severe conductive hearing loss — varies from 15 to 35 dB, depending on the thickness and amount of fluid in the middle ear cavity
- Sensation of fullness in the ear
- Popping, crackling, or clicking sounds on swallowing or with jaw movement
- Echo during speech
- Vague feeling of top-heaviness.
  Chronic otitis media:
- Thickening and scarring of the tympanic membrane
- Decreased or absent tympanic membrane mobility
- Cholesteatoma (a cystlike mass in the middle ear)
- Painless, purulent discharge.

CLINICAL TIP

If the tympanic membrane ruptures, the patient may state that the pain has suddenly stopped. Complications may include abscesses (brain, subperiosteal, and epidural), sigmoid sinus or jugular vein thrombosis, septicemia, meningitis, suppurative labyrinthitis, facial paralysis, and otitis externa.

Diagnostic tests
- Otoscopy
- Pneumatoscopy
- Culture of the ear drainage
- Tympanocentesis
- Tympanometry
- Acoustic reflex measurement
- White blood cell count.

Treatment
- Antibiotic therapy
- Myringotomy — insertion of a polyethylene tube into the tympanic membrane
- Inflation of eustachian tube by performing Valsalva maneuver several times a day
- Nasopharyngeal decongestant
- Aspiration of middle ear fluid
- Concomitant treatment of underlying cause, such as elimination of allergens, or adenoidectomy for hypertrophied adenoids
- Treatment of otitis externa
- Myringoplasty and tympanoplasty
- Mastoidectomy
- Cholesteatoma, requires excision.

CLASSIFICATION AND COMMON COMPLICATIONS OF OTITIS MEDIA

Classifications

Otoscopic view

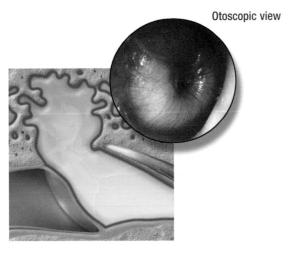

Acute otitis media
- Infected fluid in middle ear
- Rapid onset and short duration

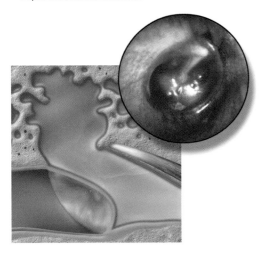

Otitis media with effusion
- Relatively asymptomatic fluid in the middle ear
- May be acute, subacute, or chronic in nature

Complications

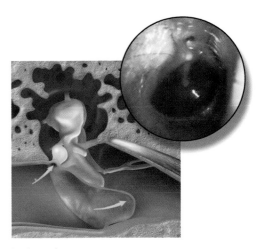

Atelectasis
- Thinning and potential collapse of tympanic membrane

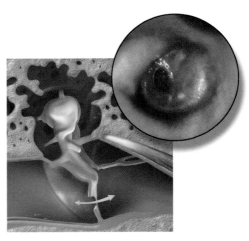

Perforation
- A hole in the tympanic membrane caused by chronic negative middle ear pressure, inflammation, or trauma

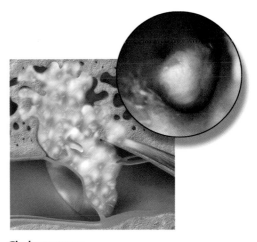

Cholesteatoma
- Mass of entrapped skin in the middle ear or temporal lobe

APPENDIX, GLOSSARY, SELECTED REFERENCES, AND INDEX

Types of cardiac arrhythmias

ARRHYTHMIA AND FEATURES	CAUSES
Sinus tachycardia	
• Rhythm regular • HR >100 beats/minute • Normal P wave preceding each QRS complex	• May be a normal physiologic response • Left ventricular failure, cardiac tamponade, hyperthyroidism, anemia, hypovolemia, pulmonary embolism, anterior wall myocardial infarction (MI) • Atropine, epinephrine, isoproterenol, quinidine, caffeine, alcohol, or nicotine
Sinus bradycardia	
• Rhythm regular • HR < 60 beats/minute • Normal P waves preceding each QRS complex	• Normal in well-conditioned heart • Increased intracranial pressure • Increased vagal tone • Anticholinesterase, beta blocker, digoxin, or morphine
Paroxysmal supraventricular tachycardia	
• Rhythm regular • HR > 160 beats/minute • P waves usually not visible; difficult to differentiate from preceding T wave • Sudden onset and termination of arrhythmia	• Intrinsic abnormality of atrioventricular (AV) conduction • Physical or psychological stress, hypoxia, hypokalemia, cardiomyopathy, congenital heart disease, MI, valvular disease, Wolff-Parkinson-White syndrome, cor pulmonale, hyperthyroidism, or systemic hypertension • Digoxin toxicity; use of caffeine, marijuana, or central nervous system stimulants
Atrial flutter	
• Atrial rhythm regular; 250 to 400 beats/minute • Ventricular rate variable, depending on degree of AV block • Sawtooth P wave configuration (F waves) possible • QRS complexes uniform in shape, but often irregular in rate	• Heart failure, tricuspid or mitral valve disease, pulmonary embolism, cor pulmonale, inferior wall MI, or pericarditis • Digoxin toxicity
Atrial fibrillation	
• Atrial rhythm grossly irregular; rate > 400 beats/minute • Ventricular rate grossly irregular • QRS complexes of uniform configuration and duration • PR interval indiscernible • No P waves, or P waves that appear as erratic, irregular, baseline fibrillatory waves	• Heart failure, chronic obstructive pulmonary disease, thyrotoxicosis, constrictive pericarditis, ischemic heart disease, sepsis, pulmonary embolism, rheumatic heart disease, hypertension, mitral stenosis, atrial irritation, or complication of coronary bypass or valve replacement surgery
Junctional rhythm	
• Rhythm regular; atrial rate 40 to 60 beats/minute; ventricular rate usually 40 to 60 beats/minute (60 to 100 beats/minute is accelerated junctional rhythm) • P waves preceding, hidden within (absent), or after QRS complex; inverted if visible • PR interval (when present) < 0.12 second • QRS complex configuration and duration normal, except in aberrant conduction	• Inferior wall MI or ischemia, hypoxia, vagal stimulation, or sick sinus syndrome • Acute rheumatic fever • Valve surgery • Digoxin toxicity
First-degree atrioventricular (AV) block	
• Rhythm regular • PR interval > 0.20 second • P wave precedes QRS complex • QRS complex normal	• May occur in healthy persons • Inferior wall MI or ischemia, hypothyroidism, hypokalemia, or hyperkalemia • Digoxin toxicity; quinidine, procainamide, or propranolol

ARRHYTHMIA AND FEATURES	CAUSES
Second-degree AV block	
Mobitz I (Wenckebach)	
• Rhythm irregular • Atrial rate exceeds ventricular rate • PR interval progressively, but only slightly, longer with each cycle until QRS complex disappears (dropped beat); PR interval shorter after dropped beat	• Inferior wall MI, cardiac surgery, acute rheumatic fever, or vagal stimulation • Digoxin toxicity • Propranolol, quinidine, or procainamide
Second-degree AV block	
Mobitz II	
• Rhythm irregular • P-P interval constant • QRS complexes periodically absent	• Severe coronary artery disease, anterior wall MI, or acute myocarditis • Digoxin toxicity
Third-degree AV block	
(Complete heart block)	
• Rhythm regular • Ventricular rate slow and regular • No relation between P waves and QRS complexes • No constant PR interval • QRS interval normal (nodal pacemaker) or wide and bizarre (ventricular pacemaker)	• Inferior or anterior wall MI, congenital abnormality, rheumatic fever, hypoxia, postoperative complication of mitral valve replacement, Lev's disease, or Lenègre's disease • Digoxin toxicity
Premature ventricular contractions	
• Rhythm irregular • QRS complex premature, usually followed by a compensatory pause • QRS complex wide and distorted, usually > 0.14 second • Premature QRS complexes occurring singly, in pairs, or in threes, alternating with normal beats; focus from one or more sites • Ominous when clustered, multifocal, with R wave on T pattern	• Heart failure; old or acute MI, ischemia, or contusion; myocardial irritation by ventricular catheter or pacemaker; hypercapnia; hypokalemia; or hypocalcemia • Drug toxicity: digoxin, aminophylline, tricyclic antidepressants, beta blockers, isoproterenol, or dopamine • Caffeine, tobacco, or alcohol use • Psychological stress, anxiety, pain, or exercise
Ventricular tachycardia	
• Ventricular rate 140 to 220 beats/minute, regular or irregular • QRS complexes wide, bizarre, and independent of P waves • P waves not discernible • May start and stop suddenly	• Myocardial ischemia, MI, or aneurysm; coronary artery disease; rheumatic heart disease; mitral valve prolapse; heart failure; cardiomyopathy; ventricular catheters; hypokalemia; hypercalcemia; or pulmonary embolism • Drug toxicity: digoxin, procainamide, epinephrine, or quinidine • Anxiety
Ventricular fibrillation	
• Ventricular rhythm rapid and chaotic • QRS complexes wide and irregular; no visible P waves	• Myocardial ischemia, MI, untreated ventricular tachycardia, R-on-T phenomenon, hypokalemia, hyperkalemia, hypercalcemia, alkalosis, electric shock, or hypothermia • Drug toxicity: digoxin, epinephrine, or quinidine
Asystole	
• No atrial or ventricular rate or rhythm • No discernible P waves, QRS complexes, or T waves	• Myocardial ischemia, MI, aortic valve disease, heart failure, hypoxia, hypokalemia, severe acidosis, electric shock, ventricular arrhythmia, AV block, pulmonary embolism, heart rupture, cardiac tamponade, hyperkalemia, or electromechanical dissociation • Cocaine overdose

Glossary

Acidemia Abnormal acidity, or low pH, of the blood

Acidosis Condition due to accumulation of acid or depletion of the alkaline reserve in the blood and body tissues

Acinus Any of the smallest lobules of a gland

Acromegaly Abnormal enlargement of the extremities of the skeleton due to hypersecretion of growth hormone from the pituitary gland

Acropachy Soft tissue swelling accompanied by underlying bone changes where new bone formation occurs

Acyanotic Not characterized by or accompanied by cyanosis

Adenomyosis Invasion of the muscular wall of the uterus by glandular tissue

Afterload The force opposing ventricular contraction

Agranulocyte Leukocyte (white blood cell) not containing granules or grains; includes lymphocytes, monocytes, and plasma cells

Akinesia Absence or loss of power of voluntary movement

Alkalemia Abnormal alkalinity, or high pH, of the blood

Alkalosis Abnormal condition of body fluids resulting from accumulation of base or from loss of acid without comparable loss of base

Allele One of two or more different genes that occupy a corresponding position (locus) on matched chromosomes; allows for different forms of the same inherited characteristic

Amyloidosis Disorder of unknown cause, in which insoluble protein fibers become deposited in tissues and organs, impairing their function

Anaphase Third stage of division of the nucleus in meiosis or mitosis

Anaplasia Loss of differentiation of cells; a characteristic of tumor cells

Aneurysm Sac formed by localized vasodilation of the wall of an artery or vein

Angioedema Localized edematous reaction of the dermis or subcutaneous or submucosal tissues

Angiography Radiographic examination of vessels of the body

Anion Ion carrying a negative charge

Anisocytosis Presence of erythrocytes with abnormal variations in size

Ankylosis Immobility and consolidation of a joint, often in an abnormal position; caused by disease, trauma, or surgical procedure

Anorexia Lack of or loss of appetite for food

Anovulation Absence of ovulation

Anoxia Absence of oxygen in the tissues

Antibody Immunoglobulin molecule that reacts only with the specific antigen that induced its formation in the lymph system

Antigen Foreign substance, such as bacteria or toxins, that induces antibody formation

Anuria Complete cessation of urine formation by the kidney

Areflexia Absence of reflexes

Arnold-Chiari syndrome Congenital anomaly in which the cerebellum and medulla protrude through the foramen magnum into the spinal canal

Arousal State of being ready to respond to sensory stimulation

Arteriosclerosis Group of diseases characterized by thickening and loss of elasticity of the arterial walls

Arthralgia Pain in a joint

Arthrodesis Surgical fusion of a joint

Ascites Abnormal accumulation of serous fluid in the peritoneal cavity

Aspiration Inhalation of mucus or vomitus into the respiratory tract; suctioning of fluid or gas from a body cavity.

Asterixis Motor disturbance marked by intermittent lapses of assumed posture; also known as liver flap

Atelectasis Collapsed or airless state of the lung; may involve all or part of the lung

Atopy Clinical hypersensitivity or allergy with a hereditary predisposition

Atrophy Decrease in size or wasting away of a cell, tissue, organ, or body part

Autoimmune disorder Disorder in which the body launches an immunologic response against itself

Autoinoculation Inoculation with microorganisms from one's own body

Autosome Any of the 22 pairs of chromosomes not concerned with determination of sex

Azotemia Excess nitrogenous waste products in the blood

Babinski's reflex Reflex action of the toes, normal during infancy. It's elicited by rubbing a firm substance on the sole of the foot, which results in dorsiflexion (upward bending) of the great toe and fanning of the smaller toes. After infancy, normal response is downward bending of all toes on the foot.

Bacteria One-celled microorganisms that have no true nucleus and reproduce by cell division

Bactericidal Destructive to bacteria

Bacteriostatic Preventing bacteria from multiplying or growing

Bacteriuria Bacteria in the urine

Balanoposthitis Inflammation of the glans penis and prepuce

Barotrauma Injury due to pressure

Benign Not malignant or recurrent; favorable for recovery

Biopsy Examination, usually microscopic, of tissue removed from the living body

Blepharospasm Spasm of the orbicular muscle of the eyelid that completely closes eyelids

Bone Hard, rigid form of connective tissue constituting most of the skeleton

Bone marrow Soft organic material filling the cavities of bones

Bradykinin Nonpeptide kinin formed from a plasma protein; a powerful vasodilator that increases capillary permeability, constricts smooth muscle, and stimulates pain receptors

Bronchiectasis Chronic dilation of the bronchi and bronchioles with secondary infection, usually of the lower lung lobes

Bronchiolitis Inflammation of the bronchioles

Bruch's membrane Support structure on the inner side of the choroid

Brudzinski's sign In meningitis, bending the patient's neck usually produces flexion of the knee and hip

Bulla (pl. bullae) Spaces filled with air or fluid

Bursa Fluid-filled sac or cavity in connective tissue near a joint; acts as a cushion

Cachexia State of marked ill health and malnutrition

Carcinogen Any substance that causes cancer

Carcinoma Malignant growth made of epithelial cells; tends to infiltrate surrounding tissues and metastasize

Cardiac output Volume of blood ejected by the heart per minute

Carphology Involuntary picking at the bedclothes, seen in states of great exhaustion and grave fevers

Cartilage Dense connective tissue consisting of fibers embedded in a strong, gel-like substance; supports, cushions, and shapes body structures

Cation Positively charged ion

Cell-mediated immunity Immune response that involves effector T lymphocytes and not the production of humoral antibody

Cercaria Final, free-swimming stage of a trematode larva

Chemonucleolysis Injection of the enzyme chymopapain (a chemolytic agent) into a herniated intervertebral disk

Chemotaxis Response of leukocytes to products formed in immunologic reactions, wherein leukocytes are attracted to and accumulate at the site of the reaction

Cholangioma Tumor of the bile ducts

Cholangitis Inflammation of a bile duct

Cholecystectomy Excision of the gallbladder

Choledochostomy Creation of an opening into the common bile duct for drainage

Cholestasis Stopped or decreased bile flow

Cholesteatoma Cystlike mass filled with desquamating debris frequently including cholesterol, which occurs most commonly in the middle ear and mastoid region

Chondrocalcinosis Deposition of calcium salts in the cartilage of joints

Chorea Rapid, jerky involuntary movements

Choriocapillaries Capillary layer of the choroid

Choroid Thin membrane that covers the eyeball and supplies blood to the retina

Chromatin The substance of the chromosomes, composed of DNA and basic proteins

Chvostek's sign Spasm of the hyperirritable facial nerve induced by tapping the facial nerve in the region of the parotid gland

Claudication Pain in the calves due to reduced blood flow to the legs

Cognition Process by which a person becomes aware of objects; includes all aspects of perception, thought, and memory

Commissurotomy Surgical separation of adherent, thickened leaflets of the mitral valve

Complement system Major mediator of inflammatory response; a functionally related system of 20 proteins circulating as inactive molecules

Congenital Present at birth

Constipation Condition in which feces in the bowel are too hard to pass easily

Cor pulmonale Right ventricular hypertrophy with right-sided heart failure due to pulmonary hypertension secondary to disease of the blood vessels of the lungs

Corrigan's pulse Jerky pulse with full expansion and sudden collapse

Cremasteric reflex Stimulation of the skin on the inner thigh retracts the testis on the same side

Crepitus Crackling sound in the joints, skin, or lungs

Curettage Scraping or collecting tissue from the wall of a body cavity

Cyanosis Bluish discoloration of the skin and mucous membranes due to reduced hemoglobin in the blood

Cystitis Inflammation of the urinary bladder

Cytokines Nonantibody proteins, secreted by inflammatory leukocytes and some nonleukocytic cells, that act as intercellular mediators

Cytology The study of cells, their origin, structure, function, and pathology

Cytotoxic Destructive to cells

Debridement Removal of all foreign material and diseased and devitalized tissue from or adjacent to a traumatic or infected lesion until surrounding healthy tissue is exposed

Decortication Surgical removal of the thick coating over an organ, such as lung or kidney

Demyelination Destruction of a nerve's myelin sheath; prevents normal conduction

Diabetic ketoacidosis Complication of diabetes mellitus that results from by-products of fat metabolism (ketones) when glucose is not available for a fuel source in the body

Diaphoresis Perspiration

Diarrhea Frequent evacuation of watery stools caused by rapid movement of intestinal contents; results in poor absorption of water, nutritive elements, and electrolytes

Differentiation Process of cells maturing into specific types

Diffusion Spontaneous movement of molecules or other particles in a solution

Diplegia Paralysis of like parts on either side of the body

Diploid Cell with a full set of genetic material; a human diploid cell has 46 chromosomes

Diplopia Double vision

Disjunction Separation of chromosomes during cell division

Divarication Separation into two parts or branches; bifurcation

Diverticula Pockets of tissue that push out from the colon walls

Dominant gene Gene that produces an effect in an organism regardless of the state of the corresponding allele

Dressler's syndrome Post-MI pericarditis that develops weeks to several months after MI or open heart surgery

Dysarthria Imperfect articulation of speech due to disturbances of muscular control

Dyscrasia Condition related to a disease, usually referring to an imbalance of component elements

Dysphagia Difficulty swallowing

Dysplasia Alteration in size, shape, and organization of adult cells

Dyspnea Labored or difficult breathing

Dysuria Painful or difficult urination

Eclampsia Potentially life-threatening disorder of pregnancy characterized by hypertension, generalized edema, and proteinuria

Ejection fraction Measure of ventricular contractility

Embolism Sudden obstruction of a blood vessel by a foreign substance or a blood clot

Empyema Accumulation of pus in a body cavity

Endocrine Pertaining to internal hormone secretion by glands

Endogenous Occurring inside the body

Endolymph Fluid within the membranous labyrinth of the ear

Endotoxin Toxin associated with the outer membranes of certain gram-negative bacteria

Epistaxis Hemorrhage from the nose, usually due to rupture of small vessels

Erythema marginatum Nonpruritic, macular, transient rash on the trunk or inner aspects of the upper arms or thighs, that gives rise to red lesions with blanched centers

Erythrocyte Red blood cell; carries oxygen to the tissues and removes carbon dioxide from them

Erythropoiesis Production of red blood cells or erythrocytes

Estrogen Female sex hormone

Exacerbation Increase in the severity of a disease or any of its symptoms

Exanthem Rash or skin eruption

Exocrine External or outward secretion of a gland

Exogenous Occurring outside the body

Exotoxin Potent toxin formed and excreted by a bacterial cell, and found in the surrounding medium

Extracellular fluid Fluid in the spaces outside the cells

Fetor hepaticus Musty, sweetish breath characteristic of hepatic disease

Fubernaculum Fibromuscular band that connects the testes to the scrotal floor

Fulguration Destruction of tissue by high-frequency electricity

Fungate Funguslike growth or growing rapidly like a fungus

Fungus Nonphotosynthetic microorganism that reproduces asexually by cell division

Furunculosis Occurrence of furuncles serially over weeks or months

Gait ataxia Unsteady, uncoordinated walk, with a wide base and the feet turned out, coming down first on the heel and then on the toes with a double tap

Gap junctions Channels through which ions and other small molecules pass

Gastrectomy Excision of the stomach or a portion of it

Gastrostomy Creation of an opening into the stomach for the purpose of administering food or fluids

Genome Total of all genetic information included in a set of unreplicated chromosomes

Gibson murmur Continuous murmur heard throughout systole and diastole in older children and adults due to shunting of blood from the aorta to the pulmonary artery

Gland Organ composed of specialized cells that produce a secretion used in some other body part

Glomerulopathy Any disease of the renal glomeruli

Glomerulosclerosis Glomerular disease characterized by hardening of focal and segmental areas of the glomerulus

Glomerulus Network of twisted capillaries in the nephron, the basic unit of the kidney; brings blood and waste products carried by blood to the nephron

Glucagon Hormone released during the fasting state that increases blood glucose concentration

Gluconeogenesis Formation of glucose from molecules that are not carbohydrates, such as amino acids and glycerol

Glycogenolysis Splitting of glycogen in the liver, yielding glucose

Glycosuria Presence of glucose in the urine

Goblet cells Mucus-secreting cells of the epithelial lining of the small intestine and respiratory passages

Granulocyte Any cell containing granules, especially a granular leukocyte (white blood cell)

Granuloma Any small nodular aggregation of mononuclear inflammatory cells or a similar collection of modified macrophages resembling endothelial cells, usually surrounded by lymphocytes, often with multinucleated giant cells

Hamartoma Benign tumor-like nodule composed of an overgrowth of mature cells and tissues normally present in the affected part

Haploid Having half the normal number of chromosomes

Heberden's nodules Small, hard nodules on the distal interphalangeal joints of the fingers in osteoarthritis

Hematemesis Vomiting of blood

Hematoma Localized collection of blood, usually clotted, in an organ, space, or tissue

Hematopoiesis Production of red blood cells in the bone marrow

Hematuria Blood in the urine

Hemochromatosis Disorder of iron metabolism with excess deposition of iron in the tissues, bronze skin pigmentation, cirrhosis, and diabetes mellitus

Hemoglobin Protein in erythrocytes that transports oxygen

Hemolysis Red blood cell destruction

Hemostasis Complex process whereby platelets, plasma, and coagulation factors interact to control bleeding

Hepatojugular reflux Distention of the jugular vein induced by manual pressure over the liver

Hepatoma Any tumor of the liver

Heterozygous Genes having different alleles at the same site (locus)

Hirsutism Abnormal hairiness

Histamine An amine found in all body tissues that induces capillary dilation, which increases capillary permeability and lowers blood pressure, causes contraction of most smooth muscle tissue, increased gastric acid secretion, and increased heart rate; also a mediator of immediate hypersensitivity

Homeostasis Dynamic, steady state of internal balance in the body

Homologous genes Gene pairs sharing a corresponding structure and position

Homozygous Genes that have identical alleles for a given trait

Hormone Chemical substance produced in the body that has a specific regulatory effect on the activity of specific cells or organs

Humoral immunity Form of immunity in which B lymphocytes and plasma cells produce antibodies to foreign agents (antigens) and stimulate T lymphocytes to attack them (cellular immunity)

Hyperplasia Excessive growth of normal cells that causes an increase in the volume of a tissue or organ

Hyperpnea Increase in depth of breathing, which may be accompanied by an increased respiratory rate

Hyperreflexia Exaggeration of reflexes

Hypertonic Having an osmotic pressure greater than that of the solution with which it's compared

Hypertrichosis Excessive hair growth

Hypertrophy Increase in volume of tissue or organ due to enlargement of existing cells

Hypervolemia Abnormal increase in the volume of circulating fluid in the body

Hypoplasia Incomplete development or underdevelopment of an organ or tissue

Hypotonia Abnormally low tonicity or strength

Hypotonic Having an osmotic pressure lower than that of the solution with which it's compared

Hypovolemia Abnormally low volume of circulating fluid in the body

Hypoxia Reduction of oxygen in body tissues to below normal levels

Idiopathic Occurring without known cause

Ileal conduit Use of a segment of the ileum for the diversion of urinary flow from the ureters

Ileus Failure of appropriate forward movement of bowel contents

Immunodeficiency Disorder caused by inadequate immune response; due to hypoactivity or decreased numbers of lymphoid cells

Immunoglobulin Serum protein synthesized by lymphocytes and plasma cells that has known antibody activity

Intention tremor Tremor occurring when one attempts voluntary movement

Interphase Interval between two successive cell divisions

Interstitial fluid Fluid between cells in tissues

Intertrigo Erythematous skin eruption in such areas as the creases of the neck, folds of the groin and axillae, and beneath pendulous breasts

Intracellular fluid Fluid inside each cell

Intrapleural Within the pleura

Ion Atom or group of atoms having a positive or negative electric charge

Ischemia Decreased blood supply to a body organ or tissue

Isotonic Solution having the same tonicity as another solution with which it's compared

Jaundice Yellow discoloration of skin, sclerae, mucous membranes, and excretions due to hyperbilirubinemia and deposition of bile pigments

Joint Intersection of two or more bones; most provide motion and flexibility

Karyotype Chromosomal arrangement of the cell nucleus

Kernig's sign Sign of meningitis in which a patient in supine position can easily and completely extend the leg; patient in sitting position or lying with the thigh flexed upon the abdomen can't completely extend leg

Ketones Byproducts of fat metabolism when glucose is not available

Ketonuria Excess of ketones in the urine

Koilonchyia Abnormally thin nails that are concave from side to side, with the edges turned up

Korotkoff sound Sounds heard during auscultation of blood pressure

Kupffer's cells Large, phagocytic cells lining the walls of the hepatic sinusoids

Kussmaul's respirations Dyspnea characterized by increased rate and depth of respirations, panting, and labored respiration; seen in metabolic acidosis

Kussmaul's sign Increased jugular venous distention on inspiration; occurs due to restricted right-sided filling

Kyphoscoliosis Forward and lateral curvature of the spine

Lasègue's sign In sciatica, pain in the back and leg elicited by passive raising of the heel from the bed with the knee straight

Leukapheresis Selective removal of leukocytes from withdrawn blood, which is then retransfused into the donor

Leukocyte White blood cell that protects the body against microorganisms causing disease

Leukocytosis Increase in the number of leukocytes in the blood; generally caused by infection

Leukopenia Reduction in the number of leukocytes in the blood

Leukotrienes Group of compounds derived from unsaturated fatty acids; extremely potent mediators of immediate hypersensitivity reactions and inflammation

Lichenification Thickening and hardening of the skin

Ligament Band of fibrous tissue that connects bones or cartilage, strengthens joints, provides stability, and limits or facilitates movement

Locus Location on a chromosome

Lymph node Structure that filters the lymphatic fluid that drains from body tissue and is later returned to the plasma

Lymphadenitis Inflammation of one or more lymph nodes

Lymphedema Chronic swelling of a body part from accumulation of interstitial fluid secondary to obstruction or surgical removal of lymphatic vessels or lymph nodes

Lymphocytes Leukocytes produced by lymphoid tissue that participates in immunity

Lysozyme Enzyme that can kill microorganisms or microbes

Macroglossia Excessive size of the tongue

Macrophages Highly phagocytic cells that are stimulated by inflammation

Malignant Condition that becomes progressively worse and results in death

Megakaryocyte Platelet precursor; the giant cell of bone marrow

Megaloureter Congenital ureteral dilation without demonstrable cause

Meiosis Process of cell division by which reproductive cells are formed

Menorrhagia Heavy or prolonged menses

Merozoite Stage in the life cycle of the malaria parasite

Mesorchium Fold in the tissue between the testis and epididymis

Metabolic acidosis Acidosis resulting from accumulation of keto acids in the blood at the expense of bicarbonate

Metabolic alkalosis Disturbance in which the acid-base status shifts toward the alkaline because of uncompensated loss of acids, ingestion or retention of excess base, or potassium depletion

Metaphase Stage of cell division in which the chromosomes, each consisting of two chromatids, are arranged in the equatorial plane of the spindle

Metaplasia Change in adult cells to a form abnormal for that tissue

Metastasis Transfer of disease via pathogenic microorganisms or cells from one organ or body part to another not directly associated with it

Metrorrhagia Episodes of vaginal bleeding between menses

Microembolus Embolus of microscopic size

Micturition Urination

Mitosis Ordinary process of cell division in which each chromosome with all its genes reproduces itself exactly

Monocyte Mononuclear, phagocytic leukocyte

Monoplegia Paralysis of a single part

Monosomy Presence of one chromosome less than the normal number

Morbidity Condition of having a disease

Morphea Condition in which connective tissue replaces skin and sometimes subcutaneous tissues

Mortality Ratio of the total number of deaths to the total population

Mucolytic Agent that acts by destroying mucous

Muscle Bundle of long slender cells, or fibers, that has the power to contract and produce movement

Mutation Permanent change in genetic material

Myalgia Muscle pain

Myectomy Excision of a muscle

Myelomatous cells Increased number of immature plasma cells

Myolysis Degeneration of muscle tissue

Myomectomy Removal of tumors in the uterine muscle

Myotomy Cutting or dissection of a muscle

Myxedema Condition resulting from advanced hypothyroidism, or defiency of thyroxine

Nausea Unpleasant sensation with the tendency to vomit

Necrosis Cell or tissue death

Neoplasm Abnormal growth in which cell multiplication is uncontrolled and progressive

Nephrolithiasis Condition marked by the presence of renal calculi

Nephron Structural and functional unit of the kidney that forms urine

Neuritis Inflammation of a nerve

Neurolysis Freeing of nerve fibers by cutting the nerve sheath longitudinally

Neuron Highly specialized conductor cell that receives and transmits electrochemical nerve impulses

Neutropenia Neutrophil deficiency in the blood

Neutrophil Granular leukocyte

Nevus Circumscribed, stable malformation of the skin and oral mucosa

Nondisjunction Failure of chromosomes to separate properly during cell division; causes an unequal distribution of chromosomes between the two resulting cells

Nystagmus Involuntary, rapid, rhythmic movement of the eyeball

Obstipation Intractable constipation

Oculogyric crises Eyelids are fixed upward with involuntary tonic movements

Oligomenorrhea Abnormally infrequent menses

Oliguria Diminished urine secretion

Omentum Fold of the peritoneum between the stomach and adjacent abdominal organs

Onychia Inflammation of the nail bed

Onycholysis Distal nail separated from the bed

Oophoritis Inflammation of the ovary

Opisthotonos Spasm in which the head and heels arch backward and the body bows forward

Opportunistic infection Infection striking people with altered, weakened immune systems; caused by microorganism that doesn't ordinarily cause disease but becomes pathogenic under certain conditions

Opthalmoplegia Ocular paralysis

Optic neuritis Inflammation of the optic nerve

Orchiectomy Excision of a testis

Orchiopexy Surgical fixation of an undescended testis in the scrotum

Organelle Structure in the cytoplasm that performs a specific function

Orthopnea Ability to breathe easily only in the upright position

Orthostatic hypotension Fall in blood pressure that occurs upon standing or when standing motionless in a fixed position

Osmolality Concentration of a solution expressed in terms of osmoles of solute per kilogram of solvent

Osmolarity Concentration of a solution expressed in terms of osmoles of solute per liter of solution

Osseous Of the nature or quality of bone

Osteoblasts Bone-forming cells

Osteoclasts Giant, multinuclear cells that reabsorb material from previously formed bones, tear down old or excess bone structure, and allow osteoblasts to rebuild new bone

Osteotomy Surgical division and realignment of bone

Ostium primium Opening in the lower portion of the membrane dividing the embryonic heart into right and left sides

Pancarditis Concurrent myocarditis, pericarditis, and endocarditis

Pancytopenia Abnormal depression of all the cellular elements of blood

Panmyelosis Proliferation of all the elements of the bone marrow

Papilledema Inflammation and edema of the optic nerve; associated with increased intracranial pressure

Paracentesis Surgical puncture of a cavity for the aspiration of fluid

Parametritis Inflammation of the parametrium

Paresthesia Abnormal burning or prickling sensation

Paronchyia Inflammation of the folds of tissue around the fingernail

Paroxysmal nocturnal dyspnea Respiratory distress related to posture (reclining at night) usually associated with heart failure and pulmonary edema

Pericardectomy Surgical creation of an opening to remove accumulated fluid from the pericardial sac

Pericardiocentesis Needle aspiration of the pericardial cavity

Perilymph Fluid in the space separating the membranous and osseus labyrinths of the ear

Periosteum Specialized connective tissue covering all bones and possessing bone-forming potential

Perseveration Abnormally persistent replies to questions

Petechia Minute, round purplish red spot caused by intradermal or submucous hemorrhage

Phagocyte Cell that ingests microorganisms, other cells, and foreign materials

Phagocytosis Engulfing of microorganisms, other cells, and foreign material by a phagocyte

Phlebectomy Removing a varicose vein through small incisions in the skin

Phlebography Radiographic examination of a vein

Photoplethysmography Plethysmographic determination in which the intensity of light reflected from the skin surface and the red cells below is measured to determine the blood volume of the respective area

Pilosebaceous Pertaining to the hair follicles and sebaceous glands

Plasmapheresis Removal of plasma from withdrawn blood and retransfusion of the formed elements into the donor

Plethora Edema and blood vessel distention

Polycythemia Increase in the total red cell mass of the blood

Polydipsia Excessive thirst

Polygenic traits Determined by several different genes

Polymenorrhea Menstrual cycle of less than eighteen days

Polyphagia Excessive ingestion of food

Polyuria Excessive excretion of urine

Preload Volume of blood in the ventricle at the end of diastole

Presbycusis Progressive, symmetrical, bilateral sensorineural hearing loss, usually of high frequency tones, caused by loss of hair cells in the organ of Corti

Pretibial myxedema Nonpitting edema of the anterior surface of the legs, dermopathy

Prognathism Projection of the jaw

Prophase First stage of cell replication in meiosis or mitosis

Prostaglandins Group of fatty acids that stimulate contractility of the uterine and other smooth muscle and have the ability to lower blood pressure, regulate acid secretion in the stomach, regulate body temperature and platelet aggregation, and control inflammation and vascular permeability

Protease inhibitor Drug that binds to and blocks the action of the HIV protease enzyme

Proteinuria Excess of serum proteins in the urine

Pruritus Itching

Ptosis Paralytic drooping of the upper eyelid

Pulsus biferiens Peripheral pulse with a characteristic double impulse

Pulsus paradoxus Drop in systemic blood pressure greater than 15 mm Hg that coincides with inspiration

Pyloroplasty Plastic surgery of the pylorus to create larger communication between the stomach and duodenum

Pyrosis Heartburn

Pyuria Pus in urine

Quadriplegia Paralysis of all four limbs

Quincke's sign Alternate blanching and flushing of the skin

Recessive gene Gene that doesn't express itself in the presence of its dominant allele

Red blood cell Erythrocyte

Remission Abatement of a disease's symptoms

Remyelination Healing of demyelinated nerves

Renin Enzyme produced by the kidneys in response to an actual decline in extracellular fluid volume

Resistance Opposition to airflow in the lung tissue, chest wall, or airways; opposition to blood flow in the circulatory system

Respiratory acidosis Acidosis resulting from impaired ventilation and retention of carbon dioxide

Respiratory alkalosis Alkalosis caused by excessive excretion of carbon dioxide through the lungs

Romberg's sign Tendency of a patient to sway while standing still with feet close together and eyes closed

Rubella syndrome Exposure of a nonimmune mother to rubella during the first trimester of pregnancy

Salpingitis Inflammation of the fallopian tubes

Sclerodactyly Scleroderma of the fingers and toes

Sebum Oily secretion of the sebaceous glands

Sepsis Pathologic state resulting from microorganisms or their poisonous products in the bloodstream

Serositis Inflammation of a serous membrane

Serotonin Hormone and neurotransmitter, which inhibits gastric acid secretion, stimulates smooth muscle, and produces vasoconstriction

Shunt Passage or anastomosis between two natural channels

Specific gravity Weight of a substance compared with the weight of an equal amount of water

Status asthmaticus Particularly severe episode of asthma

Steatorrhea Excess fat in the feces caused by a malabsorption syndrome

Stenosis Constriction or narrowing of a passage or orifice

Stratum corneum epidermidis Dead top layer of skin

Stroke volume Amount of blood pumped out of the heart in a single contraction

Subcutaneous emphysema Crackling beneath the skin on palpation

Subluxation Incomplete or partial dislocation

Surfactant Mixture of phospholipids which reduces the surface tension of pulmonary fluids and contributes to the elastic properties of pulmonary tissue

Sympathectomy Excision or interruption of some portion of the sympathetic nervous pathway

Synovectomy Removal of destructive, proliferating synovium, usually, in the wrists, knees, and fingers

Synovial fluid Viscous, lubricating substance secreted by the synovial membrane, which lines the cavity between the bones of free-moving joints

Telophase Last of the four stages of mitosis or of the two divisions of meiosis

Tendon Fibrous cord of connective tissue that attaches the muscle to bone or cartilage and enables bones to move when skeletal muscles contract

Tenotomy Surgical cutting of the tendon

Teratogens Environmental agents that can harm the developing fetus by causing congenital structural or functional defects

Thoracentesis Surgical puncture and drainage of the thoracic cavity

Thrombocytopenia Subnormal number of platelets in circulating blood

Thrombocytosis Excessive number of platelets in circulating blood

Thrombus Blood clot

Thymoma Tumor on the thymus gland

Tinea cruris Fungal infection of the groin

Tinel's sign Tingling over the median nerve on light percussion

Tophi Accumulations of urate salts; occur throughout the body in gout

Torticollis Abnormal contraction of the cervical muscles, producing torsion of the neck

Transcription Synthesis of RNA using a DNA template

Transient ischemic attack Brief episode of neurologic deficit resulting from cerebral ischemia

Translocation Alteration of a chromosome by attachment of a fragment to another chromosome or a different portion of the same chromosome

Trisomy Presence of an extra chromosome

Trousseau's sign Carpal spasm

Truss Elastic, canvas, or metallic device for retaining a reduced hernia within the abdominal cavity

Vagotomy Surgical interruption of the impulses carried by the vagus nerve or nerves

Vasculitis Inflammation of a vessel

Ventriculatrial shunt Drains fluid from the brain's lateral ventricle into the right atrium of the heart, where the fluid enters the venous circulation

Ventriculoperitoneal shunt Transports excess fluid from the lateral ventricle into the peritoneal cavity

Virus Microscopic, infectious parasite that contains genetic material and needs a host to replicate

Vitiligo Absence of pigmentation

Wilms' tumor Rapidly developing malignant mixed tumor of the kidneys, made up of embryonal elements; occurs mainly in children before age five

X-linked Inheritance pattern in which single gene disorders are passed through sex chromosomes

Selected references

Albers, G.W., et al. "Antithrombotic and thrombolytic therapy for ischemic stroke," *Chest* 119:300S-320S, 2001.

Allessie, M.A., et al. "Pathophysiology and prevention of atrial fibrillation," *Circulation* 103:769-777, 2001.

Bisgaard, H., and Nielsen, K.G. "Immunobiology of asthma and rhinitis. Pathogenic factors and therapeutic options," *American Journal of Respiratory and Critical Care Medicine* 160:1778-1787, 1999.

Bullock, B.A., and Henze, R.L. *Focus on Pathophysiology.* Philadelphia: Lippincott Williams & Wilkins, 2000.

Cook, L.S. "A simple case of anemia: Pathophysiology of a common symptom," *Journal of Intravenous Nursing* 23(5):271, 2000.

Cutolo, M., et al. "The hypothalamic-pituitary-adrenocortical and gonadal axis function in rheumatoid arthritis," *Zeitschrift für Rheumatologie* 59(Suppl 2):66-69, 2000.

Deuschl, G., et al. "The pathophysiology of Parkinsonian tremor: A review," *Journal of Neurology* 247(Suppl 5):V33-48, 2000.

Gelband, C.H., et al. "Current perspectives on the use of gene therapy for hypertension," *Circulation Research* 87:1118-1122, 2000.

Gonzales, R., et al. "Uncomplicated acute bronchitis," *Annals of Internal Medicine* 133(12):981-991, 2000.

Hart, S.M. "Influence of beta-blockers on mortality in chronic heart failure," *Annals of Pharmacotherapy* 34(12):1440-1451, 2000.

Horwitz, R. J., et al. "The role of leukotriene modifiers in the treatment of asthma," *American Journal of Respiratory and Critical Care Medicine* 157:1363-1371, 1998.

Hussong, J.W., et al. "Evidence of increased angiogenesis in patients with acute myeloid leukemia," *Blood* 95:309-313, 2000.

Kraus, W.E. "Taking heart failure to new heights: Its pathophysiology at simulated altitude," *American Journal of Medicine* 109(6):504-505, 2000.

Manolagas, S.C., and Jilka, R.L. "Mechanisms of disease: Bone marrow, cytokines, and bone remodeling — Emerging insights into the pathophysiology of osteoporosis," *The New England Journal of Medicine* 332(5):305-311, 1995.

Menzel, T., et al. "Pathophysiology of impaired right and left ventricular function in chronic embolic pulmonary hypertension: Changes after pulmonary thromboendarterectomy," *Chest* 118:897-903, 2000.

Moraes, D.L., et al. "Secondary pulmonary hypertension in chronic heart failure: The role of the endothelium in pathophysiology and management," *Circulation* 102:1718-1723, 2000.

Price, S.A., and Wilson, L.M. *Pathophysiology: Clinical Concepts of Disease Processes,* 5th ed. St. Louis: Mosby, 1997.

Proesmans, M., and De Boeck, K. "Failure of local defense mechanisms in cystic fibrosis," *Acta Otorhinolaryngolica Belgica* 54(3):367-372, 2000.

Riedel, M. "Acute pulmonary embolism pathophysiology, clinical presentation, and diagnosis," *Heart* 85(2):229-240, 2001.

Schwartz, G.G. "Exploring new strategies for the management of acute coronary syndromes," *American Journal of Cardiology* 86(8B):44J-49J; discussion 49J-50J, 2000.

Thomas, D.J., and Harrah, B.F. "A new look at heart failure," *Home Healthcare Nurse* 18(3):165-171, 2000.

Van Soeren, M.H., et al. "Pathophysiology and implications for treatment of acute respiratory distress syndrome," *AACN Clinical Issues: Advanced Practice in Acute and Critical Care* 1(2):179, 2000.

Young, N.S., and Maciejewski, J. "Mechanisms of disease: The pathophysiology of acquired aplastic anemia," *The New England Journal of Medicine* 336(19):1365 1372, 1997.

Yucha, C.B., and Shapiro, J.I. "Acute renal failure: Recognition and prevention," *Primary Care Practice: A Peer-Reviewed Series* 1(4):388-398, 1997.

Index

t refers to table.

t refers to table.

t refers to table.

t refers to table.

t refers to table.

t refers to table.

Inflammation *(continued)*
 of hair follicles, 356, 357
 of liver, 174, 175
 of middle ear, 396, 397
 of ovaries, 314, 315
 of pancreas, 190, 191
 of peritoneum, 192, 193
 of prostate gland, 318, 319
 of tendon, 224, 225
 of tendon sheaths in carpal tunnel
  syndrome, 202
 of vagina, 328, 329
 of vertebrae, 256, 257
 of vulva, 328
 signs of, 14
Inflammatory response, 14
Inguinal hernia, 180
 detecting, in male patient, 180
 types of, 180, 181
Injury
 as disease stage, 5
 to cells, 4
Insulin-dependent diabetes, 270
Intertrigo, 366
Intertrochanteric fracture, 207
Interventricular septum, thickened, 41
Intracapsular fracture, 207
Intracellular fluid, 26
Intracerebral hemorrhage, 55
 site of, 127
Intracranial aneurysm. *See* Cerebral
  aneurysm.
Intracranial hemorrhage, symptoms of,
  118
Intrarenal failure, 352
Intrinsic renal failure, 352
Ionizing radiation as cancer risk factor,
  6-7
Iron deficiency anemia, 234
 peripheral blood smears in, 235
Irritable bowel syndrome, 182
 effects of, 182, 183
Ischemic stroke, 126, 127
Ischemic tubular necrosis, 334, 335
Isotonicity, 26t
Isotonic solutions, 28

t refers to table.

J

Jejunum, adenocarcinoma of, 159
Jock itch, 366
Jones criteria for rheumatic heart dis-
  ease, 68
Junctional arrhythmias, site of, 39
Junctional rhythm, 400t
Juvenile polyps, 156

K

Kaposi's sarcoma as AIDS-related illness, 251
Karyotype, 20
Keratoconjunctivitis, epidemic, 384
Kidney
 acute tubular necrosis and, 334, 335
 cancer of, 350, 351
 hydronephrosis and, 342, 343
 polycystic kidney disease and, 344,
  345
 renovascular hypertension and, 354,
  355
Kidney stones. *See* Renal calculi.
Knee
 deep veins of, 49
 inflamed bursa of, 201
 rheumatoid arthritis in, 261
 with osteoarthritis, 213
Kveim-Stilzbach skin test, 106
Kyphosis, 218, 219

L

Lactic acidosis in shock, 70, 71
Lacunar infarcts, site of, 127
Landouzy-Dejerine muscular dystrophy,
  210, 211
Landry-Guillain-Barré syndrome. *See*
  Guillain-Barré syndrome.
Large intestine, appendicitis and, 151
Laryngeal cancer, 390, 391
Larynx, cancer of, 390, 391
Latency as disease stage, 5
Lateral malleolus fracture, 207

Latex allergy, 254
Left atrium
 in atrial septal defect, 42, 43
 in mitral valve prolapse, 56, 57
 in myocardial infarction, 59
Left-sided heart failure, 52
Left ventricle
 in atrial septal defect, 42, 43
 in heart failure, 53
Left ventricular hypertrophy, 55
Legs, deep veins of, 49
Leiomyomas, 304
Leiomyosarcoma, 304
Lens, cataract and, 380, 381
Lentigo maligna melanoma, 374, 376
Leukemia, 236
 histologic diagnosis of, 237
 types of, 236, 237
Leukocytosis as sign of infection, 14
Limb-girdle muscular dystrophy, 210,
  211
Liquefactive necrosis, 5
Listeriosis, 16t
Liver, 153
 in cirrhosis, 155
 in cystic fibrosis, 87
 in hepatitis, 174, 175
 renovascular hypertension and, 354,
  355
Liver cancer, 184
 common sites of, 184, 185
Liver failure, 186
 in shock, 70, 71
 signs of, 186, 187
Lobar pneumonia, 96, 97
Lobular pneumonia, 96
Lordosis, 218, 219
Lou Gehrig's disease. *See* Amyotrophic
  lateral sclerosis.
Lower esophageal sphincter, incomplete
  closure of, 170, 171
Lund and Browder chart, 361
Lung cancer, 92
 tumor infiltration in, 93

t refers to table.

t refers to table.

t refers to table.

Rheumatic heart disease, 68
  sequelae of, 69
Rheumatoid arthritis, 260
  joints affected by, 261
Rheumatoid spondylitis. *See* Ankylosing
    spondylitis.
Rhinitis, 111
  allergic, 252
Ribonucleic acid, 2
Ribosomes, 2, 3
Rickettsia as cause of infection, 12
Right atrium in atrial septal defect, 42,
    43
Right-sided heart failure, 52
Right ventricle
  in heart failure, 53
  in ventricular septal defect, 44, 45
Ringworm, 366, 367
Robin sequence, 382
Rolling hernia, 176
Rubella, 18t
Rubeola, 18t
Rule of Nines, 361
Rupture. *See* Inguinal hernia.
Ruptured disk. *See* Vertebral disk injury.

S

Saccular aneurysm, 36, 37
Saccule, Ménière's disease and, 394, 395
Salmonellosis, 16t
Salpingitis, 314, 315
Sarcoidosis, 106
  effects of, 107
Sarcomas. *See* Bone tumors.
Schistosomiasis, 19t
Sclerodactyly in CREST syndrome, 263
Scleroderma, 262
Scoliosis, 218, 219
Sebum production, excessive, acne and,
    356, 357
Second-degree AV block, 401t
Secretory otitis media, 396
Seizure disorder. *See* Epilepsy.
Semicircular canals, Ménière's disease
    and, 394, 395

Semilunar valves, 73
  defects in, 72, 75
Senile cataract, 380
Senile osteoporosis, 216
Senile plaques in Alzheimer's disease,
    114, 115
Sensorineural hearing loss, 388
Sensory disorders, 380-397
Septic shock, 70
Sex, determining, 20
Sex-linked disorders, 21, 23t, 24
Sex-linked inheritance, 21
Sexually transmitted infections, 320,
    322
  effects of, 323
  manifestations of, 321
Sexual practices as cancer risk factors, 6
Shigellosis, 17t
Shock, 70
  effects of, 71
Shock lung. *See* Adult respiratory dis-
    tress syndrome.
Sickle cell anemia, 22t, 246
  peripheral blood smear in, 247
Sickle cell crisis, 247
Simple goiter, 282, 283
Sinus bradycardia, 400t
Sinusitis, 111
Sinus node arrhythmias, site of, 39
Sinus tachycardia, 400t
Skeletal muscle cells, 3
Skin cancers, 374
  types of, 374, 377
Skin disorders, 356-379
Skin in cystic fibrosis, 87
Sliding hiatal hernia, 176
Slipped disk. *See* Vertebral disk injury.
Slow-reacting substance of anaphylaxis,
    role of, in asthma, 82
Small intestine. *See also* Bowel.
  appendicitis and, 151
  in cystic fibrosis, 87
  in irritable bowel syndrome, 182, 183
Smith's fracture, 207
Smooth muscle cells, 3
Sodium, characteristics of, 27t

Somatotropin deficiency, 272
Spastic colitis. *See* Irritable bowel syn-
    drome.
Spastic colon. *See* Irritable bowel syn-
    drome.
Spermatic cord abnormality, 326, 327
Spermatic vein, varicocele and, 330, 331
Spina bifida, 24t, 144
  types of, 144, 145
Spinal cord defects, 144, 145
Spinal cord injury, 146
  effects of, 146, 147
Spine, curvature of, 218, 219
Spondylitis, ankylosing. *See* Ankylosing
    spondylitis.
Spontaneous pneumothorax, 98
Sporadic goiter, 282
Sprains, 220
  grading, 220
Squamous cell carcinoma, 374, 377
  of esophagus, 164, 165
  of skin, 374, 377
Squamous intraepithelial lesion, 296,
    297
SRS-A, role of, in asthma, 82
Status asthmaticus, 82
Status epilepticus, 128
Stiff lung. *See* Adult respiratory distress
    syndrome.
Stomach
  herniation of, 176, 177
  inflammation of lining of, 168, 169
Stomach cancer, 166, 167
Strains, 222, 223
Stress fracture, 207
Stress ulcers, shock and, 70, 71
Striated cardiac muscle cells, 3
Stroke. *See* Cerebrovascular accident.
Struvite kidney stones, 348, 349
Subacute glomerulonephritis, 340
Subacute thyroiditis, 280
Subarachnoid hemorrhage
  cerebral aneurysm and, 124
  site of, 127
Subclinical acute phase as disease stage,
    5

t refers to table.

V

Vagina, inflammation of, 328, 329
Vaginitis, 328, 329
   trichomonal, 321, 322
Vaginosis, 329
Valvular disease, chronic, in rheumatic heart disease, 68, 69
Valvular heart disease, 72-75
Valvulitis, chronic, in rheumatic heart disease, 68, 69
Varicella, 17t
Varicocele, 330, 331
Varicose veins, 76
   changes in blood flow in, 77
Vascular changes, progressive, in Raynaud's disease, 67
Vascular headaches, 132, 133
Vascular retinopathy, 55
Vasopressin deficiency, 268, 269
Venereal warts, 321, 322
Venous thrombus, 49
Ventricles, enlargement of, in hydrocephalus, 134, 135
Ventricular arrhythmias, site of, 39
Ventricular chamber
   decreased, 41
   increased, 41
Ventricular fibrillation, 401t
Ventricular septal defect, 44, 45
Ventricular standstill, 401t
Ventricular tachycardia, 401t
Vernal conjunctivitis, 384
Verrucae, 378, 379
Vertebrae, inflammation of, 256, 257
Vertebral disk injury, 148
   herniation and pain in, 148, 149
Vertebrobasilar artery as CVA site, 126, 127
Villous adenomas, 156
Viral conjunctivitis, 384
Viral hepatitis, 174, 175
Viral infections, 17-19t. *See also* Infection.
Viral pneumonia, 19t, 96
Viruses as cause of infection, 12

Vision loss as diabetes mellitus complication, 271
Vocal cord, laryngeal cancer and, 390, 391
Vulva
   cancer of, 332, 333
   inflammation of, 328
Vulvar cancer, 332, 333
Vulvitis, 328, 366

W

Warts, 378, 379
Wenckebach block, 401t
Wet gangrene, 5
Wet lung. *See* Adult respiratory distress syndrome.
Whiplash injuries of head and neck, 112, 113
Whiteheads, 356, 357
White lung. *See* Adult respiratory distress syndrome.
Whooping cough, 17t
Wrist
   fractures of, 207
   rheumatoid arthritis in, 261
   with carpal tunnel syndrome, 203

X

X-linked disorders. *See* Sex-linked disorders.

t refers to table.